MORE PRAISE FOR *POTENTIAL WITHIN'S* AGELESS PERFORMANCE

"In 10 years of professional bodybuilding I have never had a protein work this well. Plus the way my body responds to the creatine and glutamine enhanced by this insulin-efficiency system is phenomenal. I've gained amazing mass while staying leaner than ever! I rely on my liquid protein heavily, since I don't have a huge appetite for food, so I need a product that works. Franco Cavaleri's Matrix 4 has outperformed anything I've ever used and I've chosen to make it part of my regular training nutrition. Good job, Franco!"
—"KING" PAUL DILLETT, top Mr. Olympia contender

"As a longtime competitive martial artist, I faced many challenges after seven years of sedentary, rural lifestyle. I returned to competitive training after having gained 40 pounds and while coping with a painful rotator-cup injury. After only five weeks of applying Franco Cavaleri's dietary, supplemental nutrition, and supplemental training program, I reached my competitive weight with a greatly enhanced focus, concentration, speed, and power. I feel 15 years younger and I'm injury-free. I'm amazed at my consistent weight achievements amid a simultaneous strength, speed, energy, and stamina increment that still continues to improve. In fact, for the first time in my life I actually have more energy after a hard training session than when I started."
—JIM McCLARTY, black belt in tashu karate

"In June 2002 we picked up abnormalities in liver enzymes on a routine pre-anesthetic screening of a 13-year-old mixed-breed dog named Tina. Follow-up ultrasound and biopsies showed a chronic active hepatitis [liver disease] that, by August, was progressing. Initially Tina hadn't responded to more traditional medical therapies—antibiotics, vitamin E, and Ursadiol. Thus, we elected to use a therapy involving nutritional support and supplement with the help of Franco Cavaleri of Biologic Nutritional Research Inc., starting in September 2002. By November we were seeing improvements in the parameters tested and, within four months, all parameters were back to normal. We were happy with this outcome, as the diagnosis is usually chronic and active as the initial diagnosis suggested."
—HOWARD THWAITES, D.V.M., Central Langley (British Columbia) Pet Hospital

POTENTIAL WITHIN

A GUIDE TO NUTRITIONAL EMPOWERMENT

FRANCO CAVALERI, BSc

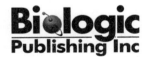

Biologic
Publishing Inc

This book is published by Biologic Publishing Inc.
115–7198 Vantage Way
Delta, British Columbia
V4K 1K7 Canada
www.biologicnr.com

Editor: Michael Carroll
Design and Production: Jen Hamilton
Front Cover Photo: Jay Shaw
Back Flap Photo: Terry Goodlad

Printed and bound in Canada by Friesens

National Library of Canada Cataloguing in Publication Data

Cavaleri, Franco
    Potential within: a guide to nutritional empowerment/Franco Cavaleri.

    Includes index.
    ISBN 0-9731701-0-7

    1. Nutrition. I. Title.
RA784.C38 2003   613.2   C2003-911196-2

Individually we are diverse, but one common factor tends to motivate all of us. We all strive for acceptance, love, and a fit within society. A struggle on this quest can become a lonely battle if we don't know where to search and we impose on ourselves unnecessary pressures to perform, achieve, and be acknowledged. To strive is healthy, but we mustn't lose sight of the fact that acceptance and love from others can be found only after self-acceptance, self-love, and self-respect have been achieved. With this discovery we're freed of fabricated stresses, our goals become more humanitarian in nature, and we begin to live with vigor, zest, and compassion. With this knowing, balance becomes a life focus that reaps more productivity and fulfillment.

As long as I can remember, I've pursued my goals with a relentless intensity that in the past has caused me to lose the present. Tamara, my life partner of 15 years, has been a constant reminder of the "now," of the real source of human power and humanitarian purpose. We've journeyed together through the trials and tribulations of competitive sports, business development, and the sobering awakening of life-threatening disease. She's my spiritual hero, lighting up my potential, helping me stay focused on my source of inner power as I press forward to deliver my potential and purpose. Tamara is an inspiration to all who meet her and I dedicate this book to her.

CONTENTS

ACKNOWLEDGMENTS

I've been blessed with the opportunity to develop a meaningful professional life rich with purpose. My passion has become my work so that I face each day with pleasure and fulfillment. I've participated in the health industry as a competitive athlete, educator, businessperson, researcher, formulator, manufacturer, and consultant.

Early on I identified my area of expertise and offered it with an open heart and was accepted in the same way by industry people who had a beautiful focus—service to humanity. The value of my journey is immeasurable and the friendships I've developed heartfelt. I thank everyone in this humanitarian health-service industry for their support and acceptance and the opportunities they've helped me create.

Potential Within has been an arduous task that I couldn't have completed without the sense of purpose I feel for this industry and the people it serves. The project developed into a mammoth 1,100 pages over several years of intense research and meticulous endeavor. However, I was able to convert the original manuscript into four individual books, of which this is the first. It's the sort of task some people would find unattainable, impossible to fathom, if they glimpsed the challenges to come. But I understood that a lot of lives could be transformed through Ageless Performance, the program in this book, and that kept me centered and diligent. Through my seminars many people applied this powerful craft even before this book was published. Their feedback has been an inspiration to me; thanks to them, *Potential Within* will reach so many more.

Immeasurable thanks go out to Tamara, my life partner, for putting up with my long days of research, typing, and proofreading, not to mention my persistent nagging to garner her valuable opinions and recommendations. Tamara's patience, support, and grounding presence allowed me to convey a message derived as much from my accumulated knowledge as from my heart. She's been a profound inspiration in my life.

I also extend thanks to my parents and my brother, Nick, who have been there to support this and all of my dreams from day one, taking time out from their own endeavors to read samples of my work upon request and assisting me to determine if my message was being delivered as intended.

To my editor, Michael Carroll, much thanks. He's truly the most painstaking person I know, and it's a good thing. His precise work has helped extract and convey a scientific message with clarity for all walks of life to appreciate and implement for better health, fitness, and performance potential. Thanks also go out to Jen Hamilton, this book's designer and production coordinator. She has patiently and scrupulously worked through the production and reproduction of this major project from cover to cover—a job extremely well done.

I commend the wonderful staff at Biologic Nutritional Research Inc. and Biologic Publishing Inc. for their loyal support of this and many other efforts. Dr. Michael Colgan must also be thanked for his vote of confidence in all that I've undertaken from the moment we first met. Long before that he was an inspiration and a silent mentor. Now, as a friend, he continues to express faith openly in my abilities and potential, instilling confidence no matter how vast the project. Dr. Colgan's belief in me has contributed to the realization of my higher goals, and I thank him for that.

NOTE FROM THE AUTHOR

The content in *Potential Within* is based on scientific research but should not be used as treatment for therapy without a clear understanding of the nature of the health condition. Since each case of disease is unique to the individual, a full review of the condition by a certified health-care professional must qualify the treatment. The purpose of the literature is to expand the knowledge of both professional and health-care recipient in order to present alternative and complementary choices that can be applied with close monitoring by a health professional. Under no circumstances are the Ageless Performance programs to be applied instead of medication or medical advice without first consulting the prescribing professional. The athletic-performance-enhancement strategies described in this book should not be applied unless a complete examination by a qualified health-care professional has first confirmed that the health condition of the individual can support the enhanced metabolic performance.

POTENTIAL WITHIN

INTRODUCTION

THE POWER OF THE ATOM

Hiroshima. In 1945 atomic power leveled an entire city in seconds. Life on Earth was changed forever without warning or discretion. Although many people believe the deployment of this innovation was justified to end World War II expeditiously, it was far from a display of harnessed might. It was more like a juvenile experiment let loose with an insidious anticipation of the unknown. Still, to this day, our understanding of atomic energy is based on the *theory* of atomic construction. No one has actually seen the components making up the atom; we've merely measured the energy dynamics that signify their existence and interaction.

The atom bomb is a crude invention of the human intellect pretending to comprehend the power of the atom—the stitch that constitutes the fabric of the universe and everything in it, including humanity. Imagine that a metal frying pan, the gold ring on a finger, the diamond in that ring, the glass in a window, the wood of a tall cedar, living flesh and blood, and the bomb that destroyed Hiroshima are all made of the same fundamental unit of matter— the atom. The only measure that differentiates the various atoms of one form of matter and another is the distinct pattern of energy each harnesses.

You and I have the ability to extract the energy potential of the atom to power our existence. The power of the atomic bomb is the same potential that fuels our cells, though our bodies are able to harness and direct it better. The relatively lifeless materials of our world don't possess this ability as we experience it, but the potential still pulsates with bounding life deep within the core of the atomic building block. The extraction of this potential within the animate system requires precise activity, which we explain in terms of chemistry, molecules, co-factors, catalysts (reaction facilitators), minerals, and vitamins. The potential that's packed within ourselves, within our genetic codes, within our atomic embodiment, is far beyond what most of us can fathom. The notion that humans can change the nature of nourishment, thus altering the cell's ability to extract atomic potential, is absurd. Not only do we not have the intellectual capability to understand the true nature of the atom but we don't possess the insight into the dynamic of nutrition that encompasses the biochemistry or bioenergy of human life.

A minute deviation from this meticulous biochemical design impairs our ability to derive the full potential from within the atom, taking the animate flesh and blood one step closer to the energetic state of the lifeless dust that constitutes our being. This is the essence of nutrient deficiency, and it's not an all-or-nothing occurrence. Nourishment delivers a dose-dependent potential for life, with optimal nutritional states promoting maximum vitality, while anything less than paramount nutrient status results in a dose-related lower state of vitality. In other words, our levels of vitality depend almost exclusively on our bodies' nutrient statuses. Every mouthful of food evokes a hormonal cascade that permeates the body, affecting each molecule. The right food choices provide a healthy hormonal wave on which we can ride to enhanced vitality. The wrong selections prompt a bioenergetic rippling much like the disruptions of a glassy pond by a stone tossed into its center. Manhandling of the food supply and environment has resulted in catastrophic consequences. In essence, it provokes a rippling interruption of cellular chemistry, interfering with the delicate dynamic of body and mind. Ageless Performance, the dietary and nutritional program detailed in this book, gets this biochemistry flowing in the right direction again. It shifts our metabolisms so that they work with us toward our goals, taking the battle out of disease prevention and therapy and elevating performance potential to completely new levels. Ageless Performance kick-starts the bioenergetic state, making it vibrate with harnessed atomic power.

The biochemistry of our nourishment was crafted over millions of years of evolutionary design. In terms of the evolutionary timeline, we've changed this carefully proportioned food chemistry in the blink of an eye with processing. Our genetic designs require specialized dietary influences that come from whole nourishment. Whole-food chemistry acts as programming for the human genome system. Our hormonal works, as well, depend tremendously on whole food's biochemical language, which also regulates its activity.

What we've done by transforming the language of this nutrient chemistry is to create an inflection point in the evolution of humanity—a shift in the internal biochemistry of human life. This shift cultivates a sort of weeding process—natural selection, survival of the fittest, a process designed to choose the genetic strains of life that will tolerate the new environmental standard.

The result of this powerful inflection point is the overwhelming escalation of disease and death whose vastness we're just beginning to grapple with. Every bite of this newly designed food chemistry evokes a foreign cascade of hormones that we try to survive. Few of us are genetically prepared to tolerate this new biochemistry, and if it weren't for our incredible medical advances, which have helped us limp along in these compromised conditions, even fewer of us would be here today.

There is hope, however. Ageless Performance can offset this biochemical shift of nourishment. That's right—it modifies genetic activity to help reestablish the body's natural biochemical performance. Taking back our health requires feeding the body many of the biochemical influences that directed its evolution, and the same is so if maximum physical and mental performance is desired. The first step toward this state is to return to whole foods as the major source of nourishment. These foods closely resemble the biochemical profiles that dictated our genetic designs. The second step is to compensate for the proven shortfalls of today's whole foods and those produced by an unnatural degree of environmental toxicity. The evidence in this book validating these strategies will overwhelm you with enthusiasm as you begin to realize that by applying this science you can control your health and level of performance.

Recent research has revealed that many of our common nutrients find their way into our genetic codes to stimulate or inhibit specific genes that are involved in the construction and maintenance of hormones, tissues, neurotransmitters, and entire biological systems. This activity permeates much deeper than the simple action of enzymes and mitochondria (the powerhouse of every cell in the body that generates adenosine triphosphate, or ATP). These recent findings indicate that common vitamins like C play a role in gene regulation, and a limitation of this vitamin results in the failure of a gene to partake in its biological role. This activity wasn't known only a few years ago.

Many other similar models have been unveiled. We've found that free radicals play a role in gene regulation, as well, and that antioxidants, which counter uncontrolled free-radical activity, are important gene regulators. Imagine that—we can actually take an active part in the regulation of our genes by modifying our diets and augmenting our dietary nutrient intakes with a strategic nutritional supplement program. It's not science fiction; it's scientific fact. The latest research has revealed how we can use specialized nutrients to activate genes that may have become dormant with age.

This amazing activation has been shown to prevent and even reverse diseases as serious as cancer, diabetes, and chronic inflammation. It has literally put a new face on medicine, health care, prevention, and athletic performance. This new age has brought nutraceuticals and the natural health industry to a new level of credibility. In fact, the synergy of nutraceutical and pharmaceutical care, which is irrefutably demonstrated in this book, will be the new wave of effective therapy.

I've seen the results of nutrient-induced gene activation and gene inhibition in the laboratory and in people outside the laboratory who have consulted me. I've witnessed firsthand, in vivo, in vitro, through personal and client trials and tribulations, the onslaught of toxicity that can so easily and inexpensively be intercepted to prevent terminal disease. Diabetes is terminal. Most diseases, although not viewed as terminal, reduce life span. Just because the process of dying that a diabetic experiences may be slower than that of an individual with liver cancer doesn't change the fact that diabetes causes death. But most cases of Type II diabetes are easily curable. The disease is only terminal because most of us choose the type of health care that allows secondary diseases to develop without opposition.

The medical practitioners who previously scoffed at these claims were mesmerized without comment when the program prompted, in mere weeks, the result they battled for years to deliver to their patients. The result I'm referring to is the reestablishment of cellular responsiveness to natural secretions of insulin in Type II diabetics—complete reversal of the disease. The same thing happened when I recovered completely from severe ulcerative colitis without any residual trace.

How was it done? In the case of diabetes it was accomplished by administering the right mix of nutraceuticals that activates the genes responsible for the manufacture of the cell membrane's glucose-transport sites. This activity literally rejuvenates the cell with respect to insulin function and, consequently, turns back the biological clock because any state of insulin resistance, even one that's pre-diabetic, accelerates biological aging. Keep in mind that this innovation is not at all like insulin compensation such as metformin, which might be required indefinitely.

Ulcerative colitis is more difficult to overcome and requires a more comprehensive program, something we'll see in subsequent pages. The point is that a state of disease can be reversed. However, Ageless Performance isn't just limited to rectifying diabetes and ulcerative colitis. It's aimed at the biochemical correction of the cellular problem that's at the root of many diseases. The chemistry of inflammation is one of these common disease-promoting denominators, and producing a sort of anti-inflammatory environment in the body is a key preventive tactic. It's not so much that Ageless Performance induces an anti-inflammatory hormonal cascade; more accurately, the program corrects the cells' chemistry to create a neutral state of non-inflammatory activity. Processed, refined foods, which tend to be insulin-straining, promote an inflammatory hormonal cascade that Ageless Performance blocks and reverses.

The solutions I'm referring to are the consequences of a complex science and relate to multiple disorders, including cardiovascular disease, chronic inflammation, dementia, asthma, and more. The simple administration of precise mixes and doses of nutraceuticals and, of course, mild dietary changes, result in profound shifts in health. This book teaches how this can be accomplished. You'll also learn how this science can be applied to maximize athletic-performance potential and to shed, with ease, unwanted pounds. It's truly an exciting time—new-age medicine and a new standard for sports performance.

We all have the ability to extract and focus this power any way we choose.

Most of us don't know that this possibility exists within us and therefore will never experience true human potential. Some of us are aware that we're filled with potential from the day we're born, but we don't know how to tap into it. Ageless Performance is designed to help release this power in a controlled manner to fuel cellular chemistry and navigate its course along the path it was designed to take.

Diseases such as dementia and other cognitive disorders; arthritis, colitis, and other inflammatory conditions; cardiovascular illnesses such as hypertension and hypercholesterolemia; and asthma, diabetes, osteoporosis, obesity, even aging are all caused and propagated by common factors. These disorders can be treated easily in one clean sweep by rectifying the cause instead of applying drug compensation for each ailment. Biochemical correction is a more logical solution. Human life was designed with a host of intrinsic genetic miracles that are geared to support life. Disease isn't a natural state. We've created it by adulterating our environment and our precisely formulated nourishment, thus polluting the chemistry of life, hindering the flow of energy within ourselves, and thwarting our ability to liberate the miracles that lie deep within our genetic codes. Ageless Performance prepares the way for the resurrection of our inherent gift of healing, recovery, performance, and life.

Most of us have heard about the frail woman who lifted the back end of a crumpled car to save the life of her gasping child. This potential didn't come from an external source. The power came from within. The uninhibited mind of that frail woman was able to dig deep into her atomic core, which embodies humanity and its genetic codes, to focus this harnessed might. We've inhibited this potential through mental, emotional, environmental, and food-borne toxicity. Extraction of this potential is next to impossible unless we free ourselves of these inhibitions.

In the face of a life-or-death ordeal few inhibiting factors are profound enough to interfere with the mind's impermeable focus. Because of the toxicity we've imposed on ourselves, it takes an extreme experience to overcome toxic interference. However, if we can accept that this atomic power is real, we can empower our minds to activate this potential day after day. Once we've released ourselves from self-imposed mental bindings, the next step is to neutralize the free-radical interference that also impedes the resurrection of this harnessed power for healing, prevention, and athletic performance, propelling us farther along the road to experiencing a programmed state of *well*-being.

Ageless Performance is about clearing the mind and guiding the way to the potential within. Ageless Performance is about neutralizing the chemistry that interferes with our genetic programming. Ageless Performance activates the path to biological self-sufficiency so that the body, mind, and soul can function in harmonized synergy to perform according to an evolutionary design programmed for vigorous life, not disease or death.

THE NATURE OF POTENTIAL WITHIN

The research-documented evidence in this book conveys how our environment has influenced gene expression (activity) in a way that throws off endocrine-hormone balance (insulin, thyroxine, and sex hormones) as well as eicosanoid-hormone balance (prostaglandins, for example). Eicosanoid or autocrine hormones, such as prostaglandins, thromboxanes, and prostacyclins, regulate multiple biological systems related to all of the epidemic diseases I've already mentioned. If you're like most North Americans, these systems are out of line. Merely addressing this biochemistry can bring the struggle with disease, including obesity, to an end easily. The prolific use of cyclo-oxygenase (cox) inhibition such as the ongoing administration of high doses of asa (acetylsalicylic acid, or Aspirin) is compensation for these hormone imbalances.

The typical nutrition-based remedies of the past such as flaxseed and salmon oils won't address the common problem of imbalance. They're only part of a comprehensive strategy. These fats need all of the essential cofactors that guide them down the biochemical path to hormone status. The solution to our epidemic problem isn't more technology and drugs; it's a series of corrections to allow the body to do what it was designed for: to heal and prevent disease, and to exist in biochemical harmony. This process involves carefully organized synergistic combinations of nutraceuticals augmented by basic food choices. The program must be easy to apply, and Ageless Performance meets that criterion.

Man-made environmental toxicity influences far more than gene integrity and gene health; it actually transforms how these genes send out their encoded instructions and can even alter the downstream chemistry or prevent it from ever being received. Translation of the genetic code involves countless biochemicals, and the modification of any single one along the extensive chain of activity can significantly change the outcome from the original instruction. Each and every one of these biochemicals must battle with the cesspool of free radicals and other forms of toxicity we impose on ourselves. Clean up the environment, and the likelihood of gene misinterpretation decreases and self-regulation is enhanced. The environment we have the most control over is our own biochemistry. *Potential Within* is a detailed description of the Ageless Performance program that will induce this biological self-regulation.

Our nutrient-depleted foods don't deliver the essentials our immune and antioxidant systems require to defend the body from this environmental assault, leaving us vulnerable to the rigors of hellion free radicals (an atom or group of atoms with one or more unpaired electrons making the free radical highly unstable and potentially toxic to the body) and chemical toxicity. This vulnerability leaves our precious genetic material open to infiltration, mutation, and misinterpretation.

The penultimate chapter of this book, "Applying Ageless Performance," details the utilization of the Ageless Performance strategy. Each of us has unique metabolic needs based on individual metabolic rates, personal activity levels, age, goals, and differing states of health. In this chapter you'll be guided to your general program template—your starting point for the program—and you'll be instructed on how to craft your personalized version from this template to meet your unique nutritional demands.

Each template is designed with the same fundamental nutritional strategy, one that instills biochemical correction and biological self-sufficiency within each cell. With this new balance the hormonal systems that make up the inner workings of the biological clock will operate with a more efficient tempo to recover, rebuild, and revitalize every aspect of the body and mind with more accuracy. In essence, biological time will slow down and the "inner clock" will be turned back to reverse biological age.

The exogenous (external) drug or nutrient doesn't cause healing. The exogenous application, whether topical, oral, or injected, is designed to give the body an opportunity to deploy its own inner healing potential, but true healing occurs only if the body's chemistry is operational. The miracle of healing, health, and outstanding athletic performance comes from within. Ageless Performance will resurrect this miracle by activating it and forming the conduit from the inner core to the surface for human experience.

The final chapter of this book contains a series of condition-specific therapies that can be applied once the Ageless Performance chemistry is in place. Ageless Performance is a powerful therapy and prevention in itself, but some cases of disease require specialized priming to guide the biochemical flow of life in the right direction. These condition-specific therapies will do just that. However, if the biochemical foundation isn't set, the therapy will have little or no effect. This could be what you've experienced in the past with incomplete nutraceutical therapies or pharmaceutical drug administration.

Faith is an integral component of Ageless Performance; it fuels the program's incorporation into our beings and facilitates successful outcomes. The power of a positive mind is critical to the triumph of any therapy. If we doubt our health practitioners' therapeutic strategies, our minds can work against the treatments. If we believe in the therapy, the powerful cellular inscription induced by the positive mind will manifest positive results more expeditiously. Belief in a program also promotes a more diligent application, and this compliance, too, contributes to a successful outcome.

The message in *Potential Within* excites me as no other message in life because it has changed me forever. It's created opportunity both personally and professionally. It has founded the passionate, healthy life I lead today. My excitement is further intensified by the chance to share this craft and show other people the way to their true inner potential.

So let's get started. Time is passing, and if you're like most North Americans, your biological clock is ticking faster than it has to. Don't worry, though, because we're about to reset that pace in short order.

PART I

PRESCRIPTION FOR AGELESS PERFORMANCE

1

UNHEALTHY STATISTICS

Do you believe you're a victim of a fixed genetic predisposition? A quick look around at closely related family members reveals common characteristics that most of us accept as our destined physical nature.

My sister battles with diabetes. Mother died from adult-onset diabetes, as did my grandfather. My father is overweight and can't shed a pound, and now I'm beginning to complain about aches and pains just as they do. There's not a thing I can do about it. My destiny is built right into my genetic code. I'm doomed.

Sound familiar?

The genes that code for the excess baggage carried around on our hips might not be much different from the code thinner people possess. Similarly we might think a genetic predisposition makes us vulnerable to diabetes, cardiovascular disease, and chronic inflammation—in effect, holding us prisoners for a good part of our lives—but that's not the case at all. Our genetic programming for athletic potential probably isn't that far off from that of athletically gifted individuals.

If disease runs rampant in your immediate and extended families, is it more likely that the cause is the genetic profile shared by your relatives? The answer is no. My investigations clearly demonstrate that we're probably not victims of our genes.

There's much more to genetic expression than genetic codes. Gene expression or gene translation requires precise biochemical conditions. We might inherit genes that code for metabolic dysfunction and disease, but until these genes are activated, life-threatening conditions can't be experienced.

However, the biochemical influences we place on our genes could be producing diseased states from these codes. In fact, many epidemic diseases today aren't caused by genetic predisposition at all. This belief simply relieves us of responsibility for our states of health, making it easier to continue on our self-destructive paths. We're responsible for the unhealthy or healthy situations our genes have created. We can also take on the responsibility to change the genetic influence and alter the outcome.

Disease can result from overstimulated genes or gene inhibition, influenced by either our environments or lifestyle habits or both. Genetic profiles were formulated to partake in a healthy biological design, but under environmental and dietary conditions that are very different from those we face today. We might not have control over which genes we inherit, but we are the masters of how these genes are expressed or translated.

Our dietary habits, the biochemical factors that mediate gene activity, also come from our parents and other family members in the form of learned traditions, customs, and lifestyle habits. These lifestyle characteristics and environmental influences are shared within the family to induce a common genetic influence. Not only do we inherit a genetic profile akin to those of each of our family members, we also impose a comparable manipulation of our inner chemistry by living in a similar environment and eating a common diet. These shared lifestyle habits are the likely cookie cutters for familial traits as much as genetic sameness is. Change the influence, change the outcome.

If you're having trouble accepting this concept, consider the following. The natural characteristics of hair, such as color and curl, are genetically programmed. The chemistry that rises out of a person's genetic code produces a specialized chemical configuration that gives hair its physical hue. Yet one can apply a chemical scalding to intercept genetic instruction and significantly transform the chemistry and the color it represents. Likewise, genetically straight hair can be easily curled, diverting it from its gene-coded physical nature; the same pertains to naturally curly hair being straightened. Artificial straightening or curling is caused by manipulating the hair's protein configuration. Again there's no actual alteration in the genetic instruction, only a massive chemical scalding to divert the downstream chemistry that derived from the original genetic code.

The message is very clear: we can shatter the mold and change the factors in your life that influence the way we look, feel, and live. If the pattern we see developing in our family members isn't acceptable, we can remove this blueprint from our life and work from one that promotes the outcome we desire. It's more than just possible; it's scientific fact. We can change immune function, hormone health, body-fat and energy levels, muscle mass, bone density, and the risk of many diseases as easy as transforming the dietary and environmental influences on our genes. We can improve our genetic potential for sport and for life the second we correct our diets and mental and emotional states.

Genes contain our destined biological age, as well, but it's not as cut-and-dried as the turning on or off of a switch that dictates when the countdown begins. The biological clock is regulated by metabolic efficiency, which in turn is controlled by hormonal health. As much as hormonal health depends on genetic health, hormone balance relies on diet and environment. Hormone therapy, for example, is totally contingent on the health status or ability of the body to receive and use the hormone signal. More precisely, the health or operational status of the cellular receptor sites, which are supposed to be triggered by an orally administered or injected hormone, is totally dependent on the nutrient status of the body.

In fact, the need for an exogenous hormone therapy might actually be caused by a nutrient deficiency that has diminished the body's ability to produce the hormone or the specific receptor site the hormone works with. In upcoming chapters we'll see various scientifically documented examples that relate to growth-hormone *resistance*, testosterone *resistance* and, of course, insulin *resistance*. Very basic mineral deficiencies result in limited hormone activity, and the solution most of our medical practitioners have been taught to apply is a megablast with powerful hormones before ever considering the possibility of the cause for this need. The megablast then throws the biological system out of kilter, and the vicious cycle of disease propagating disease is instigated.

Genes might encode for the production of an important hormone or for the cell-membrane receptor for that hormone, but unlimited supplies of nutrient building blocks, such as protein, result in unlimited production from the genes' commands. Ultimately our cells are protein factories.

Messages and cellular construction materials are all designed from a proteinacious message that rises from genetic instruction. Dietary protein is critical to optimal health and athletic performance, and the quality of this protein is a critical factor in the health equation. In order for dietary protein to be incorporated into the gene-directed synthesis of a cellular message, a multiplicity of vital nutrient co-factors must be made available. A gene might be healthy, but a restricted diet can limit its potential.

However, genetic influence by diet and environment is far more complex than these simplified dynamics. Multiple factors turn genes on and off and dictate gene-transcription rates. Today our environment has evolved drastically to deliver a scourge of free radicals that our human evolutionary design hasn't accounted for. These free radicals—altered chemicals that have become toxic—are now known to influence gene activity significantly, far beyond mere damage or mutation.

Free radicals are recognized accelerators of specific genes that are involved in the production of highly specialized enzymes and hormones. Enzymes perform very specific, very delicate operations in the body, directing the flow of our internal biochemical paths. This accelerated enzyme activity is now seen as a major factor in the development of disease.

In fact, the metabolic pathway—the biochemical process in the body—in which the enzymes we'll be focusing on are linked to today's common epidemic diseases, including obesity. Free radicals increase the risk of obesity as well as of cardiovascular disease, cognitive disorders, and chronic inflammation. We've known this for some time, but more recently it's become apparent just how the genetic chemistry is influenced by these free-radical hellions. Ageless Performance is a comprehensive dietary and nutritional-supplement program designed to neutralize this toxicity and get our genes, metabolism, and bodies to work with us toward our goals. The program extracts the potential within each of us.

Today's new-age environmental toxicity actually accelerates the production of certain hormones that are inflammatory in nature, as well. This same hormonal profile is the very one that increases the risk of blood clots and requires the ongoing administration of ASA as compensation. People who require ASA daily to prevent cardiovascular disease do so because their cellular chemistry is severely imbalanced. If balance is restored, ASA isn't necessary.

Our bodies perpetually recycle themselves with a prevalent quest for healthy restoration. From the root, for example, natural hair color will eventually grow out to replace the chemically altered hair, the hair of changed hue. In fact, the entire body is completely recycled within a year or so. However, the new tissue can be as dysfunctional as the tissue it replaced if it's produced with the same nutrient intake and amid the same environmental scalding.

Imagine, say, if from the day you were born, your mother played a horrible trick on you, placing a hair-coloration chemical in your shampoo that maintained your genetically brown hair black. When independence day came and you moved out to provide for yourself, this chemical influence would be absent from your life. Soon you'd identify light brown hair growing out from the root, and eventually your hair would be completely brown. For your entire life before setting out on your own you would have thought your genetic hair color was black, but only because of the chemical interference.

Now what if you wanted brown hair while still living with your mother's chemical influence that altered it to black and you began to dye your blackened hair brown when brown was your original hue, anyway? In this case the solution would be to remove the chemical that dyed the hair black in the first place. Instead, because you didn't know any better, you would apply a second chemical to neutralize the influence that colored your hair black, thus making it brown. Sounds absurd, doesn't it? But that's what we do when we use drugs like ASA as cardio- and cerebro-protective chemicals. That's what we're doing when we need insulin enhancers and secretors because of a toxic environment. The functional solution is to remove the toxicity or block it from interfering with the body's biochemical design. This allows the body's metabolic chemistry to grow out from the root according to the natural messages of the genes, just as hair will sprout from the root with its natural color.

The ongoing application of cholesterol-lowering drugs, anti-inflammatories, and the newer, more specific cox1 and cox2 inhibitor drugs are usually required because of chemical toxicities that interfere with the activity of our genes and specialized enzymes in a way that prevents them from functioning properly. If we remove the dietary and environmental toxicity from the equation, we alleviate strain and the necessity for these compensatory drugs. Our genetic programming isn't designed to make us fat, frail, or vulnerable to disease. It's engineered for vigorous life and vibrant fitness. The chemical influences we've imposed on these genes have turned them against us. I'm not referring to the excess calories we consume that contribute to fat stores and other diseases; I'm talking about direct chemical influences to genetic chemistry that inhibit our natural fat-burning furnaces. This influence is much more profound than the extra calories themselves. Ageless Performance is *not* a restrictive diet. To stay with Ageless Performance is *not* a struggle; battling to remain on a program is itself disease-promoting. Ageless Performance *is* carefully designed to provide the correct biological chemistry.

Type II diabetes, cardiovascular disease, chronic inflammation, obesity, cognitive disorders, and respiratory afflictions like asthma are no different. They can be cured and eliminated by neutralizing the chemical influences food and environment have on the body, in particular the effect on one special biochemical pathway that rises from a group of genes—one system common to each of these conditions.

It's hard to believe that so many of our epidemics can be linked to one metabolic pathway, but it's true. I've shown just how the balancing of this pathway is treatment for many of these epidemic diseases. The devastation of this biochemical pathway has contributed billions of dollars of profits to pharmaceutical companies whose products are designed to deliver relief from the variety of symptoms that stem from this common pathway. If the deep-seated cause is addressed, symptomatic relief wouldn't be required. But that would mean pharmaceutical profits would likely diminish dramatically, as well. And I can assure you that won't be an option offered to you passively.

Establishment of biological self-sufficiency is up to us. Clearing the way for this biochemical pathway isn't as simple as antioxidant protection from free-radical toxicity. Our diet also contributes to the free-radical load on the body and from much more than food-borne toxicity. Processed food is higher in glycemic index (easily absorbed, refined sugars) than our cellular chemistry can tolerate, and the result is today's increased frequency of insulin resistance and diabetes.

Hyperglycemia is toxic to the body, as is hypoglycemia. Disorders of glucose tolerance increase the free-radical load on the body as well as interfere with the regulation of powerful inflammatory hormones. The common North American diet imposes many destructive influences on this hormone chemistry, and Ageless Performance is meticulously crafted to offset each of these impositions, allowing our cellular biochemistry to function according to design and deliver the longevity we were born to experience.

You're not as doomed as you think you are. You can take control of genetic expression and the physical attributes that rise out of this activity. Preventing in you what you see in your family members is as easy as changing your lifestyle to a healthier program than theirs. You may have realized already that the lifestyle program you're on delivers an outcome you don't want any part of. The problem is that most of us don't know where to find a proven alternative. Ageless Performance is the answer that has come out of decades of research. It's the guide to your true potential.

Ageless Performance is a design based on the blueprint crafted by evolution, and the objective of evolution is survival. What else could work better? This program is designed to optimize insulin function, and if insulin efficiency in your body is already going downhill, it's not too late for you. Ageless Performance will rectify insulin dysfunction. Ageless Performance is powerful enough to reverse diabetes.

As a supply of balanced nutrition that with each meal evokes a healthy hormonal response, Ageless Performance actually activates an anti-inflammatory influence throughout the body. That's right—food can act just as drugs do in the body. What's more, the very fact that we pop powerful pills like ASA, metformin, and glyburide by the millions to oppose the considerable influence of our processed, high-glycemic-index diet is a clear sign our food is druglike. Change your diet and you might not need the opposing drugs.

The essence of Ageless Performance isn't single specialty supplements such as glucosamine, s-adenosyl-methionine (SAMe), and cetyl myristoleate for arthritis and soft-tissue inflammation. It's not about administering methylsulfonylmethane (MSM) for recovery from connective-tissue damage or skin wear. It's not about the treatment of cardiovascular disease with salmon oil, vitamin E, or grapeseed extract. These supplements deliver spectacular recovery and preventive potential. However, they, too, are temporary Band-Aids for cellular disarray and, as one symptom of this imbalance is treated with these nutrient therapies, another surfaces unless the root of the multiple symptoms is addressed comprehensively.

Nutraceuticals, such as the ones already mentioned, can at least permeate to a degree below the surface of the symptom to help alleviate imbalance or deficiency, but not deep enough to resolve the cause of disease completely. Many pharmaceuticals are even less effective from this standpoint, since they're generally designed to mask the symptom closer to the surface. Pharmaceuticals have a place in therapy, but only as temporary support until the biochemical cause of disease is rectified. Rely on the pharmaceutical strategy alone and you might require this compensation for life, either ongoing or sporadically, but not without consequences.

The objective with Ageless Performance is to cut and direct a healthy path for the common biochemistry each of our cells relies on for communication. Impair this communication and death and disease are possible. The right timing and proportions of nutraceuticals will navigate the precise course, and once that's established, nature will take over the role of prevention and therapy as long as the correct natural balance of nutrients is maintained in the diet.

That's how Ageless Performance differs from any other program you've previously tried. It's a supply of the vital nutrient precursors and their cofactors necessary for healthy hormonal cascade, but the design doesn't end there. A multiplicity of calculated influences are incorporated into the program to guide this chemistry from the genetic level onward, escorting the essential nutrients down the right path in every cell of the body.

Our cells' ability to cope with environmental triggers of disease is highly dependent on the condition of our cellular biochemistry, which is a direct reflection of our diets. A nutritional imbalance sets the foundation for an imbalanced metabolic response to these triggers. This imbalance gives rise to chaotic hormonal cascades and a symptomatic profile defined as disease. However, with a healthy metabolic response the symptomatic profile of disease won't develop. In effect, with the right nutritional state we become more resilient to disease.

Our evolutionary blueprint wasn't designed to face the toxic environmental assault we've created. Ageless Performance is structured to provide our cells and bodies with the essentials they require to face this new-age onslaught. Today's toxicity has prompted the need for a new variety of nourishment—a revised list of essential nutrients. What is necessary now to combat this dangerous barrage might not have been vital 80 years ago when vitamins were first being discovered. In addition, our food supply wasn't refined then the way it is now. Today's unnaturally higher levels of toxicity must be met with equal and opposite unnaturally elevated levels of antioxidants in our bodies and food. As we'll see, the kind of supplementation detailed in this book is not a replacement for a healthy lifestyle, but when it's added to the whole foundation the protective and corrective shield that results is truly powerful.

The outcome of applying these new standards is the resuscitation of our metabolisms, cells, immune systems, and lives. With this new level of activity our cells will function according to design, even amid the hazardous conditions prevalent today. Once this level of functionality is established, specialty ingredients like glucosamine, SAMe, and curcumin, as well as performance enhancers such as creatine, hydroxymethylbutyrate (HMB), and ribose, can work as expected. For many people who apply these powerful specialty nutrients the results are nominal or nil. The problem, in almost every case, is a faulty biochemical foundation. Ageless Performance optimizes this underpinning.

With this new balance our cells will operate from a functional foundation, whether for prevention, therapy, or sport, and this includes weight management. Experience tells me you won't need more prevention than Ageless Performance, you'll rarely ever face therapy again, and your performance enhancement will be a completely new experience.

MATTER OF EXPRESSION

Weighed down by traditional Italian cuisine consisting of a carbohydrate-rich diet, including an abundance of processed pastas, breads, rice, and potatoes, my efforts to define lean muscle were grueling in my younger years. More than 14 years later, when a slower metabolism should have resulted in a bulging midsection, I'm leaner than ever and now find myself striving to keep body-fat levels high enough. In other words, I have a completely different body type but possess the same genetic predisposition.

I still enjoy some of the same foods; however, the time of day I eat them and how they're combined have changed. In addition, the inclusion of a strategic supplement program to complete the plan and support my "revving" metabolism has completely transformed how my body makes use of the food I eat and altered the way my genes are expressed. Forging a new life is simple, and you can do it if you apply Ageless Performance.

A POSITIVE OUTLOOK

The mind is an extremely powerful tool that can be used to set the foundation for health or disease. If you believe strongly, it will be inscribed in your cells. The inscription can be fitness and prevention, but if you choose otherwise, you can write the code for destruction. The choice is yours. You have the ability to manifest change as well as the remarkable power to facilitate recovery from trauma and illness. If you think all this is gibberish, that a positive outlook isn't a significant factor contributing to health and fitness, you're dead wrong. If you think drug therapy will easily combat a negative mindset, you're equally wrong. The mind will always prevail.

We've all had that twisted-gut feeling or heart-in-the-throat tightness that often results from stress. This is simply the physical manifestation of mental or emotional disturbance. Emotions and mindsets release neurotransmitters and neuropeptides that relay messages to each cell. Corticosteroid and chatecholamine secretions result, as well, from the chemistry of emotion and thought influencing every molecule. Thoughts are imbedded in our cells. Believe that and then guide your thought chemistry every day to induce a positive physical outcome.

Matters of the mind will produce physical change. You can choose to manifest health and fitness or you can harbor the misconception that you have no control. The only outstanding factor that can limit positive results once the right decision is made is an inadequate supply of the right dietary fuels and building blocks your body requires to make the connection with your vision.

MOTIVATING CHANGE

Many years ago my small stature on the soccer field limited my impact in the game. My solution was to embark on a weight-training program to help build a stronger physique. I was determined to enhance my performance on the field, visualized the result, and pursued it with conviction. Soon I realized I could successfully work toward altering the way I looked. My goals quickly changed, and again I glimpsed my vision of the future with clarity and embarked on a successful bodybuilding career, sculpting a muscled, 225-pound, five-foot-six frame. With 19.5-inch arm circumference and legs that measured significantly bigger than my 30-inch waistline, I had a powerhouse body that exceeded the norm for most human beings. I saw, I applied the strategy, I believed in the outcome, and I made it happen.

Whatever your goals, whatever the reason, the ability to achieve results resides in you. If your goal is to change what you see in the mirror, grasp it. Focus the mind, strategize, and stride toward your goal.

Ageless Performance was first put to the test due to my own personal trial. Diagnosed with ulcerative colitis in 1992, I was faced with the challenge of a lifetime. I saw recovery, applied the program, believed in the outcome, and healed my condition. You, too, have this power within you.

Take action. Ageless Performance will deliver the tools you need to live a life full of health, fitness, and joy. All you have to do is believe in the program, follow the instructions, and go for it! If you need to implement change and haven't found the motivation yet, perhaps some of the alarming statistics found in sidebars in the following pages will do the trick. Don't be disheartened by what you're about to read. These statistics are presented to get your attention and help make my point; they're real, they're climbing, and you could become part of them. However, you can choose the simple strategies outlined in Ageless Performance to alter your odds, genetic outcome, or phenotype.

Health Canada Report in 2000

The prevalence of obesity in children has increased in the past decade from 14% to 24% among girls and from 18% to 26% among boys.

In 2000 Health Canada told us that approximately 23% of Canadians were overweight—almost a quarter of the country's total population! This percentage is escalating so quickly that by the time you read this book more than 35% of Canadians may have reached a state of obesity. The concern that rises from these statistics has little to do with the physical appearance associated with obesity. Plain and simple—obesity increases the risk of disease. Fat mass is susceptible to and propagates oxidation; it promotes insulin resistance and diabetes; and the consequence is excess free-radical toxicity, which wreaks havoc in the body.

Accept obesity as an inevitable part of your life and be prepared to suffer an increased risk of cardiovascular disease, cancer, diabetes, chronic inflammation, cognitive disorders, and respiratory ailments like asthma. It's common knowledge that obesity can cause insulin resistance and diabetes. Insulin resistance is a condition in which insulin fails to function at full capacity, prompting the body to require more to do the job. Ultimately the body becomes desensitized to the insulin secreted by the pancreas. In this state every meal you eat stimulates a secretion of insulin that exceeds normal levels. This extraordinary insulin secretion then induces related hormone cascades that are proportionally unbalanced. In turn, these subsequent hormones each communicate an unbalanced message. This miscommunication occurs with every meal, advancing the biochemical disarray every time.

Essentially insulin resistance is a complication of diabetes that starts out as a minor degree of cellular desensitization to insulin and progresses to a Type II diabetic state. Insulin resistance tends to increase with age. Our high-glycemic-index diets can fuel the development of diabetes and accelerate our biological clocks.

An extreme acceleration rate exacerbates a greater degree of insulin resistance at an earlier age, thus increasing the risk of Type II diabetes. A sedentary lifestyle and a processed diet contribute to this desensitization to insulin, accelerating further the development of Type II diabetes.

The risk of dangerous secondary consequences associated with insulin resistance increases with the advanced desensitization of the body to insulin. We'll soon see how this is all related and how we can easily reverse and prevent the process from occurring in our lives—how we can easily reset our biological clocks!

Recent scientific findings have unveiled the biochemical link between obesity, insulin resistance, and diabetes. Fat mass is now known to represent much more than deadweight. It's understood to secrete hormones and communicate chemically in the body in a complex manner. The fat mass of the body operates much like an organ—a larger fat mass produces and secretes greater quantities of hormones.

The adipocyte (fat cell), for example, has recently been shown to produce a newly discovered hormone labeled resistin. Early studies linked this hormone to insulin resistance as a causal factor. More recent studies demonstrate that resistin might not be the cause of insulin resistance but that it definitely has a significant influence on the way autocrine hormones function in the body. Autocrine hormones (prostaglandins, thromboxanes, prostacyclins, et cetera) are produced from essential fatty acids in the cells throughout the body, affecting localized areas. They're different from endocrine hormones (insulin, thyroxine, estrogen, and testosterone), the gland-produced variety sent out via the bloodstream to influence target cells or systems far away in the body.

Larger volumes of fat in the adipocyte will propagate the production and secretion of more resistin, which interacts in the body with tumor necrosis factor (TNF) and either directly or indirectly with insulin. TNF and insulin are implicated in common diseases that are inflammatory in nature—rheumatoid arthritis, for example. This means an unhealthy fat mass can interrupt the natural communication systems of the body through the hormones it secretes. The fat mass is an organ that must be maintained in functional form in order for general biological health to be optimal.

Health Canada Report in 2000

Cardiovascular disease accounts for 37% of all male deaths in Canada and 41% of female deaths.

American Heart Association Report in 2000

Fifty-seven percent of men and 64% of women who died suddenly of cardiovascular disease had no previous symptom of this disease.

Body fat breeds insulin resistance and insulin resistance begets body fat. You might have heard of Syndrome X and the rising number of individuals diagnosed with this mysterious disorder. Syndrome X is insulin resistance and its associated secondary diseases. Insulin resistance (lesser degrees of diabetes) and obesity have rapidly become present-day epidemics that lay the foundation for other common pandemic disorders plaguing us, the majority of which are intensified by underlying inflammation. And fat mass propagates inflammation!

The American Diabetes Association warns Americans that the incidence of obesity is on the rise in the United States. A quick look at the figures tabulated below confirms this.

Rates of Obesity in the United States

Year	Percentage of Obese Men and Women (Average)
1991	12
1994	14
1996	16
1998	18

Not surprisingly, the occurrence of obesity-related diseases is escalating, as well. The choice is yours: stick with the typical processed, high-glycemic, convenient North American diet and you'll continue to choke the life right out of you. Ageless Performance will activate and maintain natural thermogenic (fat-burning) activity without toxic, stimulatory drugs. The biochemical influence that Ageless Performance generates on the body's hormonal cascade will burn unwanted pounds away naturally, safely, and with little effort. In fact, weight loss will ensue without even requiring the energy expenditure of exercise, although exercise facilitates the process and promotes other health benefits.

Hypertension is said to be the "silent killer," affecting millions of people without their knowledge. Long-term effects include enlargement of the heart, blood-vessel occlusions, stroke, and damage to kidneys and eyes. The North American diet establishes the basis for the development of these disorders, but you don't have to contribute to the horrific statistics.

American Heart Association (AHA) statistics reveal that 24% of men and 42% of women die within one year of experiencing an identified heart attack, and every 53 seconds an American suffers a stroke while every 3.3 minutes someone in the United States dies from a stroke. Since tabulation of these statistics is a time-consuming and cumbersome process, only in 2000 were the results for 1998 determined. In 1998, 12.4 million, or 4.6% of the total population of the United States, had coronary heart disease (CHD). Ageless Performance corrects cellular chemistry so that cardiovascular-system maintenance ensues according to genetic design. Healthy cardiovascular function is a central focus of the program.

As for athletic performance, all of these factors apply. Maintaining a healthy fat mass contributes to better performance potential in many ways. It allows the body to recover from training more efficiently and frees it from an unnecessary free-radical load. A healthier fat mass maintains healthier insulin function, enhancing athletic-performance potential. Maintenance of optimal cardiovascular operation is an obvious advantage for athletics, as well. Ageless Performance prompts the body to establish maximum efficiency in numerous ways and for all walks of life.

Just think. A family of four or more, perhaps your own family, has at least one member who could die of

American Heart Association Report in 2000

Cardiovascular disease accounts for about 41% of the total mortality from all causes.... These diseases as a whole represent the number one cause of death in the U.S.

Health Canada Report in 2000

Cancer accounts for 28% of all male deaths and 27% of all female deaths.

cancer. Chances are you may battle alongside one of your loved ones and finally bury him or her after cancer has taken his or her life. If it's not someone in your family, it could be you everyone else mourns. That's hard to take, but it's a statistical fact. However, you can change your family's odds. You do have the ability to battle cancer successfully, but the most powerful strategy against this opponent begins long before you encounter the disease. Prevention before intervention! Ageless Performance is powerful prevention.

Ageless Performance molds and balances the chemistry of eicosanoid-hormone status. Studies show that the imbalance of this system produces hormones that support the development of cancer. Insulin resistance grossly distorts this system, and diabetes desecrates it. Bringing balance helps prevent cancer.

Health Canada Report in 2000

Over two million Canadians have diabetes and over 90% of these cases are Type II diabetics.

The majority of Type II diabetics develop the disease due to poor lifestyle and physical conditioning. The symptoms are something we need to be aware of: irritability, frequent urination, unusual thirst, weakness, fatigue, poor wound healing, numbness in the hands and feet, and blurred vision. Type II diabetes is now common in teens and even children. However, this trend could be stopped if nutritional instruction became part of the national education system. But it's not, and so the responsibility is ours to set by example. If you have children, you have to teach them habits they'll carry with them into adulthood. Lead by example! Break the cycle now and give them the chance they deserve.

In the United States statistics are no better for diabetes. The American Diabetes Association (ADA) states that "15.7 to 17 million people, or 5.9% of the population in the U.S., have diabetes." These numbers don't include the vast population not diagnosed. U.S. statistics further reveal that the fourth leading cause of death is diabetes, with that disease also being the major cause of blindness and kidney ailments. The ADA reports that "each year in the U.S. 12,000 to 24,000 people lose their sight because of diabetes...each year 56,000 amputations are performed among people with diabetes."

These frightening trends have made health care one of the most lucrative businesses to pursue in the United States. In Canada these statistics clearly indicate the breakdown of the national health-care system. The ADA states that diabetes is a chronic disease that has no cure, but that isn't true. Type II diabetes *is* curable; well in excess of 90% of diabetics are Type II, and Ageless Performance is the power-punch cure.

The University of Washington Orthopedics and Sports Medicine Department informs us that arthritis refers to as many as 100 different diseases affecting the area in or around the body's joints. The Arthritis National Research Foundation reports that "over 43 million Americans, or one in every seven, has arthritis." That's about 14% of all Americans! Can diet ameliorate an arthritic state? It certainly can.

Arthritis is crippling our young; it's no longer a disease of the elderly. Studies detailed in ensuing chapters demonstrate that the poor nutritional status of the body plays an immense role in the development of this disease. Obviously if the body is supplied with all the building blocks it requires for the reconstruction of tissues, its degree of degeneration might not reach levels of disease so early in life. Nutraceuticals can provide relief from inflammation and usually without the common side effects that pharmaceutical drugs deliver. Prevention, however, furnishes maintenance so that inflammation is never a factor.

The degradation of tissue develops at an even faster pace in the extraordinarily active athlete. The consequence

Health Canada Report in 2000

The incidence of arthritis and other inflammatory conditions is greater than ever.

of a more concentrated free-radical pool can be arthritis and other degenerative injuries that arise more expeditiously in the athlete. Studies are now confirming that this includes brain damage. Ageless Performance facilitates tissue recovery to maintain optimal function and maximum performance potential—a clearer mind and a stronger body for a much longer period of time.

Even rheumatoid arthritis, a disease known to be autoimmune in nature, can be relieved with sound nutraceutical strategies. Resorting to pharmaceutical strategies rarely addresses the biochemical cause of the symptom or disease. On the other hand, the application of a precise nutraceutical strategy can induce a positive, gene-directed regulation of the chemistry responsible for the inflammatory process.

The recent unveiling of the complete human genome has opened a window into the chemistry that predisposes such diseases, allowing for more precise applications of nutraceutical combinations as well as of pharmaceuticals. The exciting opportunity resulting from this unveiling is twofold: the preventive potential of nutraceuticals can now be applied with meticulous accuracy and greater potency, and the recovery or therapeutic potential of natural-remedy programs can be designed with such exact focus that the need for foreign chemistry such as common pharmaceutical drugs will decrease significantly in years to come. Consequently, and fortunately, the side effects associated with the extensive use of pharmaceuticals will also decline. Ageless Performance is a function of this new-age science— a new age in health care.

Coritcosteroids, commonly prescribed anti-inflammatory drugs, can deliver immediate relief, but they also impede the deployment of the body's natural anti-inflammatory chemistry, seeding a dependency on the drug. The nutraceutically founded strategy of Ageless Performance, very simply, addresses the biochemical imbalance, the root of disease, to allow the body to implement its intrinsic anti-inflammatory chemistry.

The program is designed to deliver potent gastrointestinal support, and in this way it protects against the unregulated systemic circulation of the microbe-loaded contents of the gut. In fact, rheumatoid arthritis might be instigated by excessive gut permeability. Gastrointestinal health is critical for recovery from arthritis and other autoimmune disorders.

Osteoarthritis, although a much different disease than rheumatoid arthritis, can also be improved with this nutritional corrective program. Most pharmaceutical drugs used to treat these conditions are analgesics (painkillers), anti-inflammatories that merely provide symptomatic relief from swelling, pain, and inflammation. But that's not enough. The cause of disease, whether physical wear and tear or biochemical assault, will continue to snip away at your connective tissue. These same factors will also chop away at your lifeline if they're not addressed. The chemical damage of cartilage tissues is truly indicative of the status of the entire body, shedding light on the biochemical festering that inevitably manifests as other disorders.

Ageless Performance is designed to stimulate widespread general healing, an inherent process that can't give rise to secondary consequences the way drugs can. It reinvigorates all of the cells to activate the healing chemistry trying to surface at all times in all of us. Most nutraceutical therapies for arthritis, for example, involve a passive supply of building blocks and, to a degree, this strategy works. Glucosamine supplementation is an example of passive therapy. It works, but the result is limited to cellular health or cellular nutritional status.

If the cells can't take up glucosamine due to dysfunctional membranes, what good is the expensive supplementation? If the cells are able to take in less than their maximum potential due to partial membrane impairment, recovery will be less than the full potential of the therapy. Studies in the past few years have demonstrated that the genes of the cartilage-manufacturing cells can become dormant, and unless they're activated, glucosamine supplementation won't work its wonders even if taken by the shovelful. If you're like most North Americans, the cause of your disease is nutrient imbalance. The cellular result is biochemical imbalance, which impairs the ability of cells to utilize building blocks like glucosamine. Nutraceuticals have been shown to stimulate the dormant genes, initiating anabolism or tissue regeneration.

The lack of nitric-oxide regulation within the chondrocyte (the cell responsible for collagen and cartilage synthesis) is now recognized as a major factor involved in the impediment of cartilage synthesis. In fact, an unnatural nitric-oxide elevation of the chondrocyte must first be down-regulated to allow these cells to utilize substrates like glucosamine and allow tissue regeneration to ensue. Nutrient deficiency leads to nitric-oxide misregulation. Today we see a lot of media hype about nitric-oxide *activators* or supplements said to stimulate nitric-oxide production in the body. These applications stem from the fact that a nitric-oxide shortfall is a central factor in the debilitation of cardiovascular function, but the model of the chondrocyte represents the exact opposite—excess nitric oxide induces impairment at this site. The obvious point is that nitric-oxide shortages or elevations aren't the causes of disease when relating to the entire human organism. We know now that nitric-oxide misregulation is thrown more out of line as we age. Regulation of this biologically universal system prevents and even reverses disease and also retards biological age.

The only way this complex nitric-oxide system can be rejuvenated is through the activation of nitric-oxide production, but only after the appropriate regulatory chemistry has been put in place to heighten the body's ability to regulate this reactive substance. Ageless Performance incorporates efficient nitric-oxide activation with precise regulation that enables us to experience better athletic and sexual endurance, better muscle pumps from physical work, more energy, and improved physical and mental health.

Recently insulin resistance and the nitric-oxide system have been identified as central to the development of multiple diseases. The resolution of our widespread debilitating diseases involves improving dietary nutritional balance, which subsequently directs the correction of cellular balance, promoting the natural enhancement of these two systems through self-regulation. Ageless Performance is high-density nourishment with highly specialized cell resuscitators that stimulate all the cells of the body and maintain their new state so they can fulfill their vital roles.

Concerning osteoarthritis, the important cells involved are chondrocytes. Activation of the chondrocyte is critical to long-term recovery from the wear on cartilage tissue. As already mentioned, chondrocytes actually utilize building blocks, such as those supplied in typical glucosamine supplements, to synthesize proteoglycans and collagen. Supplying the building blocks without first *resuscitating* these cartilage-producing cells will result in less than maximum results from a basic glucosamine-supplement strategy.

SAMe acts as a resuscitator of burnt-out chondrocytes. There are studies that compare this nutraceutical to pharmaceutical remedies, proving that the natural alternative is as good, if not better, than anti-inflammatories such as ibuprofen and piroxicam. The great thing about these advanced nutraceutical strategies is that they're able to help regenerate new tissue and provide an analgesic and anti-inflammatory result without the gut-busting side effects pharmaceuticals can deliver. SAMe induces regeneration by down-regulating nitric-oxide levels of the chondrocyte.

The majority of pharmaceuticals designed for these inflammatory disorders don't deliver the same regeneration potential nutraceuticals supply. Most pharmaceutical drugs are devised to deal with the symptom of disease. SAMe, however, even works to stimulate the synovial cells' production of synovial fluid, which fosters the recovery and reversal of the damage rheumatoid arthritis imparts. Still, SAMe and glucosamine supplementation is only part of a complete strategy. For the newly resuscitated cells to persist with their new level of functionality, they must have a sound nutritional status from which to operate, and this involves presaturation with all of the essential nutrients and requires that a whole-food foundation set a stable biochemical platform in the cells. A recovery program must address the cause of disease, and in most cases the cause is the poorly equipped cell. If deficiency isn't addressed, even if recovery is experienced with the likes of SAMe, the diseased state will reappear quickly.

This phenomenon is characterized by our acceptable cycles of remission and activity for common afflictions such as inflammatory bowel disease (IBD), colitis, Crohn's disease, multiple sclerosis (MS), and so on. If the diet and/or environmental influence that created the imbalance or deficiency isn't corrected, the disease is placed into a state of remission by a pharmaceutical or a nutraceutical. The festering will continue, and sooner or later a trigger will bring the underlying imbalance to the surface in the form of the same disease or perhaps another.

TAKING THE RIGHT PATH

There are so many products, nutraceutical and pharmaceutical, that claim to deliver one benefit or another and, in some cases, the boasts are valid. However, the purveyors of these remedies may apply incomplete strategies to meet saleable prices. An ingredient scientifically proven to provide results might be found in a nutritional product, but the recommended doses on the label might not be high enough to support the claims indicated in the research.

The formula is often developed this way to prevent the application from being cost-prohibitive. A manufacturer may use this strategy when hyped research is brought to consumer awareness by the media. Unsuspecting consumers might not know that MSM is required in 3 to 10 g daily doses to furnish significant results. However, the hype has prompted them to buy 250 mg capsule doses when the correct way to take MSM is by the teaspoonful.

A certain ingredient may be included in the wrong biochemical form or without the synergistic components noted in a study. Consumers might buy citrus aurantium (CA), having heard that studies have proven it to be a great fat-busting aid, but they might not know that caffeine (a phospho-diesterase blocker) and ASA (a prostaglandin blocker) must be taken with it to release its full potential. Alpha lipoic acid is another similar example in which an expensive nutraceutical is often recommended by a product label to be taken in 50 mg doses daily to present an economical supplement when the best results are delivered by 100 to 150 mg three to four times daily. The form of this compound is also critical, since the R+ isomer is the biologically active type while other forms can interfere with the active isomer and even produce ill effects. Armed with reliable information, the kind you'll find in this book, you'll be able to choose the best-quality ingredients, the most effective products, and the right therapeutic path.

When it comes to pharmaceuticals, research is often incompletely reported and side effects are rarely clearly conveyed, but the consequences these drugs can impart can be far more profound than those imposed by common nutraceuticals. Most of us don't know where to turn amid this confusion, so we leave all the decision-making to health-care professionals. However, medical professionals don't get the training needed to appreciate the value of nutraceutical prevention and therapy programs, while naturopathic doctors don't receive the thorough pharmaceutical education conventional practitioners acquire. This is a problem because these two realms become separate courses of action for therapy, and the complementary value of each is rarely applied. Health care isn't about pharmaceuticals versus nutraceuticals. Health care is one science.

The healthy solution is to find a health-care professional who is well versed in both pharmaceuticals and nutraceuticals, with nutraceutical applications being the primary therapy of choice. The best solution is prevention, and that requires self-education.

By the time osteoporosis is evident, the degenerative results are well advanced and the effects are far deeper than the bone mass. Turning the condition around isn't easy, but it is possible. Contrary to popular belief, recovery means much more than just calcium supplementation and a great deal more than combination treatments involving calcium, magnesium, and vitamin D. This condition most often results from poor dietary and lifestyle habits that have persisted for decades.

Osteoporosis is another disease that arises from poor metabolic health. Ageless Performance is intended to transform dysfunctional metabolism into a functional state and then support this status. The program will facilitate recovery from osteoporosis simply by enhancing the biochemical operation of the cells responsible for resorption and mineralization of bone, delivering an unlimited supply of the many building blocks essential to bone-matrix construction.

Ageless Performance involves a nutraceutical tuning of the highly specialized osteoclasts and osteoblasts, cells engaged in the regulation of bone mass. You don't have to wait for disease to appear before you apply this remarkable plan. More than likely you won't even know osteoporosis is brewing until it's too late, so get on the program now and take a strong stand against this debilitating disease.

Health Canada Report in 2000

Osteoporosis affects one in four women of age 60 or more. Although it's found to be more frequent in women, it can develop in any one of us for various reasons.

Asthma is usually caused by triggers or allergens that irritate the airways, forcing them to constrict. I say it's "usually caused" by these external triggers because much of the time our cells are hypersensitized by imbalances that fuel the hyperactivity leading to the attack. We're all exposed to similar triggers, especially with the level of pollution we encounter today. However, we all respond in different degrees and in variable ways to these triggers due to the unique condition of our individual intracel-lular biochemistries, which profoundly influence our immunogenic responses to environmental toxins.

Our biochemistries in turn are directed by our profiles of nourishment. In other words, our food intakes have a significant influence on the status of asthma. As with arthritis and other inflammatory conditions, asthma involves nitric-oxide regulation, insulin activity, and eicosanoid and other hormone cascades that have gone haywire but can be guided back to regulation. In short, we can take control of an asthmatic condition by changing our dietary chemistries.

The American Lung Association (ALA) reports that pollution in our outdoor air is a growing concern, but the answer to this problem isn't tightly insulated homes to barricade us from this assault. In fact, reports convey that our houses and apartments might be as toxic as our workplaces and the outdoor air we all share. Combustion products from stoves, furnaces, fireplaces, heaters, and cigarette smoke are major sources of car-cinogenic and irritating pollution. Other household irritants include pet dander, mites, pollen, and molds, as well as organics from paint, glues, adhesives, asbestos, cleaning agents, pesticides, disinfectants, and deodorizers. Surveys show that American adults spend about 90% of their time indoors. The triggers for asthma are impossible to avoid, but managing our biological responses is something we can achieve.

The ALA estimates that "asthma is the number one cause of school absences amongst children. It's the second leading cause of hospitalization amongst children…some data suggests that asthma accounts for a third of emergency room visits…. The cost of asthma in the year 2000 in the U.S. was estimated to be 12.7 billion dollars." The American Academy of Allergy, Asthma and Immunology offers a September 2001 article (Canada NewsWire via Comtex). The article reveals, based on statistical data, that "worldwide asthma rates are rising by 50% every 10 years and more than 180,000 people die from asthma each year around the world." Ageless Performance opens the airways and oxygenates our bodies.

INVESTIGATE FOR YOURSELF

The next time you visit your local grocery store do a little investigation. Take a close look at the shoppers around you. The objective will be to assess their perceived state of health by visible inspection and then link your conclusions to the contents of their shopping carts. The best place to do this is at the checkout counter. Peer into your fellow shopper's eyes to look for clarity. Is there a dark ring around them? How does his hair look? Is it dry and brittle, or is it healthy and lustrous? Does he walk with a limp? Is he in pain? Does he seem arthritic? How is his skin tone? Is it pale and pasty, or does it have a healthy color? Is his skin dry and flat or glowing with life? Is the person slouching, leaning, or lacking energy? Is he vibrant and full of life? Does he have muscle tone?

The above is a long list, but you don't have to itemize everything. You can usually get a pretty good idea of a person's state of health and general vitality with only an extended glance.

Now make your assessment of each person. Very simply categorize them: are they Healthy, Unhealthy, or Can't Tell. Then look at the contents of their carts. The Healthy category of people will likely have smaller carts filled with more whole foods such as fresh vegetables, grains, and fruits, as well as healthy meats like fish and free-range chicken. The Unhealthy type will usually possess full carts crammed with boxes, cans, premixes, sugary breakfast cereals, bread, chips, pop, candy, and other high-glycemic-index, processed foods. The number of people making it into the category of "shallow cart consisting of whole, fresh, unprocessed foods" is likely to be small.

Dare you look at yourself with the same scrutiny? You'll be better equipped to assess the value of food after you finish reading this book. However, I suggest a preliminary self-examination now so you can compare your results with a similar evaluation after you've learned a lot more about nutrition.

You've probably noticed that supermarkets are packed with many of the foods you and your loved ones should avoid. In fact, since most of these disease-instigating, processed foods reap big profits for businesses, they're well marketed. Good salesmanship involves product positioning and visibility in stores. Which products are most visible? Which ones are at eye level for adults or their pleading kids?

Cereal marketers craftily tempt innocent children with sugar-coated disease in colorful boxes. They first attract a child's attention through television commercials, then place the poison at low levels in stores where children will recognize the advertised product. This vicious attack on our youth is unforgivable.

North Americans are being poisoned with these refined, high-glycemic, additive-laden foods. Consumer demand ensures these products take up the majority of shelf space in convenience stores and supermarkets. But you can change all that by creating a different, healthier demand by making healthier choices.

DEFINING THE PICTURE— THE OTHER END OF THE SPECTRUM

People in pursuit of leaner measures have been the targets of marketing campaigns since the inception of the health-and-fitness industry. Although being lean is the healthy way to go, extremely lean measures can lead to disease. The images fashion statements portray have resulted in unrealistic, unhealthy goals for those who fall victim to the messages.

Many people hastily strip unwanted pounds, and to do so they employ fad diets and rigorous training to work out their bodies to the bone. Having reached these excessive goals through methods that fail to preserve nutrient status, these individuals set themselves up for a rebound that often leads to more than just the original weight restored. This rebound can also result in an increased risk of the diseases mentioned earlier.

Not only have I seen this rebound in family and friends, I've personally experienced it. Obsessive competition can result in an unhealthy lifestyle as the quest to make a weight class and define muscle for the event can cause extreme leanness that makes an individual fall below healthy levels. For me, peaking for a bodybuilding competition meant that body-fat percentages could drop as low as 3%, a condition that made me feel lethargic until a safer minimum of 8% to 9% was reestablished after the show.

Although this feeling of malaise is alleviated within a week of competition—the time it usually takes to restore healthy body-fat levels—the underlying damage isn't as quickly reversed. Healthy body-fat levels for women differ from those of men. Typically women shouldn't drop below 16% body fat, since extreme lows often interrupt ovulation cycles. There are some atypical individuals in both genders who seem to function normally at drastic lows. However, even these people may experience dire consequences due to acute leanness, consequences, in fact, similar to those related to obesity.

Reducing body-fat levels quickly and to dangerous lows can result in an imbalance of the cells' essential fats and the specialized compounds produced from them. The cellular disarray that develops from this extremely lean conditioning isn't that different from the havoc created by the nutrient-scant, processed diet many North Americans indulge in. This costly strategy produces the severe imbalance of cell-membrane fats and the fats required for eicosanoid-hormone synthesis, which leave cells disconnected from one another, puts the body into a kind of metabolic hiccough, and lays the foundation for grave consequences.

VITAL FATS

Special fats and their derivatives constitute the fundamental structure of every cell membrane in the body. These derivatives are additionally used as precursors or building material for powerful hormones that regulate many important processes that influence the cardiovascular system, insulin function, inflammatory response, cognition, weight management, and more. In my case every time I peaked for a bodybuilding event, this imbalanced state advanced. After several years of competition, the implications were quite serious, with each year having a cumulative effect. Eventually I succumbed to chronic inflammation, which led to ulcerative colitis. But Ageless Performance was developed through years of trial and tribulation and painstakingly compiled, documented research to address this disease, and for nine years or more ulcerative colitis has been nonexistent in my life—gone for good!

This biochemical phenomenon is common today because these very fats are lacking in our diets. Such fats are also reactive and susceptible to degradation or deactivation by the processing methods currently used. The deactivation of these fats in our processed foods is another way our North American manner of eating interferes with the route to healthy hormone status.

Yo-yo dieting is no different from the recipes some athletes employ. Every time we reduce body-fat levels quickly and to extreme lows a state of imbalance is established—and we don't have to sink to 3%. Furthermore, the common binging that takes place between restrictive periods often results in consumption of foods that contain the wrong fats, which can be inserted in place of the correct fats in the previously depleted cell membranes. All of this damage can be avoided if a nutrient-dense diet, limited in caloric value, is adhered to. Ageless Performance is nutrient-rich and calorie-restricted, and it's easy to stay with because *you* become the hormone regulator rather than let yourself be controlled by hormone fluctuations. The solution to our common problem is quite simple: we must return to whole, unprocessed, nutrient-dense foods for sustenance. But this alone isn't enough; we must also do something about the nutrient-depleted state of our food supply.

The evolutionary process took place with food of higher density than our current whole food's potential. In addition, we are now subjected to unbearable environmental toxicity. The only way to survive this cesspool is to provide higher-than-*normal* antioxidant protection. This goal requires the meticulously crafted plan Ageless Performance delivers, but again the program involves much more than mere antioxidant protection.

HISTORICAL DEVELOPMENT OF AGELESS PERFORMANCE

Ageless Performance is based on sound scientific principles. My studies from performance nutrition to therapeutic and preventive nutrition were motivated by personal goals and my own struggle. The early years of my research focused exclusively on the biochemistry of cellular efficiency geared for athletic performance.

Major events in my life changed this research concentration and opened my eyes to a new perspective and a different way of life. Sports and performance are still big parts of who I am, but so are the science of nutraceutical therapy and the extraction of our inherent healing and preventive processes.

Some time ago my studies revealed that the same cellular efficiency underlying athletic performance serves as the foundation of immune-system performance. These discoveries propelled me to another level of understanding of cellular biochemistry. One day, while overwhelmed by the anguish from uncontrollable disease, it became clear to me that many of the concepts I had applied in sports were common to the protocols required for recovery from disease. This was a true turning point in my life.

The common factor in most cases of disease, I soon confirmed in my research, is the biochemical process propagated by inflammation. In the cases of cardiovascular illnesses or cognitive and neurological disorders such as Alzheimer's and multiple sclerosis, the underlying factor in the mediation of their development is inflammation. Aging, as well, has an inflammatory basis.

Regulation of the body's inflammatory process helps keep disease at bay. Inflammation, as we'll see, is ultimately caused by oxidative stress (free-radical toxicity) and this presents a very difficult situation. While oxidative stress promotes inflammation, the damage engendered by the latter triggers immune activity, which in turn leads to more oxidative stress, creating a vicious cycle of disease propagating disease that's extremely hard to terminate once initiated. What's more, oxidative stress converts biologically important nitric oxide into a destructive compound—the dreaded peroxynitrite free radical—as well as into other nitrites and nitrates. These substances inflict carnage on the chemistry, cells, and genes of the body. The most powerful way to remedy this problem, however, is to regulate the inflammatory process before it's knocked out of control, and this can be achieved through proper diet and strategic supplementation—the essence of prevention and life extension.

Oversecretion of insulin promotes degenerative free radicals, inflammation and, of course, aging. Take control of this inflammatory chemistry and the years will pass you by while your biological clock ticks at a slower pace.

SLOWING THE AGING PROCESS

In ensuing chapters you'll be shown just how vital a complete antioxidant strategy is to the regulation of inflammation and the prevention of disease. The imposition of the free radical on the body permeates at various levels. It damages the delicate cell membranes and, as already mentioned, it interferes with biological enzymes, hormones, and gene expression or translation. The result of this interference is disease and an accelerated rate of aging. How can we neutralize free radicals? With antioxidants, but not just any old one.

Judith M of Toronto, Canada, left a message with my answering service to tell me her fight with diabetes was over after 30 years of battling with the disease. I finally spoke to this elated woman to get the whole story. She attended one of my seminars in Toronto and applied my recommendations, and in a matter of weeks experienced complete recovery. Judith M explained that her case was a difficult one in which pharmaceutical drugs couldn't help. She turned to naturopathics and experienced better results, bringing her fasting serum-glucose levels down to 8 to 9 millimoles from an astronomical high. With this historical success she became the central focus of a case-study series that was written up in textbooks to detail her pseudo-recovery.

After listening to my lecture, Judith M presented her notes to her health-care professional and insisted that she be put on my program. She terminated all naturopathic and pharmaceuticals which, of course, I don't recommend anyone should do without a professional's guidance. Judith M's health-care professional monitored her progress on Ageless Performance. Within weeks of applying the strategy exclusively, Judith M experienced normal blood-sugar readings—fasting serum-blood-sugar levels of 4.5 to 5.5 millimoles. After 30 years of unnecessary struggle, Judith M achieved a miraculous recovery in merely weeks and maintained this state. She also managed to alleviate her chronic arthritis at the same time. Miraculous indeed, but it wasn't my miracle.

The miracle is built right into our genetic programming. We only have to learn how to extract it. Ageless Performance leads us down that path. Improved athletic performance can be ours, too. The possibilities are deep within us. We simply need to instill cellular efficiency to the point where genetic potential is allowed to surface.

I have yet to see a fitness or competitive nutritional program that's complete. Incomplete programming results in less than maximum performance, both athletic and immune. Incomplete programming results can also cause further degradation of the body. The power source for sport is deep within us waiting to emerge. People who think they're at their full potential without having applied complete nutritional support are dead wrong. Ageless Performance extracts our full potential to propel us to new levels of skill.

GET WITH THE PROGRAM

Many different facets of health and fitness are covered by Ageless Performance. The objective of the program is to initiate biological efficiency and optimize the function of each of the different systems that need to work in co-dependent synergy. With this efficiency the immune system can employ an impermeable shield, every cell of the body can perform at full capacity, the metabolism will burn at a proper rate, weight management will become effortless, and you'll be vitalized with a new outlook and, consequentially, a new "outer look."

Every single one of us is exposed to environmental assault from toxins such as pesticides, pollution, and man-made synthetics. Your test will come when your immune system is called upon to battle disease, and the odds dictate disease *will* come your way. Statistics inform us that one in every two of us will die of cardiovascular disease. Obviously your chances of long-lived health can be significantly improved if you evade this affliction alone. One in every three of us is expected to die of cancer. Regardless of your perceived health today, tomorrow can be a turning point for which you must be prepared. Maximum nutrient status of the body prepares you for a successful battle. If you give Ageless Performance a chance, you'll reduce the risk of cancer ever successfully infiltrating your body.

In subsequent chapters you'll learn more about studies that confirm conclusively that pre-exposure to antioxidants such as grapeseed extract and other special antioxidant concoctions will reduce and even completely prevent damage from exposure to toxicity. Control subjects who *did not* administer these protective shields experienced irreversible tissue and organ damage from the same exposure. That's what prevention is all about. If you're like most people, not only are you ill-prepared but you're contributing to disease.

Health and fitness require *knowing*. This *knowing* is two-dimensional. The first dimension is *knowing* your true potential. Know it's in you and know you can develop it. The second dimension is knowing how to feed and fuel a healthy outcome. Whether you're battling illness or boxing in the ring, you'll start to lose the second your faith in your ability to win falters. You have atomic power packed deep within you just waiting to emerge. Know it's there, harness it, and take delivery of this potential to serve your needs and those of your fellow humans.

Believe and you will achieve!

2

PEERING INTO THE PROGRAM

IN DAYS OF OLD, GRANDDAD SAID...

In days of old, specifically the late 19th and very early 20th centuries, vitamin supplementation was unheard of and natural food was the only source of nourishment. However, once upon that same time hardworking farm folk plowed their fields and sowed their own futures. Physical work wasn't feared; it was a way of life and a conditioner of health. Chemical fertilizers were uncommon then, and automated labor was hard to come by. Your grandparents and their parents, if they lived on a farm or in a small town, might not have had a car, and perhaps they didn't have conveniently piped-in running water carrying lead, copper, and other toxic metals. But those days of old are gone, and there's nothing we can do to detoxify completely the cesspool we find ourselves in.

The need for vitamin and mineral supplements might not have been as critical in former days. The environment wasn't as poisonous as it is today, and fruits and vegetables were grown organically, harvested and eaten freshly picked, and dense with nourishment. Chemical pesticides and growth facilitators didn't exist, and the demand for neutralizing phytochemicals (plant chemicals) and antioxidants wasn't as great as it is today.

Antibiotic-, pesticide-, and hormone-free animal stock were fed local hay, corn, grain, and fresh grass. Meat, poultry, eggs, dairy products, and fish were fresh. Cooking oils such as olive and flaxseed were locally pressed without the need for deactivating long-term storage. Manual harvesting and commuting by foot and bicycle provided for natural-resistance work-load and cardiovascular conditioning. This is the very lifestyle many of us are trying to revert to now, but escape from our new-age pollution is impossible.

The reckless manhandling of nature has caused sickening global consequences. Our efforts to increase crop yields and prolong the shelf life of our food have resulted in frightful ramifications that have long been recognized but are only now beginning to be understood and addressed. The very chemicals that have boosted crop yields to help meet demands for food supply have instigated serious health concerns. This imposition has intensified free-radical toxicity, consequently amplifying the body's need for vitamins, minerals, and other phytonutrients (plant nutrients) at a time when they're less available in our food.

Recent research has revealed that these impositions permeate far deeper than the damage they deliver to cell surfaces. The destruction is even more profound than gene damage, which can usually be repaired by built-in DNA-maintenance systems. This toxicity influences gene activity, stimulating some and blocking other genes. The net result of this uncontrolled gene modification is metabolic havoc and disease. But the genes and gene modifiers involved have now been identified to allow us to focus our counterefforts with great precision. Ageless Performance delivers these cutting-edge countermeasures.

Deficiency in vitamin and mineral status results in modification of gene activity at multiple levels. At one level vitamin and mineral antioxidants can neutralize the unnatural modification that toxins may impose before they get a chance to deliver their altering effects on genes, thus alleviating some of the strain. Another level of activity is much deeper: various vitamins and phytonutrients stimulate or help regulate the operation of genes. They can even reactivate codes that may have become dormant over time and with toxic chemical influence. This newly discovered nutrient activity is a more direct gene modification, a powerful remedy that supports the application of various orthomolecular strategies with new scientific evidence. Minerals and vitamins are also essential co-factors for hormones and their cell-membrane receptors. A mild shortfall in these mediators and protectors of cell chemistry results in a mild downfall in the chemistry of life.

It's unfathomable that our government-regulatory efforts pull many of our protective supplemental nutrients out of an over-the-counter status and into a prescription-only system. In this reactive situation these supplements aren't available to us unless disease is diagnosed which, of course, means the incidence of disease will rise. The most successful application against disease is the preventive potential of supplements. Supplementation with doses of vitamin C that exceed 2,500 mg daily is an example of the orthomolecular influence we can impose on gene activity. But a question we have to ask ourselves is whether or not this dosage level is, in fact, orthomolecular, or a normal requirement amid today's free-radical-laden environment.

Vitamin C, for instance, influences the activity of the chondrocytes, the cells responsible for proteoglycan and cartilage synthesis. Conventional thinking has misinterpreted this activity as pharmacological, and the question of whether such applications are drugs is now an issue. However, in this case the positive activity associated with the vitamin might not be pharmacological at all and is likely a result of making an essential nutrient available in doses that allow it to reach the chondrocyte at a level of concentration that's effective. It might take such high doses to permeate the cellular sludge of oxidation we experience in this age of toxic overload. In essence, the prerequisite for nutrients such as this one to overcome free-radical loads and then deliver its biological potential to our genetic codes is probably much higher today than several decades ago. Thus the minimum daily requirements of these antioxidant co-factors are higher than they used to be, necessitating supplementation in order for demands to be met. Positioning our essential nutrients as pharmacological agents that require prescription for administration is an absurd notion that pushes us even deeper into a failing, reactive health-care system.

Megadosing vitamin C alone, however, might not allow this gene modifier to target specific genes efficiently, either. Other factors synergize its activity and navigation to the site, and that's why many people fail to experience results from common supplements. Grapeseed extract also supports cartilage-tissue regeneration and anti-inflammatory activity and, as we'll see in the reference-supported chapters to come, this is due in part to grapeseed's maintenance of vitamin C in its antioxidant role, allowing the vitamin's levels to be raised high enough in the body to provide a positive influence on cartilage regeneration in the chondrocyte. In this combination lower intakes of vitamin C can produce the results of higher levels of C taken without grapeseed. Precise synergy and exact dosages are critical to a successful outcome. The natural synergistic combinations have been undermined by our food processing and unnatural fertilizing methods, as well. It's easy to see how we've developed a dependence on daily use of plant extracts. Lower doses of our vitamins in our diets give rise to the need for herbal extracts such as grapeseed's as ongoing enhancers. It all sounds complex, but in the end you'll get the proven, distilled program to apply.

Incomplete fortification of overused agricultural plots and premature harvesting have led to lower nutrient values in our foods when we need them most to combat environmental assault. As though these inadequacies weren't enough, aggressive processing of our life-sustaining nourishment further degrades its value to human health. This malnourishment has left our genes in a state of disarray. Our genetic profile is designed to react and be activated by a natural nutrient profile that doesn't exist in the 21st century no matter how hard we try to deliver it through a non-supplemented diet.

Nature has carefully formulated and bundled up packages of nourishment that, over millions of years, have developed concurrently with human evolution to sustain our existence. These profiles carefully crafted our genetic design. However, we've taken these nutritionally complete and nutrient-dense foods for granted and in a very short time, in relation to the evolutionary timeline, have altered them significantly to suit our own purposes. Hydrogenation, purification, debittering, decaffeination, extraction, isolation, hydrolysis, bleaching, genetic engineering, and many more processes strip raw foods that would otherwise supply complete and live nutrients.

These nutrient and environmental alterations have seeded and cultivated illnesses such as cancer, arthritis, asthma, diabetes, gastrointestinal disorders, skin diseases, and obesity. We have arrogantly chosen to apply more technology to treat our symptoms, but as soon as we admit our wrongdoing, we can address the causes of our uncontrollable afflictions.

You can choose to correct your direction right now. Change the food chemistry in your life and you'll immediately change your cells' biochemical makeup.

The irrefutable correlation between the world's increased rate of disease and the rapid acceleration of ecosystem and nourishment manipulation has created the basis for a research focus that scientists are now beginning to embrace. With the recent human genome work, the acceptance of nutraceutical science has become indisputable. What has been accomplished thus far in this new direction is the type of care we must adopt quickly if we're to survive our more toxic future. Health-care systems have failed to combine the nutraceutical and pharmaceutical factors into *one* program with *one* focus. Profit has become the all-consuming goal of the health-care equation and has interfered with the delivery of the right message and the correct treatment for those in need. It's time to wake up to the facts.

FREE-RADICAL STRESS AND THE PERILS OF NITRIC OXIDE

In the previous chapter I discussed how dangerous free radicals are. They rip away electrons within atoms in our bodies and change their chemical nature, thus damaging them. This havoc causes a chain reaction that flashes through our bodies, creating more unstable free radicals and more devastation. And that's why antioxidants are so important: they donate electrons to the unstable free radicals to stabilize the *hyper*activity and preserve and protect our functional atoms, cells, tissues, and genetic codes from damage.

Our environment is a cesspool of naturally occurring and man-made reagents that react with our complex biochemical systems, giving rise to free radicals. We are extensions of one another and our environment, and there is no escape from the wrath we've set ourselves up to be assaulted by. Your body is a vessel that carries on the environment's chemical reactions; free-radical activity bolts through you and into the universe as if no dermal barriers existed.

A multitude of chemicals such as synthetic drugs, pesticides, and pollutants can cause direct cellular damage as well as secondary oxidative stress from the free radicals they generate. In addition, free radicals inevitably born from normal metabolism of essential fuels will also contribute to the bombardment of tissues, DNA, and vital biochemicals to alter their functionality. Free radicals promote free radicals in an exponential manner similar to the way a secret can travel from one friend who tells two close friends and each subsequently tells two of their close friends and so on. Free radicals aren't science fiction; for a long time now they've been implicated as a major cause of aging and a significant facilitator of disease. Protection against these ravenous piranhas, however, isn't completely out of our control, but it's not as easy as we've been led to believe, either.

Oxidation is the process that slowly degrades our bodies, but we also depend on it for life as it ignites the fuels in our cells much as the spark in a combustion chamber ignites the gas that powers an engine. This energy-producing oxidation, however, is regulated in our cells. Given the many factors that influence oxidation and free-radical generation, directing the process to eliminate "uncontrolled" oxidation is likely impossible. Still, nature has provided us with miraculous substances with which our cells have been able to infuse some degree of protection. Like armor, antioxidants of plant origin that our cells can't synthesize join our internally manufactured antioxidants to shield the body from the ricocheting wildfire of rampant oxidation.

The scarcity in our food supply of these protective phyto-antioxidants (plant-sourced antioxidants), however, and the limited availability of other vital substances required by our bodies to produce their own protective antioxidants have resulted in protection that is far from impermeable. Antioxidants function as a complete system of co-dependent chemicals. The absence of one results in the incomplete neutralization of the high-energy, highly reactive free radical.

In essence, the free radical is taken down a series of steps in the antioxidant system to reduce its reactive potential to zero. If one step, or one antioxidant of the system, is missing, it's less likely that the reactivity potential will be reduced to zero or a harmless state. A complete system is more likely to reduce the highly reactive free radical to harmless carbon dioxide and water. Vitamins E and C, isoflavones, and other delicate antioxidants can be destroyed or removed by food processing, limiting the zero potential for reactive free radicals in our bodies.

Antioxidants possess powerful defensive capabilities, but they may only get to display one round of protection. They can also preserve the vegetables, grains, and fruits of which they are constituents. When foods are exposed and allowed to dehydrate for prolonged periods in our extremely oxidative environment, their antioxidants attempt to shield the plant's tissues and lose "loaded" status. If this deactivated sustenance makes up the majority of your diet, you're consuming, in a sense, used or dead food. Furthermore, recooked or reheated meals usually deliver reduced nutrient activity due to much of the same damage.

Supplementing our food's nutrient supply is critical for optimum health, and antioxidants really are potent preventive agents. So powerful, in fact, that in addition to influencing genes, specific nutraceuticals help control nitric oxide, a critical regulatory compound in the body. As much as nitric oxide is important to general biological function, it is still highly reactive, and amid a free-radical-laden system it can become quite toxic.

As mentioned in the previous chapter, many health-care experts have jumped on the nitric-oxide bandwagon. Nitric oxide is now recognized as a central factor in the disease equation. Stimulation of nitric-oxide-synthase (an enzyme that manufactures nitric oxide in the body) activity, and an inadvertent supply of nitric-oxide precursors such as the amino acid arginine, might not be a good idea unless biological regulation of this reactive molecule is concurrently implemented. The same is true for insulin regulation. Supporting efficient insulin activity and preventing insulin resistance are critical to the maintenance of optimal health, athletic performance, and youthful biological age, but efficiency isn't a function of stimulating the production of more insulin in the body above the normal baseline or by administering the hormone exogenously as many blind specialists recommend. Nutraceuticals and precise diet protocols have been recognized as significant strategies for improving insulin function and diminishing associated secondary diseases— powerful enough even to *reverse* a diabetic state within weeks. And insulin control is now seen as critical to nitric-oxide regulation.

The point is that addressing one isolated biological system of the body doesn't necessarily result in overall improved health. Paying attention to the multiple common systems that make up the biochemical Internet of human life *will* instill a positive outcome. Ageless Performance is a hormone regulator, a nitric-oxide optimizer, a gene modifier, and a biological network coordinator. It truly is the new face of health care, fitness, and athletic-performance facilitation.

The first step that Ageless Performance takes us through is the consumption of a whole, fresh-food diet to increase nutrient density and enhance the natural supply of protective antioxidants. Additionally the elimination of refined foods will itself contribute to insulin efficiency and reduce free-radical generation within the body. This simple step alone will contribute to better glucose tolerance and reduce any predisposition to inflammation. Remember, as mentioned earlier, that the chemistry of inflammation is the foundation for many of our epidemics. Furthermore, the inflammatory cascade can be seeded by insulin resistance or, more accurately, by hyper-insulinemia (excessive insulin secretions). You'll reduce and even eliminate this activity with Ageless Performance.

The next step of the program will be to supplement this more biologically active nourishment with a specialized formulation of antioxidants and building blocks. Our bodies have the ability to produce powerful antioxidants, but they require the right building blocks to do so. Our food supplies these building blocks, but it's up to us to make them available from whole, unprocessed sustenance. You wouldn't expect your car to run without fuel, and you know that same vehicle won't operate at full potential with gas that's diluted by water or contaminated. Usually a higher-octane fuel delivers better performance due to its greater concentration of combustibles. Nutrient supplements are much like the octane boosters we add to our gas, allowing the fuel to burn with greater efficiency and letting the body properly vent the toxic residue of combustion.

A car designed for high-octane gas won't operate as proficiently with lower-octane fuel. In fact, its engine is likely to wear out faster if a lower-grade fuel is used with each fill-up. Whole, concentrated nutrition delivers the same potential to our bodies, while compromised nourishment results in reduced performance and accelerates the rate of degeneration as our bodies knock and ping through the workload of life. The harder we push our bodies amid this uncontrolled combustion, the more damage we do to their internal mechanisms. Rigorous exercise or competitive sport wedded to a compromised nutrient intake is a prescription for disease.

FAT FACTS

The focus on essential fats as health-promoting supplements has recently become intensified. The therapeutic value of strategic polyunsaturated fatty-acid supplementation is inconceivable, but what's becoming clearer is the preventive potential these fats bring to the table. This potential isn't derived from some mystical property; it's due to the fact that these fats are delivered in imbalanced proportions or are completely missing from the diet. Supplementation simply offsets the diet's shortfalls.

Our bodies can't manufacture essential fats that are critical for hormone communication and cell integrity. These essential fats, like antioxidants, are easily destroyed by exposure to our harsh environment and are further deactivated by processing. Choose a processed diet and you're selecting food that's devoid of antioxidant activity and full of rancid, lifeless, disease-instigating fats.

One objective of food processing is to remove the factors that contribute to spoilage. Our processed food can last on shelves for longer periods before going bad. The alteration of the fat chemistry in such food causes a loss in reactivity, enhancing the shelf life of the nourishment but also undermining its effectiveness in our bodies. The very reactivity of these fats is the biological activity we depend on for life, yet we have purposely removed this activity to maintain commercial viability. Absurd, isn't it? Consume these "preserved" foods as our major source of sustenance and we *will* succumb to the Health Canada statistics displayed in the previous chapter. Ensuring that the diet supplies these essential fats in their active form guarantees that the body's cells will receive the tools they were designed to use for normal operation. Without this sufficient supply cells simply hobble along and attempt to fulfill their roles. Supplementation with these fats ultimately ensures delivery of one category of building blocks essential to the chemistry of life. But this one category depends on an immeasurable amount of biochemical support, which Ageless Performance provides.

The "right fats in the right proportions" is the focus of Ageless Performance. However, in order to maintain activity of these fats, in order to direct these fats to the right biochemical pathway, in order for the body to metabolize them efficiently, the program must be followed in its entirety.

Supplementation with essential fats alone such as flaxseed oil just doesn't cut it. Augmentation with fish oils such as salmon oil instead of or in conjunction with essential-fat sources like flaxseed oil won't fix an unbalanced biochemistry, either, unless these special nutrients are properly escorted and protected in the body. Essential fats (supplemented through flaxseed oil) such as linoleic and alpha linolenic acids, and omega-3 fats (supplemented through marine oils) like eicosapentaenoic acid, or EPA, and docosahexaenoic acid, or DHA, are only part of the comprehensive strategy. They are a major component of Ageless Performance, but they are useless without the rest of the program. Nutrient co-factors literally act as navigation factors, and without them the course these fats are designed to take in our cells is impossible to steer through.

Taking these specialized oils in aggressive supplemental doses is like getting into a high-performance, 500-horsepower super car and putting the pedal to the metal before realizing you have bad brakes, poor handling, a broken suspension, and no steering. The extraordinary high speed is uncontrollable. The exceptionally unstable activity of these fats without the right guidance by the rest of the program is no different; the highly reactive nature is uncontrollable and cellular damage is inevitable.

Experts with good intentions will advocate supplementation of these fats for therapy and prevention, but the expected benefits are usually minimal or nonexistent. Why? Because these fats are very unstable, highly reactive, and susceptible to oxidation, which means they won't make it through the free-radical load commonly produced by a diseased state. Disease itself propagates free-radical proliferation. The immune system actually uses free radicals to destroy foreign invaders, and this can give rise to uncontrollable oxidation in the body. This free-radical density makes poorly planned polyunsaturated-fat supplementation hazardous. However, with a protective foundation in place the results are overwhelmingly powerful.

Essential and other omega-3 fats are the crux of most nutraceutical and complementary (nutraceutical plus pharmaceutical) therapies and preventive programs, but their delicate nature makes them difficult to work with. Once oxidized, these now-rancid fats lose their life-supportive activity and actually contribute to free-radical stress in the body, increasing the risk of disease and the rate of biological aging. Today disease runs rampant due to a limited supply of these important essential fats, but just as much to blame is the limitation of the co-factors required to protect the fats' integrity and mediate or navigate their metabolism. Ageless Performance supplies an abundance of these fats in the right proportions, but not before the protective and navigation systems have been installed.

The relationship between environment, lifestyle, diet, and disease is an easy one to correlate. A toxic, free-radical-laden environment, accompanied by a high-stress, fast-paced lifestyle, which itself propagates free-radical generation, increases oxidative pressures on the body beyond the antioxidant potential we're able to accomplish with a limited nutrient supply. The very nutrients that are critical to the metabolic pathway I often refer to throughout this book are among the most delicate and most vulnerable molecules at risk in this overwhelming oxidative stress. Thus the breakdown in the metabolic pathway that's at the center of multiple diseases is caused, in major part, by inadequate protection from oxidative stress and insufficient availability of the precursors (building blocks) for the system. The wrong diet not only fails to provide defenses and precursors, but it increases strain on this fatty-acid metabolic pathway.

Ageless Performance zooms in on this pathway to hone every facet of the driving force so that hormone-cellular communication is exact and biological efficiency utmost. As a result, the immune, endocrine, digestive, and detoxification systems all function vigorously. But that's not all. Later we'll see convincing data that demonstrates how efficiency in these systems supports better mood, mental, and emotional health, as well. The outcome is extraordinary immunity, preventive potential, healing power, athletic performance, and mental and emotional well-being. In essence, the extraordinary experience is not at all extraordinary. We were originally designed to function this way, but most of us don't know that, and those of us who do may not know how to achieve it.

More and more age-related diseases attack the young. Asthma, arthritis, heart disease, cognitive disorders, gastrointestinal ailments, and immune-system impairment are accepted as likely or inevitable afflictions in our lives. The reason is that we increasingly rely on processed foods and, more than ever before, our children are subjected to the predatory marketing of synthetic food.

DHA, an omega-3 fatty acid often supplemented through marine oils, is critically important for normal cognitive function. It's produced in the body from the essential omega-3 fat linolenic acid (abundant in flaxseed oil). A limitation during fetal neural development of these fats can result in serious shortcomings throughout life. However, let me reiterate, if we supplement these fats without addressing poor vitamin and mineral status, free-radical load, poor dietary protein intake, and high-glycemic dietary values, we'll get nothing but more stress out of polyunsaturated-fat supplements.

Ageless Performance primes the cells so that they produce their own requirements of DHA from essential-fat sources. In addition, the program's extra dietary DHA further augments the program because it must be made available in unlimited supply in case our internal chemistries aren't able to fulfill biological demands. DHA is a major cell-membrane fat, and its higher concentration in neural tissues and the heart lends these tissues their specialized activity. Furthermore, DHA is critical to healthy insulin activity, supports mental health, and harmonizes the body, mind, and spirit.

Mothers-to-be, listen up! This issue is of paramount importance if you're thinking about conceiving a child. Your own cellular DHA and EPA status must be optimal in order for the development of your child to progress in a healthy fashion. Cellular saturation with these fats prior to conception, during pregnancy, and even after birth will ensure an adequate supply for normal neural development of your fetus. Flaxseed oil doesn't supply these fats. Supplementation with omega-3 marine fats, in conjunction with the essentials from flaxseed oil, will facilitate the development of this healthy state more expeditiously for you and your child. The saturation objective should persist past the point that lactation ceases in order to resaturate a mother's depleted state.

If your cellular status is poor, it's likely your child will be short-supplied. If your diet is lacking, these building blocks will be extracted from your cells for fetal development until you run out yourself. Mother's milk must be rich in these building blocks, but recent studies of North American mother's milk reveal below-par levels, a consequence of the continent's diet and lifestyle. These factors have contributed greatly to our children's poor condition of health, especially their compromised cognitive state, but we can easily prevent and reverse this trend if we know the nutraceutical facts.

The consequence of limiting these fats can lead to neural and cardio-vascular shortcomings in our children. A balanced nutritional status starts in the womb, and at that point it's strictly a mother's responsibility to make sure the demands are met. Keep your eyes open for krill-oil-based supplements. In light of what I'm seeing about this oil, it will be the next fat source to make an impact in the health industry. It's loaded with omega-3 fats, important cell-membrane phosphatides, and much more, marking it a likely candidate for the perfect fat supplement for all walks of life and all ages.

EXERCISE FOR LIFE

Endorphins are opiatelike neurotransmitters that occur in the brain, deliv-ering pain-relieving properties and a feeling of well-being such as euphoria. Dietary fat can stimulate the release of endorphins and that euphoric feeling, but so, too, can exercise, remedying the need for the fat fix. I, too, feel the desire to consume fatty foods if I miss my regular training sessions, and you've likely experienced the same when you skip your usual exercise routine. Exercise provides multiple health benefits: expenditure of excess calories, modification of cravings, maintenance of lean body mass, activation of natural fat-burning furnaces, attainment of improved cardiovascular health, achieve-ment of better glucose regulation, and production of healthy mental and physical energy. Exercise also helps pump cellular debris out of our bodies.

We all have active systems that deliver oxygen and nourishment to our tissues. Our hearts pump nutrient-rich blood to our cells, but the removal of metabolic waste relies ultimately on our lymphatic systems, which are propelled by working muscles. Sedentary lifestyles result in our cells being bathed in metabolic wastes for prolonged periods, which contributes to cellular toxicity. We'll discuss some of the benefits of regular exercise later in this book, outlining some nutritional strategies that will maximize the results from your training program with the least amount of effort.

Ageless Performance resets cellular biochemistry so that calorie expenditure during exercise is optimal and, as much as possible, fat is the source of these spent calories. As a result of facilitated fat oxidation, weight management and the maintenance and building of lean muscle become much easier. This is the program that helped make me a North American bodybuilding champion.

Timing of foods and the proportions of a meal have profound influences on hormone responses. The meal can be modified to produce biochemical outcomes that support our physical goals. The right program stops your body from using muscle as an energy source during activity, a phenomenon that's very difficult to eliminate, especially with exercise programs that exceed 35 minutes and involve high intensity. The correct plan can assist in building muscle and shedding fat with a lot less effort. The wrong diet and its poor timing can make all efforts a hellish struggle. Although you'll receive a multitude of pointers concerning food and supplements, their timing, quantities, combinations, and proportions around your training programs, instructions on exercise won't be extensive. This topic could constitute a book on its own. You must appreciate, however, that an active lifestyle is a vital factor contributing to the whole, healthy body, mind, and spirit. It relieves stress, maintains muscle mass, and removes toxic waste.

Muscle mass is akin to a functional organ in the body, and although it shouldn't be used as a reservoir for immune-system fuel, it will be the tissue the body falls back on during an emergency. As we age, our lean-muscle mass tends to diminish. This decline is so reliably consistent that muscle mass is, in fact, one of the markers utilized to help assess biological age. Lose muscle and we raise the risk of disease and lower our potential to recover from it.

If exercise isn't part of your lifestyle today, you must start immediately, even if it's just one brisk 20-minute walk each day. If exercise is already incorporated into your lifestyle, you might want to take a close look at a recent book that's caused a buzz in the marketplace. It's called *The Power Program* and was written by a colleague of mine, Dr. Michael Colgan.

I suggest you make it a goal to work toward including a resistance-training program if it's not part of your daily protocol already. There's much more to skeletal muscle than meets the eye; exercising the skeletal muscle mass works the bone mass, and this, too, helps maintain healthy bone density.

We'll discuss the metabolic value of this lean mass in more detail in upcoming chapters.

Contrary to conventional thinking, exercise is important even if you're contending with disease, arthritis included. The endorphin secretions induced by exercise actually help alleviate pain, raising your threshold to help you cope. The alternative is to resort to dietary fat for immediate relief of pain because it, too, induces the release of endorphins. This is the easier, more common choice these days, one that inevitably presets multiple grave consequences. In the long run the resulting body fat promotes inflammation, insulin resistance and, of course, the rest of the diseases mentioned in the previous chapter.

If you participate in a regular exercise program and eat the right polyunsaturated fats, your natural anti-inflammatory and painkilling processes will be activated as will your built-in regenerative processes. Even an arthritic condition will improve! The difficulty will be in getting started to change the direction your chemistry is flowing in. This is like altering the course of a large supertanker. It's a slow process; you'll have to fight to make the turn, but once you begin moving in the correct manner, you'll find it harder to get off course. As soon as you've established this healthy state, even if you cheat or deviate on occasion from the Ageless Performance plan, your healthy metabolic momentum will keep your internal chemistry gliding along the right anti-inflammatory path. Ageless Performance is designed to force this positive change in your cells expeditiously. It's not a supply of passive nourishment; it's a strategy that actively promotes the cellular shift to a new status of cell life.

GETTING THE MOST OUT OF SPORTS SUPPLEMENTS

Ageless Performance sets the biochemical foundation that allows adjunctive sports supplements such as creatine to deliver the results you expect. Countless athletes fail to experience what they want from proven performance-enhancing supplements like creatine, but with a simple change in diet results can be outstanding. I use creatine in cycles, and every time I go back on a cycle, *bwam*, it delivers a surge in muscle cell volume that's extraordinary. And that, believe it or not, can happen in just two or three days and often without a saturation phase.

For most people a saturation phase requiring higher-than-typical daily doses might take five and even 10 days. Creatine works at maximum potential for me because each of my cells functions at top efficiency, sucking up creatine quickly and allowing it to deliver its benefit without interference.

Believe me, I've tried many scientific and theoretical nutraceutical applications to experience a wide spectrum of results, from metabolic dysfunction to my present-day strategy. I've even reached states where enhancers had little or even negative effects because of a biological system that backed up and choked when these enhancers attempted to deliver their influence. Choking is caused by a cellular foundation that isn't ready for action. Without a solid foundation you can forget about applying the enhancer with success.

Athletic performance might not be your reason for applying Ageless Performance, but other system enhancers depend on the same efficiency. Only after Ageless Performance has been established can echinacea deliver its maximum immune-enhancing potential; Tribulus terrestris provide its intense libido- and fertility-boosting effects; arginine supply its big libido, cardiovascular, and other system enhancements; or isoflavones and ipriflavones contribute their optimum bone-building properties.

Struggling to stay with a nutritional-intake program for any goal is an unhealthy endeavor that often leads to failure. Ageless Performance isn't a restrictive diet, and you won't feel as if you're struggling. Sticking with the program will be easy. As much as these strategies are powerfully effective, the greater part of the results won't be noticed immediately. Survival of the program is critical, but I'm confident you'll have no problem remaining on the course.

Unlike most pharmaceutical drugs, the remedies in Ageless Performance are aimed at rectifying the problem, correcting the biochemical imbalance, and/or enhancing nutrient status. Pharmaceutical drugs are typically designed to relieve the symptoms of disease, and results are often immediate but short-lived. Understand that imbalances and deficiencies in nutrient status, and the consequential compromised cellular efficiency, don't just appear after one day, one week, one month, or even one year of poor nutrition and poor lifestyle. These developments are often caused by years, even decades, of unhealthy habits. Ageless Performance needs to be applied for some time to produce results.

The program will deliver all you need to beat the odds and run the human race of a lifetime. By reconstructing the body cell by cell with these new building blocks, you'll allow your body to perform with renewed functionality. Our bodies are constantly turning over nutrients, cells, and tissues. Skin, in fact, can be completely replaced every two weeks, lean muscle every six months. This turnover requires massive volumes of building blocks, and not just any type, either.

Our genetic plans call for highly specific materials, and we have to supply them with precision to support this perpetual construction. You can expect dramatic shifts in health when you administer functional nourishment, but the results are limited to the rate of your body's turnover. As new functional cells with balanced systems replace withered, limping ones, a new vitality will be instilled so that the body can perform according to design. However, these revitalized cells must still contend with the slower pace of the limping ones they depend on for synergy, the ones that haven't yet been recycled.

The degree of deficiency, level of imbalance, and intensity of toxin and free-radical imposition all dictate how long recovery and optimal metabolic efficiency will take, whether it's three weeks, two months, or one year. Although you can experience enhancement from Ageless Performance within days, the full impact might not be possible for several months.

Rectifying these cell-deep anomalies takes a lot more time and effort than the results apparent on the surface indicate. These topical successes may develop within weeks in some people and should serve as motivational factors to persevere with the program. But even if we stick with the correction until deep cellular balance has been achieved, does this justify a return to the unhealthy habits that caused disease? Of course not! Ageless Performance is a lifestyle, one you'll undoubtedly never leave once the high-voltage results of its application are experienced.

PERFORMANCE NUTRITION
RAISES THE BAR

Training to accomplish an Olympic dream requires a program that's a full-time commitment. In fact, it necessitates a dedication to a unique lifestyle that incorporates strategic training, visualization, and high-performance nourishment, a plan that ultimately brings cohesiveness to the body, mind, and spirit. The physical and mental demands create above-average nutritional needs that can't be met by food alone.

Competitive athletes are well aware that their full genetic potential is out of reach without the use of a comprehensive supplement program. Surprisingly most athletes I've interviewed and consulted, even those of Olympic status, have no comprehension whatsoever of how to implement a viable plan. For those who attempt to supplement their diets, the programs are often so rudimentary that benefits are likely minimal, possibly nonexistent.

Let me make it *very* clear right now. If you're not on a strategically designed nutritional supplement program and you're a competitive athlete, you haven't experienced your true genetic potential. In fact, without such a program you're probably causing significant damage to connective tissue, the brain, and other important life-support systems such as the immune system and gastrointestinal tract. Payback for that kind of punishment is only a matter of time!

If today your main concern is athletic performance and you think you can survive without optimal immune and gastrointestinal function, think again. Not only does nutrient deficiency make you susceptible to tissue injury, it leaves you vulnerable to disease. With a greater intensity of training the potential for nutrient deficiency increases. Nutrient depletion and metabolic inefficiency become even more pronounced as we age and are at the heart of the age-related decline in performance potential.

Even acute colds and influenzas can result in downtime from training to affect your final performance, which means maintaining optimal immune status is critical to maximum athletic achievement. The few days leading up to a track meet, for example, are likely to be more stressful than the average day. Don't be fooled: your calm and collected demeanor may not be indicative of the underlying biochemical unrest that anticipation may conjure up. In combination with physical training this "pre-performance anxiety" can take its toll on nutrient stores as catabolic hormones overtake the body. This destructive process can take bites out of your painfully acquired arsenal for competition.

Track star Donovan Bailey can tell you from his experience at the 2000 Sydney Olympics that illness can nip at the heels during periods of duress. As fast as he was, Bailey lost his Olympic race to a bronchial pneumonia virus, and although he was on a supplementation program, it was meager because, to my astonishment, the understanding of these protocols by the majority of trainers and athletes who need them most is nil.

When I spoke to high jumper Mark Boswell weeks before the Sydney Olympics, he complained of an ankle injury that haunted him from time to time. He made known a lack of understanding for the importance of supplementation and seemed to pay little attention to my message. He's no different than most. At his young age he's shown us remarkable genetic potential. However, I'm confident that the administration of a strategic supplement program, even a basic plan, will raise the bar for this gifted athlete to extract the full genetic potential that lies semi-dormant and just waiting to leap out at the world.

If your goal or dream isn't as extreme as those of Donovan Bailey or Mark Boswell, don't belittle it. Reaching a personal objective is a lesson, and every time you achieve one you strengthen your self-esteem. If you feel physically fit, you act physically fit, and the confidence that comes with this conditioning can help you succeed in other facets of your life. Being physically fit doesn't mean you have to have 8% or 14% body fat with a physique of a Greek god or goddess.

It does mean, however, that you need to be fit enough to feel healthy and perform whatever it is you do with confidence. Physical fitness contributes to mental and emotional health, and mental and emotional health lead to physical fitness. The circle is based on a functional nutrient status in the body that communicates this state throughout. Apply Ageless Performance, believe in your vision, and propel your way to the top!

IRON WILL

I'd like to share my personal evolution as an athlete and student, a very ill patient in distress, and a scientific researcher. By doing so I'll give a greater understanding of my trials and tribulations, the origin of my passion, and the role Ageless Performance has played in my life.

Ageless Performance is more than a foundation for health created from research. It's the result of my experiences, an extension of my life, a product of purpose and personal growth. My motivation to research this vastly underestimated field was sparked by a competitive nature. As a youngster, my dream of competing at elite levels as a bodybuilder was so vivid that I made it happen.

Performance nutrition had already become a topic of intense research in the early 1980s, and it was becoming big business very fast. Weider Publications displayed the awesome physiques of Larry Scott, Bill Pearl, Samir Banout, Arnold Schwarzenegger, and Franco Columbo, all endorsing the use of supplements: casein, soybean, and egg protein powders; freeform amino acids such as arginine and ornithine; complete amino acid blends; and vitamins and minerals.

The selection of supplements at the time was minimal, and the technology pales in comparison with that of today. Weider and Twin Lab Nutritional products dominated the market. I recall early in my bodybuilding career that what mattered most was weight gained, and the only proof of results of any worth were those from a rickety old scale at the hard-core, window-less Vancouver pit called the Western Gym.

Although it's known that genetics play a major role in athletic success, I was keen enough to realize early in my journey that, undoubtedly, nutrition would influence significantly to what degree those genes could be expressed. However, what we've discovered in the past few years of research about nutrient-related gene activity makes me look back and chuckle at the programs we applied even 10 years ago.

The iron will to succeed took on yet another dimension. In 1984 I was accepted at the University of British Columbia in the disciplines of bio-chemical and then nutritional sciences and soon became my own guinea pig. My research in the ensuing years confirmed many of my theories and negated others. I soon added to my résumé a powerful scientific arsenal.

Quickly I veered off into my own research to integrate Eastern practices, which included the power of herbs. I merged these fundamentals with the biochemistry of vitamins, minerals, and phytochemicals, extending my studies into pharmaceuticals, as well. Many drugs are plant extracts or analogues of naturally existing molecules. In many cases it was possible to trace back the source of these drugs to find natural extracts that would act in much the same manner. Frequently natural compounds proved to be more effective than pharmaceutical drugs designed for the same symptoms. More often than not, these plant sources were available on the market. However, finding quality standardized extracts that would induce the expected pharmacological effects was quite a task.

In other cases it was possible to track down Eastern remedies that affected biochemical pathways precisely the same way that pharmaceutical drugs did without the equivalent side effects. One such case is that of arachidonic-acid conversion to the inflammatory eicosanoid hormones or prostaglandins. You'll see later just where this activity takes place in the biochemical pathway and how crucial its influence is to the Ageless Performance program. Creating efficiency in this pathway results in optimal biological performance.

Aspirin or ASA simply blocks the conversion of this cell-membrane fat to slow down eicosanoid-hormone production and alleviate inflammation. Curcuminoids, extracted from a natural herb called turmeric, deliver comparable results, as does alpha lipoic acid, but their method of activity is different than that of ASA. Proanthocyanidins from grapeseed extract and Pycnogenol from pine-bark extract have similar anti-inflammatory and regenerative properties, as well. However, these applications must be precisely used and synergized. Most people in the nutraceutical field don't apply them correctly and don't use the right forms of these substances. When they're employed appropriately, they're extremely effective.

This was my introduction during the mid to late 1980s to the biochemistry of cellular modification, an initiation into the dynamics of natural inflammatory and anti-inflammatory activity. By taking advantage of these scientific principles, I was able to advance in my chosen sport in leaps and bounds and recover from disease in a way health professionals perceived to be unexplainable. The more evidence I uncovered, the more excited I became. I knew I was on the right track, and going in even deeper I realized that I was onto much more than just athletic-performance enhancement.

Disproportionate yields of autocrine hormones—prostaglandins, prostacyclins, thromboxanes, and leukotrienes—are a direct result of dietary imbalances that include overconsumption of high-glycemic-index carbohydrates, fried foods, hydrogenated fats, alcoholic beverages, poor-quality protein, and much more. The very corticosteroid drugs that we so freely use to treat inflammation also impair enzymes of this system and the resulting hormone actually interfering with our natural ability to control what we're trying to alleviate. This creates lifelong dependency on pharmaceutical drugs.

Early on, inflammatory control became a passionate focus in my studies. The level of training intensity that's required to reach extreme athletic goals such as the one I was entering upon takes you close to and often past the point of injury. Regulating inflammatory activity and facilitating expeditious recovery from daily training with nutraceuticals gave me a significant advantage over my competitors. Similar research was available on tissue anabolism in trauma patients, hormone therapy, and more. I applied these, as well.

I was fortunate to have the chance to explore this controversial field to bring together calculated science, theory, a competitive iron will, personal sacrifice, and dedicated physical work, merging them into a carefully balanced, astute strategy. In 1984 I competed in junior bodybuilding events, and in 1986, still at a junior level, I began winning, scoring first place in my class in the British Columbia Junior Championships. I was well into my university research by then, and I was already developing Ageless Performance. In 1988 I scored first place in my class and overall in the Iron Ore Classics. Two years later, at the B.C. Championships, I again placed first in my class and overall. That same year I did likewise in the Western Canadian Championships, and in 1992 I finished first in my class at the International Federation of Bodybuilding (IFBB) North American Championships, achieving professional status.

FROM PASSION TO DESPERATION

My struggle with a relentless case of chronic tendonitis, which resulted from an injury sustained in a 1990 automobile accident, caused me to immerse myself more deeply in the study of inflammatory prostaglandin hormones to find a coping mechanism. This impediment kept me from the 1991 North American Bodybuilding Championships, but another setback to come could have ended my competitive dreams completely.

In 1991 I was diagnosed with a severe case of ulcerative colitis. Shortly after diagnosis, I was admitted to hospital, anemic and barely able to walk from the general inflammatory assault on my joints, a secondary symptom of this gastrointestinal disease. After two weeks of aggressive corticosteroid therapy, I shrank from over 220 muscular pounds to 170 pounds—more than 50 pounds stripped away in 14 days! Still, there was no sign of remission, and the next inevitable step, I was told, was surgery: the removal of the nonresponsive large intestine.

My gastroenterologist prepared me for the worst. "Not only is your bodybuilding career over, Franco," he insisted, "but you'll have to prepare yourself for a completely new way of life." For those who don't know about ulcerative colitis, let me say that it can be a bloody disaster! The disease is characterized by an uncontrollable inflammation of the large intestine that leads to blood loss and infection so severe that death is imminent unless drug treatment down-regulates the inflammation or surgery removes the unresponsive large intestine. The disease, they say, is lifelong and surgery is inevitable.

After a few days of wallowing in a my hospital bed, I began to think about the studies relating to inflammation that I had pursued so intensely—scientific research motivated by a competitive iron will. I was quick to recognize the common ground between the two realms of athletic performance and physical healing. However, there were many unanswered questions. The incentive by now had moved from passion to desperation.

With a spark of hope and an immediate attitude change, I accepted my physical condition but revoked my sentence of death or lifestyle change. The body has the ability to manifest miraculous outcomes, but it all starts with positive instruction from the mind. We've surrendered the power of absolute healing to medical professionals and have allowed their sentencing to drive disease, as well. If you can be convinced of a tragic outcome, it's likely to occur. On the other hand, if you believe with conviction that you can manifest recovery, you will.

Don't think for one minute that the many pharmaceutical drugs heal the body of disease. On the contrary, these drugs set the stage to promote healing, providing a small window of opportunity for your inner potential to prevail. If you believe in your doctor's therapy, your body will take advantage of this window of opportunity. If you fall victim to a death sentence, however, you'll die a slow death.

In my case I had a head start. I believed in my internal ability to drive biological performance long before disease challenged me. Throughout my bodybuilding career I had employed the potency of visualization and meditation alongside powerful nutraceutical-performance enhancement to help materialize the muscled outcome that brought me to championship bodybuilding form. The mind always plays a central role in health and fitness, and I was lucky to realize this early in my life.

I already knew that much of the research done with sports-nutrition products originated in a clinical setting designed to unveil their therapeutic potential on victims of disease, trauma, and surgical intervention. Glutamine, whey protein, branched-chain amino acids, HMB, methoxyisoflavone, ribose, chrysin, and many others were proven to be powerful facilitators of recovery from disease. Today creatine is also recognized as a nutrient that supports general health; it's activity includes anti-inflammatory, antioxidant, and cognitive and neurological support.

Sports-nutrition companies embellish the research and market the potential to competitive athletes looking for an edge. The clever marketing creates a dust cloud, taking attention away from the original or more fundamental applications for these supplements—prevention of disease and recovery from physical impairment. The point is that most of these so-called sports-nutrition supplements are proven therapeutic and preventive nutrients. I studied, learned, believed, and applied these supplements in my sport.

When I became ill, there was no doubt in my mind that these applications could support recovery from my disease, as well. There was no wasted time sitting passively on the fence. I called upon my inherent healing systems, the same systems I used to facilitate muscle development and performance, systems directed by the power of a healthy mind. Relying on my unfaltering belief in this potential from within and the confidence that I could concoct the right nutraceutical program to fuel recovery, I was able to move toward wellness immediately. Weeks after my sentencing, by my own wish, I was wheeled out of the hospital barely able to walk. A passionate study of biochemistry had now turned into what I felt to be a desperate battle for survival.

My studies uncovered many answers, and the newly applied strategies quickly ameliorated my health. Less than a year after sentencing by my health-care professional, I won the prestigious bodybuilding title of Mr. IFBB North America at Redondo Beach, California, but my health wasn't 100% yet. Before that glorious victory, though, I was wheeled out of a hospital, barely able to walk, and required assistance to get into a car. It takes a human with perseverance beyond that which most of us can fathom just to qualify for this competition, let alone compete in it, let alone fight against injury and illness to make it there, let alone win it.

It's not because I'm so terrific that I was able to overcome these barriers. I succeeded simply because I believed in both my personal potential and in the potential of my therapy. Although I experienced short periods of remission during the many months of competition preparation, inflammatory bouts of ulcerative colitis plagued me from time to time.

After winning this international event, I decided to take a little time off from the energy-consuming training to focus all of my efforts on recuperation. Within a year I achieved complete recovery to the astonishment of medical professionals. Miraculous? Yes, but the miracle is a gift we all possess, a gift you can also call upon.

For those of you who know a little about ulcerative colitis, you'll understand how serious it is. For those of you who are battling disease, you've likely had your fill of the sentence you're living. More than 10 years have passed since my diagnosis, and approximately eight years have elapsed since my aggressive therapy proved successful, yet I underwent no restrictive diet, no surgery, and still today no debilitating disease. Not a sign whatsoever! You, too, can do the same.

My postgraduate research endeavors continue. All of the scientific and practical knowledge I've collected during my experiences has been incorporated into Ageless Performance, my remarkable personal program. Recent scientific findings concerning the horrific manipulation by free radicals of the genes that regulate eicosanoid-hormone balance have provided fresh evidence to support a new level of fine-tuning for the program.

Until recently all we've been able to do to compensate for these biochemical imbalances is to offset the result of accelerated enzyme and gene activity with nutraceuticals like essential fats and drugs such as ASA and other cox1 and cox2 inhibitors. This dawning era in nutraceutical science will allow us to intercept the acceleration of these genes to prevent hormone imbalance from the depths it's conceived at. Ageless Performance penetrates deeply to invigorate life with a new sense of being.

EMBRACE THE PROGRAM

Today I'm in the best physical shape and best state of health ever. In addition, those who see pictures of me that were taken 10 years ago insist I now look younger! My metabolism revs with controlled energy. Body-fat proportions are easy to maintain at healthy levels. My program has proven to be a powerful therapeutic, preventive (weight management included), and anti-aging strategy for all the people who have applied it. You, too, have the opportunity to reverse disease, to take control of your health, to prevent disease, and to reach your goals and live life in a state of perfect health.

Ageless Performance is new-age medicine that serves as a basis for a new era of health care. The upcoming chapters are your entry into this remarkable realm. You may encounter some technical biochemistry along the way, but don't fret. Read through the scientific foundation and each point will be clarified in order to gain your confidence in the strategy and its potential. The facts go beyond supporting natural remedies as possible preventatives. They prove that these naturally derived medicinals aren't merely alternatives, that these substances are powerful primary curatives.

And if drugs *must* be applied, the ensuing chapters will show that complete recovery can't be achieved unless these nutraceutical corrections are concurrently administered with whatever pharmaceuticals your doctor deems necessary.

In some cases of disease this complementary strategy reduces our need for high doses of unnatural pharmaceutical chemicals, therefore minimizing possible side effects. However, the most exciting application for these new-age nutritionals is their preventive potential. You'll be convinced that age isn't a matter of time. You'll understand that youth, longevity, and ageless performance are within your grasp and that you do have the ability to extract your potential and block negative influences.

You, too, can maintain youthful and fully self-sufficient function of your neurological, cognitive, cardiovascular, immune, respiratory, sexual, and general maintenance systems. If you apply the easy-to-administer, scientifically proven strategies of Ageless Performance, *you will* maintain a youthful predisposition, *you will* create self-sufficiency, *you will* extract your full potential in life. The active component of this entire program is *you*, and only *you* can apply the strategy!

PART II

BODY OF EVIDENCE

3

HISTORY DOESN'T HAVE TO BE REPEATED

THE CASE FOR NUTRIENT DEFICIENCY

The nutritional sciences have attracted worldwide attention with a research initiative that permeates far beyond the scope of the government's recommended daily minimums. Yes, you read that correctly, "recommended daily *minimums*."

Research long ago confirmed the essential need for a wide array of vital substances required to prevent the onset of diseases such as scurvy, beriberi, pellagra, kwashiorkor, and others. In Third World countries these diseases may still be an issue of concern. In the more developed world nutrient deficiencies and their related diseases have been eliminated, so we think, through mass-awareness campaigns and government-implemented food-fortification programs.

Although we've successfully eliminated the clinical signs of these diseases with the vitamin levels we've determined sufficient for prevention, there's a factor we don't account for. Have we eliminated the underlying subclinical biochemical dysfunctions caused by lesser degrees of deficiency that we can't readily measure? In other words, are there lesser degrees of these debilitating diseases that cause slower rates of death that we can't attribute directly to deficiency or associate closely with these identified diseases?

The answer is a very likely *yes*. Our ecological and social environments have become more toxic today, leaching more nutrients from our bodies to increase the risk of development of these subclinical symptoms. A subclinical symptom is related to a disease, but it's so mild that we don't recognize the symptom; it sort of festers. As a result, the mild dysfunction persists without diagnosis and might not itself cause death directly but could very well contribute to the demise of other biological systems, precipitating disease and death.

In this case the identified cause of disease could be the secondary system that fell due to the primary dysfunction. Let me give you an example. Beriberi is caused by thiamine deficiency. Thiamine deficiency, if it persists, gives rise to neurological disorders, coma, and eventually death. What if a given thiamine deficiency didn't reach clinical levels? Could lesser degrees of it result in compromised neurological function that couldn't be diagnosed as thiamine deficiency? If so, extended periods of this mild deficiency could induce symptoms of disease similar to one of the common dementias—the primary cause, nutrient deficiency, never assumed to be an issue in the equation.

Those who say diseases like Alzheimer's and Parkinson's have no relation whatsoever to nutrient deficiency have closed their minds to a possible preventive program. A diet with a minute thiamine deficiency could still sustain the operations of the neurological system and eventually cause a system seemingly independent of thiamine to fail, and this second system would then be implicated as the factor involved in the pathology of Alzheimer's. In this instance a thiamine deficiency might never be implicated as a contributor to disease.

Parkinson's is associated with an accelerated degree of degeneration of the substantia nigra. Postmortem studies suggest that free-radical toxicity plays a huge role. Interestingly, degeneration of this system tends to progress with age regardless of general health and lifestyle to result in the age-related cognitive diseases we're familiar with. An acceleration of this deterioration results in the disease we've named Parkinson's, manifesting the symptoms at an earlier age or before failure of other life-support systems such as the cardiovascular. Although we're still looking for triggers of the disease, we now know that nutrient deficiency can contribute to its advancement, and antioxidants can block various factors that culture it.

In fact, implicated triggers include dopamine-blocking pharmaceutical drugs such as those used to treat psychoses like schizophrenia. These drugs might create vulnerability to Parkinson's down the road.

The point is, we shouldn't rely exclusively on drugs for relief from every ailment under the sun and we can't rule out nutrient deficiency as a possible contributor or cause even if it doesn't seem likely. Vitamin C deficiency results in scurvy, which is also characterized by psychological manifestation among many other symptoms. Deficiency in essential fatty acid results in cognitive disorders. The elderly are often found to have low serum ascorbate levels (vitamin C in blood) usually due to poor dietary habits. A serious lack of essential fats and thiamine is common among the elderly, as well. The compounding results of these deficiencies could lead to dementia, or at least to many of the symptoms we relate to dementia.

Although scurvy is rarely diagnosed, a marginal vitamin C deficiency could contribute to many diseases prevalent today. The combined subclinical effects of multiple marginal vitamin, mineral, and other nutrient deficiencies could be difficult, if not impossible, to pinpoint as a cause of disease. As a result, these diseases are ignored as unsolved mysteries as we seek to resolve the problem with more technology and more drugs: an absurd compliance when the research irrefutably demonstrates that technology can contribute to the problem.

In the 21st century we live by old-fashioned nutritional standards established by research in the early 20th century. Even if we could maintain this old nutrient status, with today's nutrient-depleted foods we couldn't combat the environmental toxicity assailing us, hence today's epidemics. In a frenzy of competitive research to develop the patentable magic cure, scientists often completely overlook the fundamental cause of disease, just as they did decades earlier.

You and your health-care professional might not even realize that most of our modern epidemics have been linked to nutrient deficiencies, imbalances, and poor lifestyle. As with the diseases of yesteryear, such as beriberi and scurvy, these modern epidemics can be minimized and even eliminated with new-age nutritional standards. The solution isn't much more complicated than the answer established for diseases of the past. Fortifications of deficient nutrients resulted in what were then miraculous "cures."

Today we take for granted these commonsense solutions as we search for the unknown symptom-relieving technology that itself is likely to breed more disease. The cures have been in our backyard the whole time, so close that we stumble over them while trying to focus on technology we can't see or understand with any clarity. At the same time we're unable to discern impositions, such as the toxic environmental chemistry we've created, that have become so much a part of our adopted ways.

Food scientists are preoccupied with food-borne microbes and microbe-propelled disease, and rightfully so. Mad cow disease, foot-and-mouth disease, and other such headlined epidemics are the results of the commercialized "bigger is better" attitude that infects society. Furthermore, government regulations aren't as strictly enforced in rapidly growing agro-industries, due possibly to a lack of manpower. As a result, manufacturers are given latitude to self-regulate, applying safety protocols they themselves design. Too often the bottom line doesn't take into account public safety. Agriculture is now a huge industrialized and centralized business, and although today's experts assure us the risk for food-borne disease is much lower than ever before, they can't guarantee they can protect us from outbreaks.

Agricultural products are harvested, prepared, packaged, and transported so quickly that contaminated food can reach every corner of the globe before contamination is even identified. At the rate microbes mutate nowadays, new strains can be spread around the world in a flash to launch attacks on our defenseless systems before we know what hit us. Although contamination *might* be less likely today, just one incident can have a profound impact. The mad cow and foot-and-mouth outbreaks are clear examples but pale in comparison to what's on the horizon.

Food-borne microbes and the associated diseases, however, aren't the biggest concerns that commercialized agriculture and fast foods present. Nutrient-compromised, calorie-rich foods are part of the problem, as well. Every day that we fuel our bodies with commercialized, processed fast food, unnecessary calories pile on and biological efficiency falls. We've taken the remarkable resilience of the human body for granted. Most of us can tolerate the abuse of incomplete nutrition for decades, and when disease manifests itself we blame it on a decline in biological operation due to age. However, disease has nothing to do with chronological aging.

Sadly billion-dollar agro- and fast-food businesses boldly confuse the issue of nutrient deficiency with aggressive public posturing. Advocates of processed and fast foods, for example, implicate organic farming as a cause of high-frequency e.coli contamination in attempts to divert attention from their own toxic ways. As much as this might have some statistical truth, the point is ridiculous.

Don't listen to all the claptrap you hear. The future of health care is self-care, and self-care is about prevention. Prevention is the implementation of a program that offsets the imbalances the typical North American lifestyle produces. Execution of this program is your responsibility. You must take an active role to inform yourself from different perspectives, taking the information found here and elsewhere to create the perfect fit that makes sense to you.

But beware! Researchers can consciously as well as subconsciously present their information with a twist to make their arguments. Consider all "facts" carefully and use common sense. What you may hear or read about e.coli contamination is a good example. The rationale is partially based on the fact that organic farming involves fertilization with animal fecal matter. Fast-food proponents argue that this creates a greater likelihood that organic agricultural products are contaminated with e.coli, while fast foods that are cooked and processed ensure that all toxic bacteria are eliminated.

Certainly farmers who fertilize with fecal matter from animals that are strictly hay-fed may expose their produce to e.coli. Studies show that hay feeding enhances shedding of the bacteria (1). This poses a higher risk for contamination of produce that may come in contact with this fertilizer.

E.coli contamination can occur on an organic farm or any other kind of farm, for that matter. However, an e.coli outbreak originating at an organic farm is likely to be restricted to an isolated or limited market, since organic farms normally supply locally. Even though the frequency of contamination *might* be higher on organic farms, the effects of such contamination originating in a fast-food chain are far more serious and widespread simply because of the ubiquitous nature of those who peddle burgers, fries, chicken, and the like.

The main health concern related to processed fast foods, however, goes beyond the potential of microbial contamination. Compared to the influence that nutrient deficiencies have had on human health, the risk from something like e.coli is minimal. Cardiovascular disease, chronic inflammation, diabetes, cognitive disorders, asthma, insulin resistance, obesity, and many of today's other common killers have reached epidemic proportions because we choose to ignore the facts that indicate the simple solution. Sedentary lifestyle and poor diet, which includes nutrient-deficient, processed fast foods, set the biochemical foundation for these afflictions. The emotional duress we've imposed on ourselves with today's frantic lifestyles further plagues our antioxidant-starved, helpless bodies with more stress-hormone-induced free radicals. The four-dimensional defense system presented in Ageless Performance—whole-food foundation, planned dietary supplementation, regular physical activity, and emotional and mental exercise—rises out of these facts.

The solution is obvious, but getting people to change lifelong habits is an incredible challenge, especially when multibillion-dollar industries have a lot to lose. Educating and motivating change amid the onslaught of propaganda and temptation seems almost impossible, but with Ageless Performance on your side, it can happen!

MODEL FOR PREDISPOSITION

Allow me, in a very basic manner, to depict the state of "predisposition for disease" and the development of disease from this vulnerable state. Our cells work arduously to build, repair, replace, manufacture, and support life at all times. Our genes are coded for health and survival. This is the objective you and I were born with.

This fastidious bustle of biochemical activity requires order, balance, and an unlimited supply of raw materials. And not just any raw materials we deem fit. The raw materials and their proportions required are nature's design. The human being is a natural design programmed to operate using nature's nutrient profiles—natural, unprocessed foods.

We—our cells—have a threshold level at which, if disarray occurs, disease surfaces. We have a baseline from which cellular activity is supposed to operate. At this baseline our cells have the ability to absorb strain and dysfunction. However, if our cells are forced to perform at levels above this baseline strain due to toxicity, stress, or deficiency, biological disarray is pushed beyond the threshold point more easily even with minute levels of trauma. The result is disease. (See Figure 1 on page 82 for a visual representation of the baseline theory.)

In other words, if your cells are functioning at a level other than the baseline, you're closer to your threshold for disease. If environmental strain is imposed on you while you're operating at this less-than-optimal level, you're brought nearer to the threshold than you would have been if you were performing at a healthy baseline capacity. If, now, you add emotional stress to the environmental strain, you're raised even closer to the threshold. Add to these two pressures a few weekend binges with alcohol, poor eating, and lack of sleep, and sure enough, you're headed even faster toward the disease threshold.

If your level of biochemical inefficiency had begun to incline from a healthy baseline level toward threshold thanks to the weekend binges only, it would be a lot more difficult to attain and surpass threshold, in effect, reach a state of disease. You can alleviate the stressors to allow for recovery from these impositions and lower the cells' level of operation closer to the healthy baseline but never to baseline levels unless you resort to the natural nourishment for which your evolutionary design calls. Poor nutrition itself raises cell function from the baseline nearer to that threshold for disease.

Multiples of these stressors may be composed of few, each with enormous impositions on your body, or many, each with small negative impacts. Either way the result could easily add up to surpass the threshold point and manifest disease.

By addressing one form of strain we can create resilience. By tackling two different types of compounding strain such as environmental toxicity and emotional stress, we achieve even more resistance to disease. Healthy dietary habits help alleviate the strain from various sources by delivering antioxidant activity, which can neutralize the free radicals that arise from emotional chemistry, environmental toxicity, and metabolic imbalance.

Supplementation instills resilience to disease. If you apply these sound nutritional strategies and actively control emotional and mental health through meditation and introspection, prevention of disease can become far more effective. Ageless Performance is designed to bring your level of biochemical operation down to baseline activity and your resilience to disease to optimal levels.

Without a healthy nutritional foundation in place, it's very difficult, if not impossible, to attain mental, emotional, and physical health. Nutrition is the conduit for the merging of body, mind, and spirit. A missing link impairs each system and severs their connection. Ageless Performance is the basis for the development of a healthy body, mind, and spirit and the glue for their union.

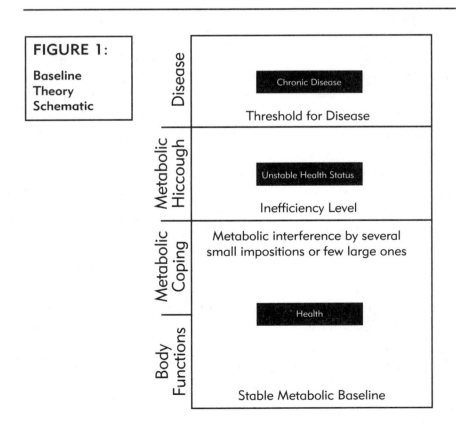

FIGURE 1:

Baseline Theory Schematic

Disease

Chronic Disease

Threshold for Disease

Metabolic Hiccough

Unstable Health Status

Inefficiency Level

Metabolic Coping

Metabolic interference by several small impositions or few large ones

Health

Body Functions

Stable Metabolic Baseline

THE MARVEL OF THIAMINE

Casimir Funk's research in the early 20th century led to the isolation of the first vital microchemical to be recognized as essential for life—vitamin B_1 (thiamine). Before then the recognized essentials for life and "normal" growth were water, some minerals, and the macronutrients (carbohydrates, protein, and fat). The eventual discovery of B_1 motivated the search for more of these life-sustaining, mystical chemicals, and a multitude of compounds were soon recognized.

However, the significance of this essentiality is still not truly appreciated. Additionally the therapeutic value of orthomolecular doses, or doses higher than those deemed to be requisite, are rarely valued by medical practitioners. (Orthomolecular treatment refers to the treatment of disease using naturally occurring molecules, nutraceuticals, as I prefer to call them.) Since most of us have placed our complete trust in the conventional medical profession, these alternative therapies are rarely considered as an option. Drug therapies are the first choice of defense. It's really a shame, because orthomolecular medicine is a powerful remedy with extensive explainable science to support it.

Vitamin C, for example, in much higher than commonly recommended doses, has been shown to prevent cancer (2). Thiamine, whose molecular structure was discovered by Funk in 1936, was found to play a critical role in energy metabolism in every cell. Imagine that: a deficiency in the B vitamins can limit energy availability, yet your dietary intake of these vitamins would be the last place your medical professional would look if you complained of chronic fatigue (3). In addition, deficiencies in thiamine can result in disease of the brain (encephalopathy), consequently producing cognitive and motor dysfunction (4). Has your health professional ever requested a detailed description of dietary intake?

In North America we may consume an adequate quantity of food and more than enough calories; however, the processed nature of this food limits its vital micronutrients such as the B vitamins. These micronutrient-depleted foods still require vitamin co-factors like the B vitamins for metabolism of the inherent protein, fats, and carbohydrates they deliver.

Processed foods deliver damaged macronutrients, as well, and this includes more than just fatty-acid damage. Few people are aware of the consequences associated with the processing of protein. The majority of our concerns regarding food processing involve the damage to polyunsaturated fats, deactivation and stripping of vitamins and antioxidants, and losses of minerals and fiber. However, the alteration that protein experiences can be profound.

Extreme heat can damage protein, preventing thorough enzymatic digestion in the intestine (5). Alkali treatment of protein can produce lysinoalanine complexes. This is the complexing of two amino acids, rendering them both nondigestible and nonabsorbable. Browning reactions, which occur when amino acids from protein react with sugars to form nondigestible, nonabsorbable complexes, ensue when carbohydrate sources are combined with protein and are heated or put away for storage. Combining carbohydrates with protein is a common practice in the supplement industry. The resulting complexing involves the formation of fructose-lysine and carboxymethyl-lysine—in other words, a loss of bioavailability for lysine (6, 7). The North American diet is now recognized to be limited in bioavailable lysine, and the processed, less-than-fresh nature of our food plays a huge part in this deficiency. These reactions to common processing methods prevent the body from extracting and using protein from a dietary source expected to be available.

This nonenzymatic reaction, the glycation of protein, also occurs in the body. Such is the case with the Alzheimer's patient's brain in which proteins react with reducing sugars to form an advanced glycosylated endproduct (AGE) such as the complexes just described. Carboxymethyl-lysine is an AGE that also accumulates in the presence of uncontrollably high serum-glucose levels (blood glucose), a degenerative phenomenon caused by insulin resistance and diabetes.

The lysinoalanine complex (amino acid-amino acid complexing) that can result from extensive processing of protein is also believed to be a factor in severe growth retardation. We're well aware of these problems but turn a blind eye to the welfare of our children who consume these cardboard foods as staples. Alkaline treatment of corn prepared for tortilla flour and hominy can result in up to 15% losses in arginine and cysteine. These two amino acids are integral elements in human biochemistry.

Commercially prepared tortillas, due to their preparation method, contain the lysinoalanine complex, which concentrates itself in the cortex of the kidney, producing irreversible cell damage (8). Our children are being fed compromised nourishment that will actually retard their mental and physical development and reduce their potential in life. It's up to parents to make the right choices for their children. They're being ensnared by the well-planned, predatory marketing of manufacturers of palate-tantalizing, addictive foods. As such, I strongly advocate the consumption of protein supplements that are devoid of added sugars, including the omission of maltodextrin and especially fructose.

Keep eating fast-food burgers, fries, and processed pies and your body will receive an abundance of carbohydrates, altered protein, deactivated rancid fat, and calories, but it will have to extract the nutrient co-factors (B vitamins, vitamin C, vitamin E, essential fats, minerals) from various systems in your body in order to metabolize the dead food you eat. Much of our food is designed by nature to carry most of its micronutrient requirements for the metabolism of its inherent macronutrients (protein, fats, and carbohydrates). Processing strips the well-proportioned micronutrients out of the balanced equation.

As your body attempts to process this compromised food day in and day out, the internal debt of vitamin and mineral co-factors gets bigger and bigger. Eventually the damage goes deeper and deeper and has a significant impact on vital systems. As a consequence, biological age begins to progress beyond the chronological more rapidly. Nutrient depletion triggers feedback mechanisms that are designed to motivate feeding. Your body tells you to eat more when these stores become depleted. Obediently you eat more dead nourishment and the cycle is perpetuated.

Processed foods are grossly deficient in thiamine. But even today with all we know through irrefutable science, if the symptoms of beriberi arise, do you think health practitioners will consider this disease as a possible cause of the symptoms? Not likely, because beriberi isn't common in 21st-century Western society, and nutrient-deficiency diseases are far from a primary component of the education our health-care professionals receive.

Did you know that Alzheimer's, for example, is not conclusively diagnosable? Furthermore, did you know that the diagnosis of Alzheimer's can't be correctly determined until an autopsy is performed? In other words, we may be treating various conditions with drugs even before knowing for sure the cause of the disease. Will a doctor thoroughly assess the nutritional status of a patient with symptoms of neurological disease like those related to Alzheimer's? Not likely. It's also not probable that he or she will prescribe the use of specific antioxidants that can protect the brain from amyloid plaque formation—plaques that are now known to be central to the pathology of Alzheimer's.

With our ever-growing reliance on processed foods and the increasing oxidative stress we're exposed to, varying degrees of serious diseases are likely to develop, degrees that may be so slight they're difficult, if not impossible, to diagnose accurately. Instead of nutritional correction as a primary course of treatment, the action most often chosen is a synthetic drug applied to, in a sense, deaden the symptom. But a symptom is a sign of imbalance, and to mask it without investigating possible nutritional deficiencies simply obscures the root of the ailment, leaving the true cause of the problem to fester.

Beriberi was first recognized in East Asia where white rice at one time provided approximately 80% of the energy intake for people in that part of the world. The polishing of rice removes the hull, creating a clean-looking white product that is still a staple in East Asia. But the discarded hulls contain important fibers, minerals, and vitamins, including an abundance of thiamine.

The symptoms of beriberi are indicative of neurological and muscular damage, including that of the heart. Physical impairments consist of general degeneration of health, poor muscular movement that inhibits walking and hand-eye coordination, eventual paralysis, and even death. Researchers at first expected the cause of beriberi to be a microbial infection of the nervous system, and for years the vast death toll escalated while scientists looked in all the wrong places. Eventually the culprit was found to be thiamine deficiency.

The beriberi model is a textbook case and is part of the university nutritional science curriculum, yet it's completely forgotten in the face of today's epidemics. Processed white rice, pasta, bread, crackers, and other dead foods make up a large portion of our diets. The effect all this has isn't much different than what happened with white rice in Asia, and fortification of our deficient foods with vitamins and minerals to compensate for processing isn't the fix-all solution.

Ironic, isn't it? We've implemented mass-fortification programs to prevent the development of disease associated with nutrient deficiency such as that caused by thiamine deficit, and most of these shortages are caused by our manipulation of food to begin with! The logical solution to our epidemics is to stop processing food. When we know the cause of diseases related to nutrient deficiencies, we fortify our foods with the appropriate vitamin, but what about the nutrients we haven't yet linked to disease? Are there natural biochemicals that haven't been recognized yet as nutritive? The fact is there are many we've recently identified and quite likely many more we haven't.

Beriberi is far from eliminated in North America. Alcoholics, for example, are susceptible to the development of the disease for various reasons. But beriberi isn't just a problem for alcoholics. To prevent the disease the Food and Nutrition Board, National Academy of Sciences (U.S Research Council), recommends that all ages consume a daily intake of 0.5 mg of thiamine for every 1,000 calories consumed. Logically there are accommodations for physical stages and states such as pregnancy and lactation, but these accommodations aren't enough.

Studies show that the maximum possible absorption for thiamine is 5 mg per day (9). However, there are many factors that influence the stability, absorption, and requirements for this essential nutrient. Thus, what might meet demands for one person isn't an immediate fit for another with a completely different lifestyle. For example, thiamine is relatively resilient to cooking temperatures if the food is acidic (low pH). In an alkaline solution of food, however, heat can more easily destroy thiamine (10, 11). If you're counting on 5 mg of thiamine daily to meet your needs, optimal health won't be achieved. As for maximum athletic performance—forget it! Supplementation is your best insurance plan and with doses closer to 50 mg daily.

Let's continue with the role of thiamine in the body as a model from which we can gain an appreciation for the complex activity of these nutrients in our bodies and the co-dependence that our nutrients display in our biochemical works. This account is not about gaining and memorizing a thorough understanding of thiamine's role. The goal here is to deliver a message about every essential nutrient and about the co-dependence of these nutrients in the body through this model.

With a limitation of just one factor, complete havoc develops and disorders, discomfort, and diseases that we treat with pharmaceutical drugs surface without obvious causes. Chronic fatigue syndrome is one likely case of such misdiagnosis. It's a label that's established after other possibilities have been eliminated.

The probable cause of energy impairment is biochemical irregularity instigated by dietary imbalance, microbe infiltration, or both. Poor nutritional status may impair immune function to allow Candida or other microbes to infiltrate the body and take it over. It may be that a deficiency in protein, fiber, one of the B vitamins, or even essential fats is the root of the problem. All of these deficiencies can impair immune-system function and the processing of cellular energy, and all of them can be linked to the processed North American diet. The typical symptoms of so-called chronic fatigue syndrome are swollen lymph nodes, mild fever, and fatigue, but that can also be a catalogue of the hallmarks of immune-system failure. The immune system depends on a rich supply of nourishment. Limit this supply and you restrict immunity. Ageless Performance revs up the immune system to powerful levels, but it also increases immune-system accuracy.

Various foods and beverages contain anti-thiamine factors (thiamine antagonists) such as caffeic acid and other chemicals found in tea, coffee, and rice bran. Ironically whole rice, containing the B vitamins, also delivers B vitamin antagonists. Regular consumption of tea and/or coffee may reduce the absorption potential of active thiamine (12, 13).

Acid secretions in the gut also aid thiamine absorption (14). You can see how poor energy metabolism and neurological impairment can be facilitated in older people by what may seem to be an *insignificant* deficiency of stomach acid. Yet we accept neurological impairment as an expected age-related phenomenon. But deficient acid secretion is easily preventable if we supply the body with the right fuels and building blocks it needs to maintain "youthful" activity.

Consuming supplemental doses of one nutrient will automatically raise the requirements for others. If we look deep into the cell's biochemistry, we see that all of the essential nutrients ultimately depend on one another at some point in cellular chemistry. Supplementing with one often results in a limitation of another somewhere along the extensive biochemical chain of events. Ageless Performance, however, is a complete design.

The ingestion of supplemental levels of alpha ketoglutaric acid (AKG) or protein, for example, requires a proportional increase in dietary thiamine for metabolism. AKG has become popular among athletes as has protein supplementation, but their contribution to health, fitness, and athletic performance are highly limited if the co-factors they depend on are unavailable from the diet.

Interestingly thiamine plays a major role in the conversion of AKG to alpha lipoic acid, and alpha lipoic acid is also linked to carbohydrate metabolism and energy manufacturing. The more carbohydrates you consume, the more thiamine you require (15). This means, typically, with more physical activity, more dietary thiamine is required. It's easy to see that thiamine requirements will vary significantly from one individual to another, which makes it impossible for one daily blanket requirement to fit the different stages and variable circumstances each of us may be exposed to. A dose at the high end is safe insurance with such water-soluble vitamins as the Bs. Ageless Performance incorporates well-planned, reliable vitamin supplementation.

I'm not about to go into detail for each and every essential nutrient we require, but I do want to express my position in regard to the recommendations our government agencies insist are appropriate. I don't believe these national and international nutritional standards are conducive to supporting maximum health. These recommended nutrient minimums might be enough to sustain human life, but the consequential immune-system disarmament, given the brutal environmental assault we all face, will take a huge toll.

The British Columbia Health Guide, distributed to the province's residents by the B.C. Ministry of Health, actually recommends the use of Tums as a source of supplemental calcium. This is absurd. First of all, calcium carbonate, the calcium source in Tums (derived from a chunk of limestone), is a poorly absorbed form of the mineral that's antagonistic to or interferes with the absorption of other minerals. Mineral-mineral antagonism is a critical factor to keep in mind with mineral supplements. If you load up on Tums daily, you can limit the body's ability to absorb minerals such as phosphates, magnesium, iron, zinc, and others. The end result is metabolic havoc.

Calcium chemically reacted or combined into special chelates like glycinates are absorbed much better than calcium carbonate, and they don't interfere with the absorption of other nutrients the way the calcium in Tums can. Additionally the buffering of stomach acids by Tums interferes with the absorption of many other nutrients, including calcium itself, thiamine, and protein.

The B.C. guide also reports that "certain vitamins found in foods have been shown to prevent some diseases." This is true, but the book goes on to maintain that "researchers are still trying to determine whether those vitamins have the same preventive effects when taken as supplements." This statement is nonsense! There is an abundance of evidence to confirm the preventive and therapeutic nature of many supplemental vitamins, minerals, and phyto-antioxidants.

There's a lot of good information in *The British Columbia Health Guide*, but the same sort of poor, uninformed propaganda concerning nutraceuticals continues to bewilder consumers. Not surprisingly, no nutraceutical organization endorses the B.C. guide. Its endorsements come from the B.C. Medical Association, the B.C. College of Family Physicians, the Registered Nurses Association of British Columbia and, of course, the College of Pharmacists of British Columbia. None of these organizations specializes in disease prevention or therapy in the way the nutraceutical profession does. The focus of each of these endorsing groups is reactive medical care that literally thrives on disease.

Vitamin supplementation, they say, hasn't been proven to deliver preventive effects. Not so. The coenzyme form of thiamine is primarily involved in tissue respiration (16). Irrefutably, levels of deficiency short of causing beriberi can have serious negative influences on energy availability, neuron development and nerve function, motor and cognitive function, cardiovascular efficiency, and more. Supplementation will reverse and prevent the disease.

Thiamine is also crucial for fat and protein metabolism but isn't ordinarily recognized for this function. The more protein you consume, the more fats including those that are essential you consume, the more B_1 you need. Thiamine, which helps regulate cholinergic activity, is also deeply involved in neurophysiology-facilitating sodium movement across the neuron cell membrane (17, 18). In short, thiamine is critical to our nerve-impulse propagation.

Impaired carbohydrate metabolism for energy production caused by a deficiency of thiamine is found to be more profound in the brain (19). Thiamine deficiency can contribute to the development of cognitive, neuro-motor, and severe cardiac muscle dysfunction. Again at what level of deficiency does impairment of, say, cognition develop without producing a common metabolic or other clinical endpoint we use as a marker of thiamine deficiency? In other words, is a mild deficiency recognizable as a cause of debilitating disease? The answer is an emphatic *no*. The preventive solution is supplementation with a sufficient dose of about 50 mg of thiamine daily. I take as much as 200 mg daily, and studies as well as my experience confirm no toxicity with this water-soluble nutrient at these levels.

So will supplementation with thiamine by an individual who is deficient and experiencing all of these symptoms help alleviate these symptoms and save this person's life? The answer is an absolute *yes* unless the subject has been led to stay away from this solution for too long, causing irreversible damage.

If your child has been placed on Ritalin by your health-care professional, has she or he first assessed your child's diet? Has she or he determined whether a nutrient deficiency is possible? Ritalin, as we'll see, isn't the answer for most cases of attention-deficit hyperactivity disorder. The activity of thiamine-related erythrocyte enzymes can be indicative of thiamine status as can urinary excretion. More than likely these steps were never taken to determine the cause of disease by deficiency in a child. Before you load your child up with vitamin B_1, however, read more about Ageless Performance.

Nutrient deficiency and imbalance *are* enormous problems in North America, though malnutrition to the point of severe emaciation, as seen in the Third World, isn't common. However, you'll soon be convinced that the underlying damage caused by our calorie-rich but nutrient-deficient diets can result in death, the kind of death associated with malnutrition cases prevalent in the developing world.

MUCH MORE THAN WE PRETEND TO KNOW

Recent research has unveiled a number of nutrients that have failed to make the category of "vitamins." But these recently discovered nutrients are just as crucial for life as the historical substances we call vitamins. The difference between vitamins and our more recent findings is simply that the latter weren't detected during the "vitamin era" and so aren't considered additions to the category.

The second factor that has distinguished these more recently discovered nutrients, or phytonutrients (plant-source nutrients), from vitamins is that their absence or limitation in the diet may not result in an immediately noticeable physiological change or disease. In fact, even with long-term omission from the diet of these phytonutrients, the development of diseases such as cancer, inflammation, cardiovascular ailments, and asthma are so slow that it is extremely difficult to correlate them with a nutrient deficiency.

Furthermore, research has revealed that a shortfall in more than one of these compounds may contribute to the aforementioned disorders, making an absolute association even harder to establish. In addition to this the toxicity level of our environment contributes greatly to these diseases in multiple ways such as gene manipulation, free-radical attack on membranes, fatty-acid oxidation, enzyme interference, and more. When so many factors are involved, scientists are wary of pointing the finger at a single or multiple cause.

Modern food-processing methods remove and deactivate vital phytonutrients, just as processing neutralizes and eliminates vitamins C and E and the Bs, as well as minerals and fibers. Research shows that phytonutrients and other more common antioxidants support immune function, cell-membrane integrity, and metabolic efficiency. We know these phytonutrients as polyphenols, catechins, flavonoids, and isoflavones. Studies demonstrate that many of these essential nutrients deliver powerful protection against cancer and heart disease and, as a result, they have become recognized as potent curative aids.

Scientists have missed the lesson! These compounds aren't curative aids as much as their deficiency results in disease. Once they're introduced into the body in required levels, disease can be overcome due to the empowerment of our inherent biochemistries. These proanthocyanidins, flavonols, catechins, citrus flavonoids, isoflavones, lignans, and others aren't considered essential by most experts. However, experts who recognize the value of these special compounds have deemed them miraculous substances that enhance longevity or display medicinal properties.

Today's nourishment fails to deliver these fundamentals in sufficient quantities, and without them the body can't carry out life-sustaining tasks. The result is a slow degradation of health that we attribute to aging, and diseases that we accept as age-related.

But these diseases aren't age-related; they're caused by a lack of essential nutrition. Scientists with barren minds may resign themselves to the concept that these special phytonutrients are conditionally essential if required at all, but I submit that today's circumstances are such that the antioxidant protection delivered by phytonutrients is indispensable. Supplementation with the antioxidant compounds found in green tea, bilberry, and grape-seed extracts; curcuminoids; alpha lipoic acid; and many more are our salvation, a natural fit to our natural chemistry. And, since as we age, the capacity to manufacture endogenous antioxidants declines, these food sources of protective antioxidants become even more critical to well-being. In other words, supplementation is far more important for the elderly. The ability of the body to generate antioxidants within cells differs among individuals, as well, and as a result each person's needs for food-sourced or supplement-derived antioxidants varies. Are you willing to take a chance and forgo the supplemental insurance program of your life?

Without pushing the body to perform at extreme levels, the metabolic and physiological limitations caused by a deficiency of these unique antioxidants might not be apparent, but when we're faced with stress the restrictions surface. When death is attributed to cardiovascular disease, for example, we don't implicate the lack of antioxidants as the cause. If the free radical is a primary facilitator of certain fatal diseases, then antioxidant protection is more than prevention and more than a cure. The antioxidant is vital for normal biological function. After all, our own definition of an essential nutrient is as follows: "A nutrient we must obtain from the diet because the body cannot make it for itself in sufficient quantity to meet physiological needs" (*Understanding Nutrition*, 8th edition, Whitney & Rolfes).

Antioxidant phytonutrients aren't producible by our bodies yet they're required protection against our hostile environments. If these antioxidants aren't supplied sufficiently, debilitating disease sets in and death is probable. Today we're witnessing health-care systems unable to cope with the strain created by a diseased populace. A larger population with a longer life expectancy is part of the problem. The fact that we're living longer, however, isn't an indication that we're on the right track when it comes to health care, fitness, and nutrition.

We may have discovered what our fundamental nutritional needs are to eliminate many diseases that once kept our population at a sustainable medium. In addition, medical technology and pharmaceutical drugs have also extended life expectancy by allowing us to overcome grave symptoms of disease as well as microbial infiltrations that in the past were lethal. The advancement of these technologies, however, won't proceed at the rate they have thus far. Even with the potential of genetic manipulation of our food about to be added to our health-care arsenal, the outcome can't be relied upon because the likelihood of disaster from this manipulation seems to be as possible if not more likely than enhancement of health.

Meeting our basic nutritional requirements such as a higher intake of quality protein has allowed us to ward off fatal disease for a longer period with the consequence of having to hobble along in our later years. Our advances have done little or nothing to change the human lifespan, which is approximately 120 years if all the conditions—genetic, environmental, and nutritional intake—are right. The odds, however, of reaching this extreme age are against us unless we take nutrient supplementation seriously.

As we bring human life expectancy closer to the maximum human lifespan, we put a greater strain on our resources, including the most valuable one—our food supplies. The very resource that we came to understand as the most important to our survival has been manipulated in such a way as to limit advancement in health care unless we take action to compensate correctly for the problem.

Why is it that the young are more frequently diagnosed with diseases that were once associated with the elderly? Those who are in their fifties or sixties today grew up in a time when food processing was scarcer and whole foods were the more likely nourishment. Such people were exposed to processed foods later in their lives, and therefore the consequences—insulin resistance, diabetes, cognitive disorders, and chronic inflammation—of this valueless food have materialized late in adulthood. During the developmental years of these people, whole foods were a bigger part of their diets and a sound nutritional foundation was set in their cells. A significant period of time would be required to offset or diminish this nutritional status.

Although individuals in their eighties today have been exposed to processed foods for many decades, the likelihood of their acceptance of these new foods isn't as great, since old habits are more liable to be maintained by them. I see this in my immediate family where my 96-year-old grandfather still eats whole, home-cooked foods and refuses to eat canned foods, fast foods, confections, and fancy desserts. His diet mainly consists of fresh vegetables and various lean animal protein sources. It's hard to break old habits.

However, my parents, who are in their early sixties, have adopted processed foods for two reasons: convenience, and the fact that the introduction of these dead foods took place much earlier in their lives than for their parents. Not only was acceptance of these foods more likely by my parents, the depletion of their nutrient status began much earlier than it did for their parents. Within two or three decades of consuming processed foods, a sound nutritional foundation has been thrown out of balance. Not surprisingly, common diseases have emerged with frequency in this generation.

With my generation, people in their thirties, the developmental years were more likely to be supported by processed and fast food, and the nutritional foundation of the body might not have been as sound as it was for our parents and grandparents. Thus, diseases, such as obesity, chronic inflammation, diabetes, and cognitive disorders, that were once more likely to develop between 50 and 70 years old manifest themselves earlier for my group as the nutritional deficiencies and imbalances reach disease-inducing states sooner.

The above information relates to the model of baseline cellular operation and thresholds previously outlined. Our parents and grandparents are more likely to have established a baseline of cellular operation that leaves more room for absorption of strain. In essence, the threshold for disease is more difficult to reach. However, people in their mid-thirties today may have adopted the typical nutrient-poor North American diet early in their development and are operating at a cellular level closer to the threshold for disease with a concomitant reduction of resilience. The longer we proceed with such a lifestyle, the closer our operating levels get to the threshold. Eventually it takes very little strain to push us over our threshold levels and manifest disease. Many people may cross that threshold and remain above it to operate at that level indefinitely and live with disease forever. The grim consequence is the necessity of lifelong drug therapy.

Ecological factors, as well, have grown from a relatively minor imposition during our great-grandparents' generation to more toxic levels in our grandparents' early days. Today the situation continues to get worse at an even faster rate. Children born in the last 10 to 15 years have parents who themselves had poor nutritional status, with mothers passing on imbalances and deficiencies to their fetuses. Such children are born with tremendous disadvantages, which is one reason why we see a greater frequency of attention-deficit disorders among them.

The developmental years of these same children are supported by foods that are processed and refined more than ever before, delivering little support for growth and development. Worse, the environmental toxicity these children face is far greater than that experienced by their parents when they were at the same stage of development. These children then function at a cellular level closer to the threshold of disease than their parents did at their age. Our children need a higher quality of nourishment than ever before to neutralize these strains and bring their operating cellular chemistry closer to that baseline level and away from the threshold of disease. Ageless Performance is the answer.

The following chapters will outline the protocols required to lay down the foundation for protection throughout the body. The evidence to come presents referenced facts about each of the protective nutraceuticals critical to Ageless Performance. The significance of this foundation is paramount, and not just as a general shield, but as an active, healing chemistry.

The foundation of the next chapters must be set in order for the central facet of the program, the carefully proportioned polyunsaturated fatty acids, to deliver their corrective potential. The antioxidant program is designed to protect the supplemental array of fats, to direct their path meticulously in the body by way of enzyme and genetic influence, to defend these newly assimilated fats in their biochemical and structural roles, and to guard the entire biology against environmental assault. The design of Ageless Performance is cutting-edge, standard-setting science that launches a new era in health care.

4

A RADICAL GENERATION

Previously I've touched on the subject of free radicals and antioxidants, but let's briefly dive into their chemistry in more detail. This will instill a better understanding of the dynamics involved when free-radical generation, oxidative stress, and antioxidants are discussed.

We so often hear about the "reactive or disease-instigating free radical" and the "neutralizing or protective antioxidant," but many of us have little or no understanding of the chemistry involved. The perceived lack of interest in this subject steers writers away from describing it more fully for fear of losing their readers' interest. However, the free radical and the antioxidant play tremendous roles in human health and disease, and a thorough understanding of their chemistry will more likely lead to complete antioxidant supplementation. Speaking on this topic in seminars, I find myself conversing with seemingly aware enthusiasts. But when I ask whether or not they understand the nature of this activity, the answer is too often *no*.

This chapter won't teach you a university-level chemistry course. The objective is to present a distilled understanding of the essence of the free radical and the antioxidant. With such knowledge each time this subject comes up in a book or in future conversations, you'll comprehend the dynamics and significance of the free radical's interaction in the body and elsewhere.

The free radical is much more than just "a bad chemical that damages our body," and the antioxidant is far more than a "good compound that neutralizes the negative reactivity of the free radical to protect the body." In fact, as previously mentioned, we rely on free-radical activity for many life-supportive processes such as immune function and oxidation of nourishment for energy production.

Because they support the immune system and protect tissues, antioxidants have a "good-guy" image. However, an antioxidant can become dangerously reactive in the body and may impart free-radical activity itself under certain conditions. On the other hand, the free radical is our savior when it works under controlled conditions with the immune system to destroy and discard foreign and damaged materials. What this means is that the "good" and "bad" definitions commonly ascribed to these entities aren't necessarily accurate.

Essential for biological health, free radicals are both facilitators and inhibitors of various biochemical systems, including hormone regulation. Nitric oxide and peroxynitrite, the nitric-oxide-derived free radical, are good examples. In some cases free radicals mediate tumor growth, but in other instances they fight tumor progression. Furthermore, free radicals are now recognized as gene modulators, a finding that differs immensely from the previous understanding of their influence as gene mutators exclusively.

The answer to this complex biological riddle is to know the functions of the different types of free radicals and identify the triggers that may turn helpful ones against us. This is central to the Ageless Performance program and the key to optimal health. If you're able to gain a genuine appreciation for the interactions and influences that our foods and the nutrients they contain have on our biochemistry, you're more likely to take my recommendations seriously and apply them as long-term lifestyle commitments. These intricacies are incorporated right into the program: you don't have to worry about applying them individually. Just follow the instructions of Ageless Performance and you'll come to understand that the complexity of this free-radical equation is built right into the nutritional formula.

ATOMIC THEORY

The hypothesized concept of the atom has been under development for more than 2,500 years, and we're still unveiling more about it. Matter, as

I've previously outlined, is made up of particles, which are invisible to us even with the tremendous technology we have at our disposal. The atom is the unit that makes up all matter in our universe. Atoms are essentially empty spaces of pulsating energy.

Particle trails, interactions, and other indicators serve as evidence for their existence and properties. Based on ingenious contributions from scientists such as Isaac Newton, John Dalton, Amedeo Avogadro, Ernest Rutherford, Albert Einstein, Max Planck, James Chadwick, and others, we've established an accepted model for the atom. This model is purely speculative, yet we base everything *scientific* on it.

Ironically our definition of science is that it's "a branch of study concerned with the observation and classification of facts with the establishment of verifiable laws." However, quantum mechanics and our depiction of the atom are based on probabilities, and probabilities aren't absolute. If we stretch this concept, we *could* say these probabilities are verifiable and are based on our ability to verify the probable events so that the depiction of the atom *is* based on fact. *Whew!*

But the concept of verifiable probabilities is in itself a paradox. Ultimately the model of the atom, the founding unit of matter, the particle constituting the fabric of the universe and our bodies, isn't conclusive at all. Yet we base our so-called science on this model.

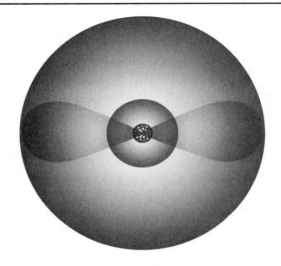

FIGURE 2:

Model of
Single Atom

The elements that make up the periodic table are essentially a variety of atoms. These elements are found in our environment in mixtures, in pure forms, and in gaseous, liquid, and solid states. Typically they can change from one form to another based on their level of atomic energy, a state that can be influenced by temperature, pressure, light, and inducement from other atoms. These energy states are reflective of electron activity of the atom in relation to the atom's nucleus. We experience these transitions in state daily such as by boiling water to produce steam and vapor (liquid to gas), or by freezing the same water to produce ice cubes (liquid to solid).

Although we can easily assert how one substance will react to temperature and other influences when it's isolated, we're far from being able to predict precisely how these atoms or the molecules they make up will respond in a soup of man-made and natural reactants. As much as we think we have a deep understanding of the atom, we haven't even scratched the surface.

However, there are many facts based on distant observations that we do know for certain. One of these is that the free radical, an atom or group of atoms, contributes to uncontrolled oxidation in the body, and uninhibited oxidation propagates disease (1). Various chemicals, those of unnatural origin as well as many that are natural byproducts, can instigate and proliferate free-radical generation to increase the risk of disease. In other words, no matter how hard we try we can't escape the free-radical assault from our environment. This activity strikes right through us like lightning.

Free radicals don't just bounce off skin as though it were a metal shield and the free radical a rubber bead. The free radical that's generated outside the body can, upon contact, damage the molecules or atoms that make up skin. The reactivity doesn't end there. It continues like a domino effect through the skin to affect molecules in contact and close proximity—an indefinite chain of reactivity.

Protection from this hazard comes in the form of cell-incorporated antioxidants such as vitamin E and alpha lipoic acid, which slow down the reactivity. The antioxidant shield acts more like a sponge or a goopy gel matrix to absorb the momentum of the free radical that ricochets our way. With this gel matrix in place the free radical can't filter through as quickly or as deeply.

However, the absorption potential of antioxidants is limited, so that the more toxicity we're exposed to, the more light from the sun and tanning beds we subject ourselves to, the more absorption potential we need. Keep in mind that once we run out of absorption potential, the ultraviolet-light, toxin-activated free radicals are allowed to infiltrate deeper into the body where, if we're prepared, they'll meet a second line of antioxidant defense guarding the core. If we're not properly fortified, though, free radicals will invade our bodies further, literally scalding us from the inside out.

Compounding this bombardment from the outside, the body produces free radicals by way of metabolic activity. Emotional and mental states drive free-radical generation, as well, as we'll see in more detail later. In addition, we all take in free radicals and other toxins through air and food. A larger intake of calories results in greater metabolic activity and more free-radical production at the body's core (2). This is the basis for calorie restriction as part of Ageless Performance; it's a good fit as a life-extension program. With more physical activity, more oxygen is metabolized, and this, as well, increases the rate of cellular free-radical generation (3).

Frankly there's no escape. Free radicals will flood your body from the outside in and the inside out. Antioxidant protection must be supplied completely to protect you from uncontrolled combustion. An effective program is much more than singular antioxidants; it's complex and comprehensive, and Ageless Performance brings it together in just the right combinations and proportions.

Without going too deeply into quantum mechanics (a theory dealing with the motion and interaction of atoms and their components—electrons, neutrons, and protons), let's briefly look at the atom and the development of the free radical.

Our basic theory of the atom involves a dense central core, the nucleus, made up of protons (positive charge) and neutrons (neutral charge). This core typically possesses a positive charge overall. Orbiting the atom's nucleus are negatively charged electrons with a relative mass of zero, offsetting the positive charge of the nucleus. An atom that has as many electrons (negative charge) orbiting it as it has protons (positive charge) within it has no net charge. In other words, the atom is neutral. Furthermore, the electrons are typically organized into distinct "orbitals."

An oxygen atom, for example, normally has eight electrons revolving around a nucleus containing eight protons and eight neutrons. The nucleus, in this case, has a positive charge of eight, which is offset or neutralized by eight negatively charged electrons. Two of these eight electrons (8^{-e}) can be easily removed from the oxygen atom if it's excited by heat, light, electricity, other electrons, or even other atoms. These two electrons are in the outermost orbit of the atom and are influenced less intensely by the positive attraction of the nucleus (the core). The loss of negatively charged electrons leaves this atom with a net positive charge. The net positive charge comes from the eight protons (8^{+p}) that still exist at the core of the nucleus ($8^{+p} + 8^{-e} = 8^{0}$ [neutral atomic charge]; $8^{+p} + 6^{-e} = 2^{+}$ [positive 2 atomic charge]).

However, the oxygen atom can also pull these negatively charged electrons into its outer orbit, since its central core has the positive force to do so. This force is similar but obviously not the same as the gravitational pull found in our solar system. The orbitals of electrons are often described as organized cloud patterns or clusters, as Figure 2 on page 100 conveys. Electrons usually exist in pairs that offset each other to impart stability. These pairings form the basis of free-radical activity.

As mentioned earlier, this *idea* of atomic structure is built entirely on speculation derived from mathematical equations and observations. The mathematical equations merely determine probabilities of what could be, where it could be, and why it should be. Are they fact or fiction? Certainly the educated guesses are based on facts, but the atom is ultimately a figment of our calculated imagination.

The oxygen we breathe is diatomic, which means that in its gaseous state it's made up of two atoms of oxygen, hence the O_2 nomenclature. These two atoms share electrons in their outer orbits. This sharing of whole atoms is called covalent bonding. When O_2 is used in the mitochondria to produce ATP, the body's universal energy source, the reaction can yield an oxygen atom with a positive charge and an oxygen atom with a negative charge as follows: $O_2{}^{0} = O_{-2} + O_{+2}$ or $O_2{}^{0} = O^{-e-e} + O_{+2}$. Incidentally the 0 in $O_2{}^{0}$ indicates a relative zero or neutral charge. The reaction can also result in the separation of the two atoms, leaving two oxygen atoms in their neutral state.

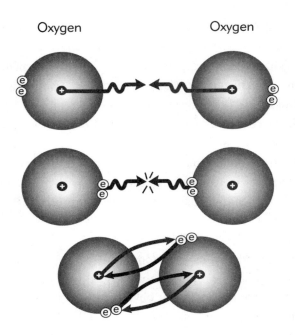

FIGURE 3:

Schematic of
Oxygen Atoms

Oxygen   Oxygen

O_2 (diatomic oxygen—oxygen we breathe)

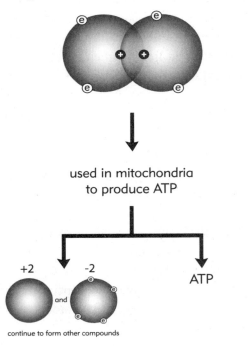

used in mitochondria
to produce ATP

+2   -2   ATP

and

continue to form other compounds

In the former case, O_{+2} is missing two of its orbiting electrons, and the other, O_{-2}, has retained the two from its partner oxygen atom, two more than it would have had in a neutral state. These charged atoms are oxygen ions; the one with the extra electrons is relatively negative and the one that has lost its electrons from the outermost orbit is relatively positive.

There is a more complex level of activity within the subatomic continuum than the above description. In addition, there are a myriad of influences from other atoms or catalysts from the biological soup of reactants in our body to produce a considerable array of interacting byproducts that include these oxygen atoms or ions.

FREE-RADICAL GENERATION

Often a chemical reaction in the body doesn't proceed as cleanly as it should. Extreme demands from intense physical exercise and disease, as well as the influence from environmental chemicals, metabolic byproducts, and dietary and stored nutrient supplies, influence how efficiently reactions ensue in our cells.

The reaction can also yield atoms with an odd number of electrons in the outer orbits, leaving behind an unpaired electron. Essentially this resulting odd-numbered entity isn't positive, negative, or neutral. In fact, it isn't even considered an ion; it's a free radical, an unstable atom or molecule with an unpaired electron in search of a companion electron. In this particular example, the free radical is a superoxide anion radical, O_2^{-e}, or it can easily form a hydroxyl radical, HO^{-e}. Both are extraordinarily vicious.

The unstable free radical requires an electron to offset the imbalance that this odd electron number imposes. It can suck an electron from another atom that makes up part of a molecule in the cells or vital chemicals of the body. When an electron is ripped away from an atom that's part of vital tissue, the atomic structure of this tissue's atom is altered and so are its chemical properties.

Ultimately this affected molecule and the tissue it constitutes are damaged. The free radical can tear away an electron from an atom of a

FIGURE 4:

Development of Free Radical from Oxygen

Noninteractive Neutral Oxygen Atoms

Interactive Neutral Oxygen Atoms

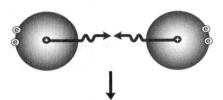

can form
diatomic oxygen
(the oxygen we breathe)

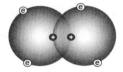

can split
(such as during respiration
for ATP production in the mitochondria)

clean reaction produces
positive and negative oxygen ions

can split in a toxic overworked or nutritionally
compromised metabolic environment to produce
free radicals

+2   -2

molecule that exists in the genetic code of DNA. The result is a mutated code that can subsequently impair cell function. This process can instigate disease if the immune system or the natural DNA-corrective chemistry isn't able to discard or fix the mutation.

Such a radical reaction isn't isolated to a single event, either. It's not slow and certainly not finite. It's more like a flash that rips through the body with lightning speed. The sacrificed molecule that neutralizes the original free radical, whether antioxidant or not, doesn't terminate the reaction. The sacrificed atom has one less electron in its outer orbit and is now a free radical itself.

Chatecholamines like dopamine and epinephrine (adrenaline) are highly reactive and initiate the production of free radicals as does hydrocortisone (4, 5, 6). While moderate chatecholamine secretions can protect the body by delivering antioxidant protection, oversecretion is oxidative, promoting free-radical generation. Prolonged periods of stress can result in incremental levels of epinephrine and corticosteroids that ultimately give rise to greater levels of free radicals. This is one way emotional and mental strains increase oxidative stress on the body and heighten the risk of disease. The stress-produced superoxide anion radical is a dangerous piranha that chews away at the body.

If your life is a scurrying frenzy, the slow-drip release of these catabolic hormones produces an ongoing flow of free radicals that munch on your tissues and undermine your health. A big part of the solution is to manage stress by changing to a less stressful lifestyle and by gaining a different perspective on the stressors. Another way, which isn't an alternative but is an essential part of the solution, is to provide complete antioxidant protection through multiple antioxidant supplementation.

Unregulated serum glucose breeds free radicals, as well. As we've seen in the previous chapter, glucose can react detrimentally with long-lived body proteins such as cartilage and other vital proteins to produce an advanced glycosylated endproduct (AGE)—a damaged protein. Free radicals play a facilitative role in this reaction, and the antioxidants making up the crux of the Ageless Performance program inhibit this damage (7, 8, 9).

You'll see later on just how glucose intolerance or insulin resistance (pre-diabetic and diabetic states) can propagate free-radical generation at both ends of the serum-glucose spike—at high- (hyperglycemia) and low-serum glucose (hypoglycemia). Ultimately the process works something like this: due to insulin resistance or diabetes (Type II), carbohydrates or other high-glycemic-index foods can raise serum glucose to an uncontrollable high. This sugar high breeds free radicals as serum sugars react in the blood (10, 11). The resulting toxicity permeates the body, whittling away at antioxidant stores such as glutathione and vitamins A, C, and E and taxing the protective matrix of your being.

A dysfunctional system and/or poor eating habits then allow blood-sugar levels to fall too low, and this in turn stimulates the body's panic response, which involves glucagon, epinephrine, norepinephrine, and corticosteroid secretions. This again can propagate free-radical generation and contribute cumulatively to an increased risk of disease. These phenomena also increase the risk of secondary diseases such as cardiovascular ailments and chronic inflammation that diabetes and insulin resistance spread throughout the body. But good eating habits and insulin health help down-regulate free-radical proliferation and reduce this danger.

You may think your skin, the mucosal lining of your gut, the walls of your arteries, and the walls of each of your organs represent barriers or confinement for these specialized systems, but they don't. Your entire body is a unit of empty space pulsating with a multiplicity of specialized energy configurations (organs and specialized tissues), each of which is made up of atoms. At the atomic level there is no barrier whatsoever within your body or between your body and the universe.

Remember, the atom is 99.9% empty space pulsating with energy, and you and I are made up entirely of these building blocks. This makes us continuous with the universe, other matter, and other beings. Ultimately we're atomic-embodied, bioenergetic patterns existing in and as part of the universal continuum.

All of our clothes and protective gear are made up of atoms, as well, but are transparent or, at best, translucent to free-radical intrusion. The best defense against chemical scalding is a tightly woven blanket of antioxidant molecules and systems, a blanket of skin profusely saturated with antioxidant protection that absorbs and intercepts free-radical lightning bolts before they penetrate deeper than the surface of the skin. This armament includes an evenly dispersed antioxidant matrix that coexists with the biochemical works of the surface of our skins right down to our cores. Ageless Performance is designed to weave this fabric.

In order for this tightly knit fabric to be maintained in a functional state, Ageless Performance must be applied daily rather than sporadically. This doesn't mean we can't deviate from the program. The occasional consumption of foods that don't fit the program's criteria can't damage this protective weave if the majority of the diet and lifestyle is healthy.

ENTER THE ANTIOXIDANT

Antioxidants such as vitamins C and E, catechins, flavonoids, and polyphenols of plant origin supply the electrons required to neutralize free radicals so that the latter don't steal electrons from the atoms that make up vital molecules, cells, and tissues. However, that's not the only activity of these powerful biomodulators.

An antioxidant readily gives up an electron to neutralize the reactive free radical, but it's left with an unpaired electron that can also become a free radical. Antioxidants work in synergistic combinations. One type, such as vitamin E, can't replace the function of another, say, vitamin C or grapeseed extract and vice versa. The claims that grapeseed extract is so much more powerful than vitamin E aren't completely true. The wide array of free radicals requires a varied arsenal of specialized antioxidants.

Vitamin E, for example, isn't able to neutralize all of the free radicals that glutathione or grapeseed extract can, but glutathione or grapeseed can't effectively counteract all of those that vitamin E can. There may be overlap in the potential of antioxidants, but there definitely isn't complete redundancy. In addition, antioxidants actually rely on one another for interaction to complete their roles. When an antioxidant becomes a free radical, it relies on its antioxidant partner to supply it with an electron to bring it down from its reactive state.

The second donor, however, becomes a free radical itself, having given up its electron, so it requires a donor of its own. Each time this co-dependent reaction takes place the free-radical reaction potential (oxidative potential or reactivity level) drops to a lower level and becomes less risky to the body. Complete antioxidant programs are crucial to the total diffusion of this destructive activity.

By limiting the availability of these antioxidants in the body, completely or in part, we become vulnerable to the original reactive free radical at the top of the chain or any of the free radicals that are left in a reactive state at the point where the co-dependent antioxidant is missing from the chain.

It's easy to induce a toxic outcome with a megadose administration of vitamin E, for example, and this is exactly what unaware scientists do when they show negative effects with supplementation of antioxidants. Typically toxicity assessments are done with extremely high megadoses. However, without the inclusion of a proportional quantity of partner antioxidants, megadoses of antioxidants give rise to a pro-oxidative (free-radical generation) situation and, therefore, increase the risk of disease. Upon reporting these findings without completely disclosing all of the facts, irresponsible scientists contribute to the confusion and doubt among consumers concerning antioxidant supplementation at a time when we need this protection more than ever.

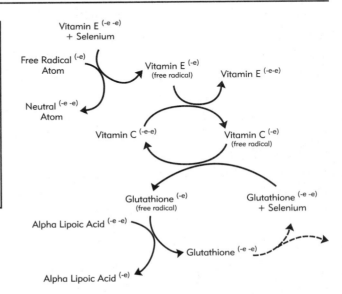

FIGURE 5:

Simplified Example of Co-Dependent Interaction Between Antioxidants

Notes:
12, 13, 14, 15

Vitamins C and E and beta-carotene are three antioxidants that come to mind. Some experts report irresponsibly that these life supporters are toxic. I can assure you that if you eliminate these nutrients from your diet while wading through today's cesspool, free radicals will eat you alive. Today's epidemics are proof of this activity. Supplement with antioxidants correctly and free radicals won't be able to sink their teeth into your armor.

Ageless Performance is more than just a complete antioxidant program. In order for its central facet to be effective, however, a complete antioxidant plan must be employed. The next chapter will introduce you to the administrable program. There I'll begin to describe and justify the components of the protective foundation as well as the navigators and facilitators of the pathway crucial to Ageless Performance. Essential fats and other omega-3 fats are central to the special metabolic pathway that represents the core of Ageless Performance. Not only are these fats extremely susceptible to oxidation by free radicals, but they're vulnerable to a multiplicity of detours from their healthy path caused by free radicals, detours that are common in all of us due to our shared toxic lifestyle and environment.

Ageless Performance will keep specialized fats intact. By normalizing gene activity, it will also maintain them on course for balanced hormone production. Antioxidants can be critical navigators of hormone production, and this is the second crucial role of the distinct, carefully crafted Ageless Performance antioxidant program. Some of the information you're about to read is common knowledge, but most of it is part of a cutting-edge revolution that will completely transform the way this cellular chemistry and the antioxidants that closely interact with it will be viewed from now on.

Here's to a new era and a new path to human health and performance!

5

NATURE HOLDS THE KEYS

Like a prehistoric dinosaur, the lumbering shovel tractor digs deeper and wider, clearing the way to solid ground. Before work can begin, bedrock must be exposed to anchor the building's foundation. Construction of any kind requires a reliable base. The same holds true for the foundation we're about to erect for Ageless Performance.

This chapter presents the list of materials and the administrative instructions required to build a rock-solid foundation. All of the information found here is validated with support from common sense and science. This amazing strategy is much more than a sturdy platform, far more than structural support; it includes a series of navigational factors that mediate the flow of our chemistries.

Humans are one of the few species unable to synthesize vitamin C and, as a result, it must be supplied by the diet. Vitamin C is found abundantly in asparagus, oranges, cantaloupes, cauliflower, broccoli, grapefruit, kale, horseradish, black currants, and strawberries. Government-established recommended daily allowances, or *recommended nutrient minimums*, as I prefer to call them, can't stand up to today's relentless free-radical bombardment, and this definitely applies to the woefully inadequate recommendation for vitamin C.

The World Health Organization (WHO) Expert Committee urges a daily vitamin C intake for men and nonpregnant and nonlactating women of 30 mg. In the United States the daily recommended dose for vitamin C is 45 mg. A daily consumption of less than 10 mg of vitamin C can result in the development of scurvy.

The fight against disease results in an increased rate of vitamin C turnover in the body. A more active immune system requires additional vitamin C, and nowadays our immune-system activity is much greater than ever before. If you expect your body to perform above-average physical feats, you'll require higher levels of vitamin C to facilitate tissue repair (1). All of these factors raise the body's nutrient demands, and this involves a lot more than just vitamin C.

Synthesis of tissues such as collagen requires vitamin C, as does synthesis and activation of carnitine, neurotransmitters, and many hormones (2, 3). A 2002 German study demonstrates one of vitamin C's roles in the synthesis of cartilage, confirming, as well, how the vitamin is involved in gene activation. This study shows that vitamin C actually enters the chondrocyte (the cell responsible for the production of proteoglycans/collagen and cartilage) to stimulate the genes responsible for collagen synthesis. The form of vitamin C delivering this activity is L-ascorbic acid (4). Vitamin C deficiency can cause delayed gene response for tissue maintenance, resulting in accumulated wear and tear. The understanding that nutrients as common as vitamin C impose gene-modulating influences has changed the face of nutraceuticals in health care. These findings justify supplementation with levels of vitamin C, for example, that far exceed the recommended allowances, especially in the case of osteo and even rheumatoid arthritis.

Face it. Your healthy genetic constitution may be sitting idle waiting for its specific activation factor in order for its instructions to be unleashed. In other words, your arthritic condition might not be a function of poor genetic predisposition and could more likely result from a lack of vitamin C, the gene activator.

We know that vitamin C is a powerful antioxidant and that its free-radical neutralizing activity is independent of the co-factor activity and gene activation it delivers for molecular biosynthesis. The dietary minimums of vitamin C we adhere to today, if we make them at all, are based on documentation from long ago. While vitamin C fulfills its duty as a co-factor for the synthesis of tissue and immune-system and chondrocyte facilitator, it must concurrently execute its role as general antioxidant in the body. It's easy to see how today's increased oxidative imposition (such as free-radical toxicity) raises the nutrient requisites for all antioxidants. In fact, this oxidative stress intercepts vitamin C to keep it from our genetic codes, which can increase the level of vitamin C required to prevent the onset of scurvy as well as maintain normal gene activity. Yesterday's essential nutrient minimums don't cut it at all, and the case of vitamin C is merely a model for all other nutrients.

The active individual encounters additional strain, further increasing nutrient demands. With more activity, more oxygen is consumed, larger quantities of toxins are created, more tissues require repair, and more calories must be consumed to sustain the activity. All of these factors contribute to oxidative imposition on the body and a higher demand for vitamin C. The damage and subclinical inflammation that exercise can cause involves immune activity and therefore a greater turnover of vitamin C.

Many nutrients, such as vitamin C, are now more accurately recognized as essential keys for genetic activity and vital activators of the genetic potential within all of us. If you're even nominally undernourished, you're living short of your maximum genetic potential for life or sport. However, the majority of us are grossly overfed while largely undernourished, which compounds the threat: excess calories translate into more free radicals, and concurrent with antioxidant nutrient scarcity, the result is grave danger.

A University of Oxford report in 2000 concludes that oral vitamin C shows tremendous promise for improving atherosclerosis, hypertension, and hypercholesterolemia, all of which have reached epidemic status (5). This is old news, but what is novel is the interesting method of vitamin C activity discovered in this study. Vitamin C is now recognized as an important regulator of nitric oxide.

Nitric oxide is involved in the regulation of processes throughout our bodies, controlling organ function, enzyme activity, blood pressure, neuron function, respiration—you name it! *Mis*regulation of nitric oxide leads to *mis*regulation of biological systems and the development of disease. As I've mentioned earlier, many of our pharmaceutical drugs induce their tissue-specific, symptom-relieving activity by helping to direct nitric-oxide systems gone awry.

Researchers strongly believe that as our bodies age our ability to produce and regulate nitric oxide declines and, in part, this promotes biological dysfunction, propelling oxidative stress in the body. Nitric oxide is highly reactive and gives rise to toxic nitrites and nitrates under uncontrolled conditions. The brain is highly vulnerable to this toxicity, but the damage permeates throughout and is a likely cause or contributor to heart disease, chronic inflammation, and even autoimmune dysfunctions like rheumatoid arthritis. These findings have clearly demonstrated that we can have preventive and restorative control over what may seem to be an inevitable decline in health as we age.

Generally we possess very efficient internally manufactured regulation systems for nitric oxide. Primarily this involves antioxidants such as alpha lipoic acid, catalase, superoxide dismutase, and glutathione peroxidase, which play central roles. However, each of us has different genetically programmed capacities to produce these protective substances, and therefore we all possess different levels of internally manufactured disease prevention.

We can even the score by administering strategic oral supplementation that complements endogenous (internal) antioxidant systems. As we age, our supplemental regimens can be augmented to offset a progressive natural decline of internal antioxidant biosynthesis by administering a more aggressive oral antioxidant program. This is one way we can take control of our health and our rate of biological aging. It's actually quite easy, and Ageless Performance makes it even simpler to apply each facet of the anti-aging strategy.

Interestingly nitric oxide and the free radicals it can cause have been recently recognized as the factors involved in the decline in pineal gland function. The pineal gland, a small appendage projecting from the top of the midbrain, is responsible for natural melatonin secretion. The gland's emission of melatonin, a powerful antioxidant and hormone, initiates healthy circadian rhythm (natural rhythmic flow) of hormones, stimulating a cascade of multiple biological processes. Impair the pineal trigger and the entire body is thrown out of whack. In fact, as we age, this impairment and the subsequent biological arrhythmia that rises from it advances until the body cycles out of its vital rhythm. As a result, the body begins to backfire, degenerate, and succumb to a slow death—otherwise described as natural biological aging.

It's easy to appreciate the complexity this cycle represents. Unregulated nitric oxide impairs the pineal gland, inhibiting normal secretion of the protective melatonin, which causes biorhythm problems. Melatonin is a recognized regulator of nitric oxide, as well. When nitric-oxide production flails out of control with age, pineal gland function and melatonin emissions decline, perpetuating the damage and allowing the rate of biological aging to accelerate (6). The pineal secretion protects and resets the entire body, but it also guards the pineal gland against the factor that injures it. It's easy to see that once the destruction is initiated, it's difficult to halt. Supplemental melatonin at bedtime slows the progression of arrhythmia, so the sooner you intercept this pineal damage in life the better.

The pineal gland is a sort of biorhythm regulator that manages human existence and synergizes it with the cycles of the universe. There may be more to that astrological link of humanity than you think. As daylight diminishes and darkness ensues, melatonin is pumped out to begin a new cycle of recovery, regeneration, and free-radical control during sleep. Often the hormone is employed as a supplement to promote sleep in cases of insomnia. When daylight hits the eye in the morning, the biochemical reaction again influences the pineal gland to reset the biological and bioenergetic systems of the body in preparation for the day.

The day-night cycles and the daylight changes that occur with seasonal shifts have a profound effect on our hormone chemistry. The transfer of rhythm from astrology to human organisms stems from pineal operation. Protecting this gland from degradation ensures the youthful activity of complex hormone cascades and keeps us in synch with the universe and with each other.

Controlling reactive nitric oxide is critical to health and longevity and can only be accomplished by the synergy of multiple antioxidants. Both vitamin C and melatonin are involved in the regulation of nitric oxide and the immediate neutralization of the toxic metabolites arising from nitric-oxide oxidation. As you'll see later, alpha lipoic acid is a powerful regulator of nitric oxide throughout the body, as well.

However, in the case of vitamin C's role, proper nitric-oxide maintenance can't proceed with supplemental daily intakes of only 100, 200, or 300 mg; 2,000 mg each day is more the answer. Many of the supplements on today's retail shelves are known to deliver health-care potential that was unfathomable until only recently. In the past few years the products haven't changed much; what has been transformed is our understanding of their pharmacology and the opportunity for more precise administration.

Today nitric-oxide stimulation has become the strategy of our time—a trend. But stimulating nitric-oxide production with arginine supplements in a body that's ill prepared to regulate it, as you'll see, isn't the answer to better health. Soy protein is now recognized as a regulator of hypertension because of its naturally high arginine content—the amino acid, arginine, promotes higher levels of nitric-oxide production required for improved vasodilation function (reduced blood pressure). However, nitric-oxide elevation is responsible for disease in other tissues, and without regulators such as vitamin C one system is enhanced by heightening nitric oxide at the expense of another biological system.

Vitamin C's protective influence in the body is enhanced further by flavonoids like quercetin, which we often discard from natural sources of vitamin C. The white, relatively tasteless material that exists between the skin and the juicy pulp of citrus fruit such as oranges and grapefruit is rich in bioflavonoids that ensure the integrity of vitamin C within the fruit as it does in our bodies. Recent research has substantiated that certain bioflavonoids are much more than enhancers of vitamin C activity and that they're essential to ascorbic-acid circulation and activity (7).

As noted earlier, when adenosine triphosphate (ATP) is produced, uncontrolled free radicals are often generated in the mitochondrial membranes. This is especially the case for athletes who metabolize more nourishment to keep up with ATP demands and as a result manufacture more free radicals. Vitamin C and the flavonoids play roles in mitochondrial longevity. The mitochondria is the essential power generator in cells, which means its unimpaired integrity translates into biological longevity. Consuming supplemental vitamin C requires that supplemental bioflavonoid levels be increased as well if the former is expected to function at full capacity in the body. A good vitamin C supplement will include bioflavonoids.

This basic display of synergy is typical of all the nutrients we depend on. Each nutrient is like a stitch in a knitted blanket. No matter how far away the first stitch is from the last in the fabric, they're still related and bound by a series of stitches that functions independently but simultaneously to maintain the integrity of the whole. As such a single missing stitch can compromise everything. Like a stitch, each vitamin, each mineral, each phytonutrient plays a role that is autonomous but concurrently dependent at one level or another; a missing nutrient, however small, will cause the fabric of our bodies and minds to be pulled apart with ease.

"FUNCTIONAL" NOURISHMENT

Vitamins, phytonutrients, and minerals are incorporated directly into enzymes that drive a myriad of processes, from the synthesis of tissues to the development of hormones. Without these activating and protective essentials the biochemical pathways that give rise to life can't be catalyzed and guarded. If greater demands are placed on the body, whether from illness or physical or mental stress, more of these activators are required to propel and steer the metabolism. Furthermore, if vitamin C intake doesn't meet demand, the level isn't functional for the complete biological system. We might deliver enough vitamin C to facilitate synthesis of collagen and other tissues, but if there isn't sufficient C for the protection of this newly built tissue, synthesis could be futile—less than a completely *functional* level of the vitamin.

Studies show repeatedly that higher serum ascorbic-acid (vitamin C) levels are associated with a reduction in the risk of coronary heart disease and stroke (8). However, one question always remains: how much vitamin C is enough? The answer for certain is not to be caught short, and the World Health Organization's 30 mg daily recommendation is definitely not enough. In addition, one dose doesn't stretch to fit everybody. Still, if vitamin C intake is increased the other synergistic essentials it relies on and lends support to must be considered with equal significance. Ageless Performance brings this synergy to the table in the correct combinations and proportions.

This very co-dependence is what makes whole, fresh, and unprocessed food critical to our survival, especially since the alternatives have been stripped of the natural balance that evolution has perfected. We might have grown up with white pasta, white bread, and white rice as staples, but we must change these predilections today!

Altered, processed, and nutrient-compromised foods can't be functional fits in our evolutionary programming. They're not part of our cellular blueprint. The changes that we've imposed on food and environment were made in a mere flash in the evolutionary timeline. But this isn't how evolution builds new strains; it's how it wipes the slate clean. In fact, many experts say this is how the dinosaurs were eradicated on the planet. An inflection point in the environment altered the conditions through which a handful of genetic variations of these prehistoric beasts had the formula to survive. A meteorite is said to have hit Earth, creating a global plume of dust that shut out the sun's restorative energy. Whatever the case, the environmental transformation was sudden, but *sudden* on an evolutionary scale doesn't imply immediate death within hours, days, or even months.

The change might have caused lung disease and a slow rate of starvation as plant life failed to regenerate efficiently. The incremental alteration in the atmospheric proportions of gases would have eventually reached unsustainable levels, but it's not as though these reptiles dropped dead all at once one dark and gloomy day. They died slowly, some resisting the likely frequent lung disease and malnourishment longer than others.

This is precisely the challenge humans are facing today. The reason why it's difficult to comprehend is that we're living through a gradual process. In addition, because of our ability to intervene with disease medically, we're able to combat some of the detrimental outcomes to mask the severity of our situation. Our only hope, while we try to clean up our act before the slate is wiped clean, is a higher density of nourishment to battle the plume of toxicity we've created, to counteract an inflection point our gene pool isn't prepared to live through without assistance.

My intake of vitamin C can reach a daily high of 17,000 mg on days when I'm run-down, exposed, or susceptible to illness. That's 17 g in one day over several small doses. Typically my C intake ranges from 10,000 to 14,000 mg daily. The administration strategy for such megadoses is an important consideration, as well. We can't just dump a megaload into our stomachs and expect full absorption. The "single-dose megapack" multivitamin/mineral strategy is old hat.

Our bodies aren't designed to absorb these excessive quantities at once. That's why two or even four daily doses are required to deliver the quantities of vitamins and minerals we may require to battle the toxic assault we've instigated. This same multi-dose strategy must be applied for the administration of the other supplementation of this or any other program. A daily vitamin C intake of 1,500 to 4,000 mg is a healthy goal you may want to strive for as long as the other synergists are included proportionately. You could start with 200 mg three times daily and slowly work up to a 1,500 to 2,000 mg total that must be divided into three or four 500 mg doses. For most people a daily dose of vitamin C in excess of 5 g (5,000 mg) will cause diarrhea, so make sure you work up to your personal maximum incrementally. Your tolerance level will increase over time.

MULTIPLE DAILY-DOSE STRATEGY IS CRITICAL

When the absorption site in the intestinal wall becomes saturated with a nutrient, any additional volume at that time will pass by the absorption site and won't be soaked up. Once past the specific absorption site, the vitamin, mineral, or phytonutrient continues along the intestinal tract to be excreted unless it's metabolized by gut bacteria to form other useful nutrients.

Successful supplementation is a strategic endeavor in which small but frequent doses are taken with food to slow the transit time of the nutrient. Supplemental vitamin C must be consumed with bioflavonoids. Proanthocyanidins, for example, from grapeseed and grapeskin extracts will enhance vitamin C efficiency and protect the connective tissues that it facilitates construction of (9, 10). Studies confirm that the main method for the cartilage-supportive activity of the grapeseed proanthocyanidin is in its ability to protect or spare vitamin C in the body. This allows C to accumulate to levels high enough to penetrate the chondrocyte and activate the genes responsible for collagen production. The type of supplemental vitamin C used is also an important factor. I've found that blends of different vitamin C sources—combinations of calcium ascorbate, magnesium ascorbate, and ascorbyl palmytate (fat-soluble vitamin C)—deliver the best results. The synergy of such precise combining alleviates the need for excessive doses of supplements; it raises nutrient efficiency and heightens pharmacological or therapeutic activity.

If, after reading about my daily 17 g dose of vitamin C, you think that Ageless Performance is a program of unreasonable extremes, don't fret. The program is built from the ground up so that you're able to find the level of participation that fits your personal goals and lifestyle. Vitamin C is one of many nutrients that must be supplemented aggressively to build an impermeable protective shield, and as we age the quantity and variety of supplemented antioxidants that must join the fight against disease has to be increased.

More research has confirmed the role of antioxidants in the prevention and reversal of damage caused by arthritis. Chondrocytes, the collagen-generating cells of our bodies, produce more nitric oxide in diseased arthritic tissue than in healthy cartilage. Excess nitric oxide breeds excess free radicals. In a 2001 Spanish study that determined the nitric-oxide dilemma, glucosamine hydrochloride, Type II collagen, chondroitin sulfate, and glucosamine sulfate were tested on the arthritic condition. These test compounds are all sold in most health-food stores as therapeutics, and the controversy over which one works better persists.

Of all the compounds tested, chondroitin sulfate displayed the most powerful effect and was the only one that demonstrated the capacity to reduce nitric oxide in arthritic tissues (11). Chondroitin is now known to be absorbed efficiently by the gut through a process called pinocytosis, delivering site-specific nitric-oxide regulation and site-specific antioxidant potential. Sulfur is a critical factor in cartilage construction, and common antioxidants and glucosamine hydrochloride *don't* contain the sulfur group.

I highlight this glucosamine issue because it's a common controversy that can be laid to rest when we consider the important antioxidant activity required to alleviate the pain and degeneration associated with arthritis. The thiol group (sulfur feature) plays two significant roles in natural therapy: it supplies sulfur, which is needed for protein cross-linking to give cartilage its rubbery, shock-absorbing characteristics; and it acts as a powerful antioxidant that helps regulate nitric oxide.

Alternative studies have shown glucosamine hydrochloride to be effective, but only if the chondrocyte is performing free of nitric-oxide interference. Glucosamine hydrochloride is a precursor or building block for collagen synthesis, and its supplementation is likely to be more valuable for younger individuals with healthy antioxidant and chondrocyte-cell status (12). However, osteo and rheumatoid arthritis are generally associated with the elderly and are probably caused or propelled by free radicals. In addition, cartilage damage is also common in athletes, and they, too, are exposed to more free-radical stress due to activity levels: glucosamine hydrochloride isn't the best source for these cases. Chondroitin sulfate delivers multiple functions: first, a pharmacological influence by down-regulating nitric oxide; second, a polymer (repeating chain) of glucosamine, delivering an abundance of the precursor for cartilage construction; and third, the required sulfur for cross-linking.

Glucosamine hydrochloride on its own can't protect the chondrocyte from nitric oxide and the byproducts of nitric-oxide oxidation (the extremely toxic and inflammatory peroxynitrite free radical), nor can it resuscitate the dormant cells the way chondroitin sulfate can. However, glucosamine hydrochloride can be effective with the addition of grapeseed extract (proanthocyanidin) and significant daily doses of vitamin C (2,000 to 3,000 mg per day) as nitric-oxide regulators. The addition of a sulfur source for complete tissue construction is also required if the hydrochloride of glucosamine is administered as a therapy. Methylsulfonylmethane (MSM) is a good supplemental source of sulfur. The additional cost for the added antioxidant activity required to accompany glucosamine hydrochloride supplementation makes chondroitin sulfate the better choice, the latter providing more of the needed components and activities.

My recommendation in order of priority, if cartilage restoration is called for, is a combination of chondroitin sulfate (1,500 mg daily), SAMe (300 mg daily), and glucosamine hydrochloride (1,000 mg daily) as an addition to the Ageless Performance program foundation. SAMe is another powerful nitric-oxide inhibitor and chondrocyte resuscitator. Much like chondroitin, SAMe is also a great pain reliever and reconstruction mediator.

The antioxidant potential of Ageless Performance requires little more antioxidant support than the program you'll apply. That's why my recommendation above doesn't include common antioxidant support. If you're on the program, just add chondroitin sulfate and SAMe for joint recovery. The Ageless Performance foundation already includes, in sufficient quantities, gene-activating vitamin C and facilitative flavonoids such as grapeseed proanthocyanidins. This program will relieve the pain and inflammation as it facilitates quick restoration. But most important, this powerful antioxidant program is preventive. It will help maintain general biological health to forestall premature degeneration and stop premature biological aging. Prevention is always the most effective therapy.

Heparin, a common anticoagulant pharmaceutical drug and a glycosaminoglycan or GAG, is a compound similar in structure and function to chondroitin sulfate. However, heparin's site of specificity is the platelet where it down-regulates nitric oxide to deactivate the platelet's clotting capacity. Many pharmaceuticals work like oxidants and antioxidants in the body. But maintaining a healthy antioxidant status can establish a healthy biological state and a youthful biochemical predisposition to intercept the need for reactive drug use. Supplementation is the key to sustaining cell vitality and biochemical balance and avoiding intervention.

Due to their cost, important nutrients such as alpha lipoic acid, coenzyme Q10 (CoQ10), glutathione, and glutamine aren't normally included in basic supplement formulas and, if they are, only at insignificant levels. In addition, government regulatory agencies fail to advocate the use of these conditionally essential nutrients in supplemental form because our bodies can manufacture them. However, the body's ability to produce these special compounds can become impaired during times of duress and as we age. The result of these nutrients' depletion is an exponential degradation of biological age that could be avoided if we practiced supplementation.

If the price of supplementation is a concern, think about the loss of income that can result from disease, think about the cost of health care, think about the cost of pharmaceutical drugs, and think about attaching a cost to your health and longevity. The choice is simple: supplement with the proven plan, apply Ageless Performance, and resuscitate your regenerative potential from within.

The deterioration in physical-performance potential experienced as we age, including athletic and immune function, results in part from a decline in the production and availability of many metabolic co-factors that we can supplement, namely, alpha lipoic acid, glutamine, coQ10, and glutathione. Additionally many of these same nutrients may not be absorbed as efficiently from food in a gastrointestinal tract that has experienced the wear and tear of time. The previously mentioned absorption impairment of thiamine in an acid-limited gut is a model for this problem.

Environmental factors create the impairment by first interfering with metabolic efficiency and therefore reducing the fabrication of endogenously produced co-factors such as alpha lipoic acid, coQ10, glutathione, and glutamine. Second, the very chemical imposition of the environmental toxin can propagate free-radical generation, which itself creates higher demands for the aforementioned co-factors. Intercepting this toxicity with precise antioxidant strategy is crucial to the creation and maintenance of health.

CAN OUR FOOD DELIVER?

Nutrients required as raw materials and metabolic facilitators for the production of these co-factors by our cells are scarce in our food today. Even if we choose whole, fresh food sources, current agricultural practices will likely ensure we're getting nourishment that's less dense than the food supply our parents and grandparents enjoyed when they were younger.

The simple fact is that we can't rely on food alone to furnish all the vital nutrients in sufficient quantities that we need, and if we do, we'll likely succumb to the common illnesses of the new millennium: insulin resistance, diabetes, cardiovascular disease, obesity, and chronic inflammation, to name just a few. The very minerals that our lives depend on are scarce in our diets, and this deficiency permeates deeply to create impairment within our cells long before diseases send out full-blown distress signals.

Each of the specialized molecules the body manufactures depends on the availability of minerals that serve as the foundation of human existence. We create many specialized compounds endogenously, or internally, such as glutamine and other amino acids and alpha lipoic acid and other antioxidants, and we deem these building blocks nonessential. However, nonessential nutrition is a figment of our misconception. Our cells *still* rely on minerals and other elements to construct so-called *nonessential* molecules like alpha lipoic acid, glutamine, and other nonessential amino acids. These cell-created molecules consist of building blocks, namely, minerals and other earthly elements, that enter our biological systems with the air we breathe, the water we drink, and the food we eat.

In other words, we're entirely dependent on our environment for fundamental units of life. At this level of thinking essential and nonessential nutrition have different connotations that convey a more profound dependence on whole nourishment and an appreciation for the reason why diseases have reached their current epidemic levels today. Put simply, food processing strips away minerals and other important elements, the molecular building blocks our cells need to produce even these so-called nonessential nutrients. Whole, undenatured nourishment is essential for life; anything less produces a compromised level of being, and supplementation of these so-called nonessential nutrients amid today's limitations is essential.

ALPHA LIPOIC ACID—ESSENTIAL OR NONESSENTIAL?

Alpha lipoic acid can be manufactured by our cells, but the levels produced may be just enough to fulfill the cells' requirements for essential metabolic activity. However, the value of supplementation with alpha lipoic acid to raise levels in excess of endogenous production capacity by hundreds of times has only recently been recognized as critical to the preservation of longevity (13). What's more, alpha lipoic acid delivers powerful antioxidant activity; in fact, in the body it does so in both lipid and aqueous tissues and fluids. This means it acts as a protective antioxidant in both fat- and water-soluble media (14).

Supplementation of alpha lipoic acid also provides potent nitric-oxide regulation that permeates the entire body (15). Furthermore, alpha lipoic acid acts as an anti-tumor agent and has now been shown to perform a central role in the preservation of the mitochondria (16). As the cell's powerhouse or lifeline, the mitochondria serves as a generator to produce fuel for physical, conscious, and subconscious activity. In fact, alpha lipoic acid supplementation can even restore mitochondrial activity that commonly declines in aging tissue (17).

Experts often refer to alpha lipoic acid as the central or universal antioxidant of the body, but the truth is that it's merely one of many that work synergistically. Interest in this central role arises from the fact that it "boosts" or facilitates the potential of other antioxidants such as glutathione and vitamins C and E. Alpha lipoic acid actually helps recycle these antioxidants once they've neutralized a free radical.

I referred to this synergy in the last chapter. Alpha lipoic acid neutralizes or works synergistically with multiples of antioxidants to reactivate their protective potential once it's been spent (18). For this reason alpha lipoic acid acts as a hub for the antioxidant system. However, its biological activity is far more profound and even more versatile than that of an antioxidant.

Although the body is able to manufacture alpha lipoic acid, it's not capable of producing the quantities required to fulfill basic metabolic requirements and ensure extensive antioxidant activity concurrently. As a result, we must rely on dietary alpha lipoic acid to top off the body's yield, but food, as a dietary source exclusively, won't do the trick. Alpha lipoic acid has even been shown to possess insulinlike or insulin-potentiating properties, facilitating clearance of glucose from blood (19, 20). My experience with various diabetic subjects indicates that supplementation of alpha lipoic acid can reduce the need for insulin and similar drugs and in some cases even eliminate the necessity of medications such as metformin. In cases of pre-diabetic insulin resistance, 500 to 600 mg of alpha lipoic acid divided into four to five daily doses can be quite effective for glucose clearance. Especially successful are *divided* doses as high as 1,000 to 1,200 mg taken daily with meals to avoid the onset of temporary hypoglycemia. These heavier amounts are required for both Type I and II diabetics.

Alpha lipoic acid may induce a mild burning in the stomach for some people if consumed on an empty stomach. Start with small single doses of 25 to 50 mg with food and work up to 100 mg and then 200 mg with each meal. However, don't switch from your professional's advocated drug program to alpha lipoic acid if you're contending with diabetes unless your professional is monitoring you.

Supplementation of alpha lipoic acid in conjunction with drugs like metformin and glyburide is frequently recommended to reduce the risk of secondary diseases that diabetes can instigate (21). Alpha lipoic acid has been shown to reduce significantly the danger of lipid peroxidation (damage to fat and membranes) as well as lessen the risk for protein glycosylation (tissue damage associated with unregulated blood sugar). These risks are normally affiliated with pre-diabetic insulin resistance and diabetes, and alpha lipoic acid protects against the catastrophic tissue damage (22, 23).

I become so frustrated and filled with anger when conventional medical practitioners insist on continuing with their pharmaceutical drugs as exclusive therapies for diseases such as Type II or Type I diabetes when complementary therapies could deliver so much more therapy and prevention of secondary disease. The so-called experts simply refute these facts without even investigating the data, for if they reviewed the research they would soon change their minds. In my opinion these shortfalls are irresponsible and highlight the need for each of us to take an active role in our personal health care. Many of these nutraceutical therapies can *reverse* the diabetic condition without the need for ongoing drug use—scientific fact and a matter of proven experience.

My personal supplement program includes 600 to 900 mg daily of R+ alpha lipoic acid, and that's not because I'm battling insulin resistance or diabetes. If alpha lipoic acid supplementation can support insulin's role as well as nitric-oxide regulation, its function in a preventive program is vital. If we look at things another way, anti-aging tactics are essentially aggressive preventive programs. One of the primary goals of the anti-aging program is to instill maximum insulin efficiency and regulate the complex nitric-oxide system. If we get a handle on these two metabolic issues, we're one big step closer to biological age enhancement.

WHY FOCUS ON INSULIN AND INSULINOGENIC POTENTIAL?

Syndrome X is the label Gerald Raven, a Stanford endocrinologist, gave to insulin resistance and its associated diseases. As we require larger volumes of insulin to compensate for insulin resistance, the risk of secondary diseases—cardiovascular illness, obesity, chronic inflammation, immune-system inefficiency, diabetes, respiratory ailments, and cognitive disorders—increases, as well. This is the essence of Syndrome X.

Insulin is crucial for optimal biological function; without it tissues would starve. It facilitates not only glucose absorption into tissues, but also mediates protein uptake by tissues and promotes cellular protein synthesis and much more. Strategic control of insulin secretions by timing and moderating meal consumption and proportions is an important preventive and anti-aging tactic, not to mention an effective weight-management strategy. Ageless Performance is developed in consideration of the timing and nutrient proportions of meals and how this influences hormone cascades in the body.

Food-derived substrates are pushed into storage from the bloodstream by insulin. If just prior to exercise, insulin levels are elevated by the consumption of the wrong food, fatty acids are directed to their storage sites for deposition instead of being available for productive oxidation (ATP energy). This can make weight management an arduous effort. A simple change in the timing and type of food eaten around the exercise program can push the body to work with us and burn fat instead of burning sugar and muscle as priority fuels.

Ageless Performance is designed to maximize insulin efficiency, and optimal insulin function is critical to general biological health.

Obesity is known to increase the risk of insulin resistance, and in a viciously cyclic manner insulin resistance has been shown to facilitate fat accumulation (24, 25, 26). Insulin resistance prompts free-radical generation, while poor insulin function, such as that found in Type II diabetic conditions, can result in extreme serum-glucose highs after meals. Unregulated serum glucose can be highly reactive, giving rise to free radicals, the cause of diabetic neuropathy (nerve damage) and many other secondary diseases. The message is that obesity perpetuates poor insulin function and free-radical stress.

The role of the Ageless Performance antioxidant foundation is protection for the core component of the program, which involves supplementation with highly unstable polyunsaturated fats. The foundation requires that an extensive antioxidant program be applied and mandates that insulin be supported to function optimally so that unregulated serum-glucose levels don't contribute to the free-radical load on the body.

This is where most programs go wrong. Poorly strategized therapeutic and preventive programs may deliver the correct fatty-acid supplementation, but the protective foundation and the factors that escort these fats down the right paths in the cells are missing. Under these limited circumstances fatty-acid supplementation, whether from flaxseed oil, fish oil, or both, can actually wreak havoc in the body and even instigate disease.

Interestingly the oxidative stress that these free radicals produce contributes to the impairment of our natural fat-burning thermogenic system. In other words, free radicals block thermogenesis, contributing to our bulging waistlines, which means antioxidants combat fat accumulation and even facilitate fat loss. To a conventional thinker this sounds absurd, but the scientific facts, as we'll see, bear out these contentions.

WEIGHT MANAGEMENT AND INSULIN

Consumption of carbohydrates prior to physical activity seems at first to be logical, since carbohydrates are known to be an efficient source of energy for the body. However, the type of carbohydrate and the amount of time before activity that it's consumed are important factors, as well.

High-glycemic-index carbohydrates cause glucose levels to rise sharply, and in response the body secretes insulin to help clear the abundant glucose from blood—more glucose, more insulin. The working muscles, though, prefer stored glycogen to fuel muscle contractions before they resort to blood glucose even during states of hyperglycemia (27, 28).

There are studies revealing that ingestion of *dilute* carbohydrate/electrolyte liquids during exercise can lead to performance benefits by way of sparing muscle glycogen for use later on in the activity, but this is *only* so during low-intensity exercise such as weight-training programs that include rest between sets (29). My suggestion, if better body fat management is a goal, is to forget about consuming carbohydrates immediately before or during activity.

It's more logical to ensure that glycogen stores within the muscles and the liver are completely saturated before activity commences. This requires carbohydrate loading far in advance of the exercise session. Carbohydrate or glycogen saturation in relation to physical activity will be discussed later.

The fact is you won't burn fat by eating carbohydrates with a high-glycemic impact before exercise because the insulin spike caused by the dietary carbohydrate impedes fatty-acid oxidation. In addition, if insulin pushes fats and glucose into storage, a pre-workout carbohydrate meal causes the energy required for activity to be unavailable and performance potential is compromised, but the physiological consequences are more profound than compromised performance.

A poorly planned diet might not restore glycogen levels in the body before activity commences. Since glycogen is a primary fuel for activity, when it runs out, the body can feed from metabolically active muscle to energize contractions and produce glucose for the brain amid the glucose low. With a better understanding of these principles, fat loss can be made easy and athletic performance progressive with each training session. Furthermore, the risk of disease isn't increased by the physical depletion caused by exercise if the body is correctly nourished. Lastly you can indulge a little if your desire for a carbohydrate treat is strong but only if you understand the timing principle. Your carbohydrate-loaded treat can be eaten immediately after your exercise session, and in this way it's not as likely to end up on your hips and belly (30).

The primary goal for fat loss must be better health. Most people who embark on weight-loss programs have a temporary vision they wish to achieve, and health is far from the primary objective. Facilitative drugs are accepted as part of the fat-loss program often without contemplation. These fat-busting drugs are required, in most cases, as compensation for poor dietary habits that lead to the suffocation of the fat-incinerating system—thermogenesis.

Allowing insulin function to decline will guarantee fat gain and makes fat loss difficult. Not only does Ageless Performance instill insulin efficiency, it also resuscitates thermogensis. It does so because the carefully proportioned macronutrient profile of the program stimulates the right hormonal cascade. This cascade prevents the overproduction of hormones that block thermogenesis, freeing the body from limitation and allowing it to burn fat independent of exercise. That means you can eliminate fat without having to do physical work!

If you're looking to work off unwanted pounds, the timing of your food intake is critical. Load up with energizing carbohydrates long before physical activity—two hours or so before exercise. If carbohydrates are to be consumed before activity, the food must have a glycemic-index value that's very low, such as that found in oranges, apples, or pears. The better recommendation is to consume a protein drink just before activity instead of carbohydrates, for instance, a whey protein drink mixed in water to eliminate the carbohydrate contribution of the pre-workout snack. Immediately after the workout you should ingest another serving of the protein source, but this time with an additional high-glycemic-index carbohydrate source in the post-workout meal.

This before-and-after strategy delivers powerful anti-catabolic protection that will help preserve lean muscle and promote fat loss. The rest of the day's carbohydrate intake will have to be carefully selected to consist of low-glycemic-index carbohydrate sources. These strategies will be expanded upon later with detailed food selections, but I'd like to impart pieces of the plan as we progress through the book in case you want to begin applying these strategies immediately.

Maintaining as much lean muscle as possible and doing away with unnecessary body fat helps maintain functional insulin activity which, in turn, lowers oxidative stress on the body. I've touched upon glycemic index a few times and you may be wondering what this concept entails, so I'll discuss the subject briefly in the next section of this chapter. For a more detailed look at the glycemic index, see Chapter 12.

READING THE GLYCEMIC INDEX

The glycemic index is a value assigned to food based on its ability to raise blood-sugar levels. A higher value indicates that, upon consumption, the food can cause blood-sugar levels to rise quickly compared to a low-glycemic-index food that would unload sugar into the bloodstream at a slower pace.

Dietary carbohydrates pack fat on your body more than you may know. The glycemic-index value of your meals will have a profound influence on the hormonal cascade triggered by the food and on the metabolism of essential fats as precursors of hormones. Carrots have a relatively high glycemic index of 90, while watermelon has a rating that can be as low as 30 if the fruit isn't too ripe. This means carrots cause blood sugar to rise quickly and insulin to follow the same pattern. Unbelievably table sugar, as sweet as it is, has a lower rating (70) than carrots, and even ice cream is lower, with a value as high as 65 to 80.

The result of snacking on large quantities of high-glycemic-index carrots as opposed to extremely low-glycemic-index watermelons, for example, is that hunger may linger and tempt us soon after consuming the former. If we think back to when we've eaten a large quantity of carrots as a snack, we might recall an overwhelming hunger that came over us not long after. In fact, the type of hunger that can develop after a carrot binge can evoke uncontrollable cravings that may be accompanied by sweating, jitters, and extreme fatigue, symptoms that characterize hypoglycemia. This often leads to another ravenous binge that will likely include calorie-dense food. So that seemingly healthy carrot nibble just might not be the appetite-control or weight-management solution we expect it to be.

Since the carrot snack isn't usually an extended grazing period and more likely to be a quickly consumed snack, the food's sugar content is dumped suddenly into the bloodstream. As this short burst of glucose goes to work, insulin comes to our rescue to normalize sugar levels. Our bodies expect that more glucose will arrive soon and attempt to clear this serum-glucose load as rapidly as possible. In doing so, a brief period of hyperglycemia is followed by an extended period of hypoglycemia.

Allow me to explain these biological developments with relatable symptoms. Immediately following the carrot snack a feeling of well-being and satiety may develop as blood-sugar levels begin to rise. However, if the pancreas isn't quick to respond with insulin secretions, or the insulin receptors of the cells are resistant to the insulin produced (more common as we reach middle age), this freshly delivered blood glucose may not be cleared efficiently from the blood and hyperglycemia can ensue. This is what actually occurs in a pre-diabetic insulin-resistant or Type II diabetic situation.

With Type I diabetes the pancreas doesn't respond sufficiently or at all with insulin production. In the Type II diabetic condition insulin may be secreted, but the receptor sites for insulin and/or the glucose-transport sites on the glucose-recipient cell membranes may not be functional. The result in either case is that glucose levels rise in the blood and wreak free-radical havoc in the body. Glycation, in which proteins are damaged and the tissues these proteins are part of are impaired, is another possible harmful result of this process. Neuropathy, or neuron degradation, is yet another probable consequence of poor sugar tolerance or insulin resistance.

Even with healthy insulin function the high-glycemic-index snack delivers an elevated serum-glucose load to spike plasma insulin and bombard the cells with free radicals. At the other end of this circumstance the clearance of the glucose spike amid insulin impairment can deplete blood sugar to the point where little is left behind for the brain. This blood-sugar low is hypoglycemia, a state the body must prevent or fight to recover from immediately in order to make glucose available to fuel the brain. That's why during a state of hypoglycemia people are driven by uncontrollable cravings that can lead to the consumption of fistful after fistful of food until serum sugar is returned to functional levels.

Low blood-sugar levels induce hunger pangs. The glucose low can also give rise to confusion, erratic behavior, and even emotional outbursts. Perhaps these are symptoms you experience occasionally yourself, or maybe you've seen them in a child who's been diagnosed with attention-deficit hyperactivity disorder (ADHD).

The development of a hypoglycemic condition is more likely to occur during exercise when high-glycemic-index carbohydrates are consumed within the hour immediately prior to exercise. The combination of physical work and insulin flux to the bloodstream clears blood glucose rapidly and can lead to tissue catabolism or breakdown as the body panics to create an energy source—feeding on itself. Understanding these principles will make fat loss easier and will also help to achieve and maintain lean-muscle-mass anabolism, or construction, and minimize tissue catabolism during and after exercise (31, 32, 33). As a consequence, biological age will be preserved at a more youthful stage as we get older chronologically.

If hypoglycemic states are frequent and are allowed to persist, whether during exercise or not, the body will compensate by going into a state of catabolism, using glycogen for energy and even breaking down functional tissues to obtain amino acids from which glucose can be created for the brain. This feeding by the brain on the body results in accelerated biological aging. Ageless Performance is designed to reduce this self-destruction.

It's easy to see how snacking on high-glycemic-index foods can initiate a vicious cycle of sugar highs and lows, free-radical generation, and insulin resistance, along with an increased risk of disease. This serum-sugar roller coaster is representative of the result induced by the average child's eating choices: hamburgers, hot dogs, french fries, pastries, soda pop, juice, potato chips, popcorn, white bread, cookies, cakes, candy bars, crackers, pretzels, dried fruit, pseudo-fruit roll-ups, boxed cereal, rice cakes, in short, a prescription for Ritalin.

A refined, sugary diet has multiple negative influences on the body. Hyperglycemia increases the rate of hepatic-lipid (liver-produced fat) synthesis and raises serum-lipid levels (fat in the blood), multiplying the risk of cardiovascular disease. The elevated blood fat also contributes to the development of diabetes (34, 35). This generates a compounding problem: the exacerbation of insulin resistance and adipose-fat accumulation. How could anyone persist with these destructive habits after being exposed to this information? The problem is that most of us read through these facts and persist with our old habits until we're forced by disease to make changes. Doesn't it make sense, though, to heed the warnings and avoid irreversible heart damage, stroke-induced paralysis, limb amputation, sight impairment, and organ damage due to diabetes?

If you've already developed Type II diabetes, you're not alone. More than two and as many as three million Canadians share your problem, along with more than 17 million Americans. Don't expect your condition to get better unless you address the cause—your lifestyle. Drugs such as metformin and glyburide essentially offset poor lifestyle for most cases of Type II diabetes. Stick with the same dietary habits that caused your impairment, however, and eventually, with or without drugs, you'll live a vastly diminished life. Furthermore, whether you're in a state of good health or not, high-glycemic-index foods will interfere with the bioprocessing of polyunsaturated fats, an influence independent of free-radical induction and one that impedes the production of critical hormones.

Dr. Andrew Weil (in books such as *Eating Well for Optimum Health* and *8 Weeks to Optimum Health*) and other experts highlight the dangers of supplementation with polyunsaturated fats, but this activity isn't dangerous at all. These claims are based on incomplete investigation of the subject. The benefits of polyunsaturated-fat supplementation are incredible if done correctly. Polyunsaturated fats are a problem if they're used incorrectly, and many people supplement them incompletely, giving rise to the problems Weil and others refer to. Ageless Performance, however, involves abundant polyunsaturated-fat supplementation in conjunction with the right co-factors.

A dietary limitation of these fats plays a huge role in the development of new-age diseases. A decision to avoid this delicate supplementation isn't the solution to our shared predicament. The problem isn't the polyunsaturated fat, but the North American diet and the environmental assault that changes how this fat works in the body. The lack of antioxidants in our processed foods leaves these fats unprotected, making them vulnerable to environmental toxicity. The lack of metabolic co-factors such as important vitamins and minerals is another aspect that impedes proper metabolism of these vital fats. The high glycemic value of the diet hinders the proper incorporation of these delicate fats by guiding them down the incorrect biochemical pathway with the wrong hormone cascade. As we've seen, this high glycemic value also promotes free-radical generation, destroying delicate polyunsaturated fats. So polyunsaturated-fat supplementation is far from detrimental. The accurate explanation is that our toxic diets set up conditions that these volatile fats can't tolerate.

The preventive and therapeutic solution is to supplement polyunsaturated fats aggressively but to defend these vulnerable molecules with concurrent antioxidant augmentation and meticulous modulation of their metabolism. This includes the consumption of a low-glycemic-index diet.

The essential polyunsaturated fats, linoleic and alpha linolenic acids from flaxseed oil, have become popular preventive and therapeutic supplements from which few who apply them experience positive results. Other polyunsaturated fats, such as those from marine sources like salmon, mackerel, and tuna oils, are also vital as supplements for the prevention of disease. These fats will eventually become recognized by all medical practitioners as cornerstones of the health-care system, but this realization by mainstream professionals will take time, something none of us can afford. It's up to us to apply the proven program now with our own prescription. However, supplementation with these fats can be a futile attempt to restore cellular balance and biological efficiency if each of the factors they depend on isn't concurrently addressed. It's this exclusive co-dependence of nourishment that's contributed to a misunderstanding about the benefits of many nutrient-based preventive and therapeutic programs. Ageless Performance is the complete and totally effective plan we all need.

DISEASE IS OUR CALL TO ACTION

Disease is a sign that change must be implemented immediately. Most of us fail to recognize the message, which doesn't necessarily mean we have to seek out medical assistance. Disease indicates that the lifestyle we've chosen isn't the right fit for us. Stick with a lifestyle that instigates disease and more problems will develop despite the administration of drug therapy. That's guaranteed. The signs of metabolic disarray arise long before clinical diseases manifest themselves. Unfortunately most people ignore the warnings.

On the other hand, if you're trying to evade disease, heed the subclinical symptoms that always precede it. They're subtle, but those feelings of "something just isn't right" have tremendous value and will help you navigate a healthier course in life. Making positive moves to prevent disease is your most powerful cure.

Step one for prevention is to minimize consumption of high-glycemic-index carbohydrates. Such indiscriminate consumption must be reduced in order to change the odds and turn back the clock. Overcoming disease requires that metabolic efficiency be utmost to facilitate recovery. A low-glycemic-index diet promotes healthier, anti-inflammatory hormone cascades, including insulin, to support recuperation from all types of diseases.

Metformin, which was originally designed for use by diabetics to restore insulin efficiency and alleviate insulin resistance, is one of the common prescription drugs used in anti-aging. This is an indication of how crucial insulin efficiency is to anti-aging, athletic performance, and the prevention of disease. However, the advancement of insulin resistance and any of its associated diseases can be stopped or at least slowed without the need for drugs by choosing healthy eating habits and preventive nutraceuticals.

Ageless Performance focuses on this strategy, applying multiple natural factors that work synergistically to induce extremely powerful additive effects on insulin efficiency and supplying without limitation the gene-promoting activity required to mediate development of the potential stored within us. This program is your much-needed change in lifestyle unless you've already got one like it in place. Ageless Performance is the easiest, least intrusive weight-management system you'll ever apply. Stressing the body into shedding pounds doesn't work; eventually you either give into cravings or your body descends into disease due to the strain.

Ageless Performance works perfectly into exercise, as well. Some experts recommend avoiding eating for an hour or so after exercise to facilitate a longer period of fat-burning. But that isn't a good strategy, since you're more likely to continue burning muscle that's metabolically active, too, with the post-workout fast. The post-workout anabolic-and-repletion potential is lost if nourishment is limited in the hour after exercise (36, 37). By failing to eat carbohydrates and protein immediately after the exercise session, not only is lean tissue lost but glycogen stores aren't as likely to be restored, increasing the risk of disease, reducing performance potential the next time, and enhancing the possibility of muscle catabolism in the subsequent training session.

Research as recent as 2002 has demonstrated the biochemical method by which exercise promotes prolonged fat oxidation, burning fat through thermogenesis long after exercise is terminated. This process can be activated in a variety of ways, but exercise is now identified as an activator of the uncoupling proteins (UCP3) that are responsible for the burning of fat to create heat.

This calorie expenditure is completely independent of the calories burnt during the work of exercise. In other words, exercise requires the consumption of ATP energy to perform the work, which can result in calorie and weight loss. But the activation of UCP3 prompts the thermogenic system to increase the heat intensity of those fat-burning furnaces so you can strip off more fat without lifting a finger for the rest of the day (38). The rise of free fatty acids in the blood, induced by exercise, has been identified as the activator of the thermogenic system.

Here's the catch, though. Research has also demonstrated that the ingestion of a carbohydrate source immediately after exercise stimulates insulin, resulting in the clearance of serum fatty acids and impeding the initiation of thermogenic-activating ucp3. In other words, insulin induction by food, protein or carbohydrate, creates suboptimal post-workout thermogenic activation and suboptimal post-workout fat loss.

So what do you do? To burn more fat I normally don't eat food or the protein-carbohydrate drink until 15 to 30 minutes have passed after the workout is terminated. Instead I consume a branched-chain amino acid (BCAA) supplement immediately after the workout, which consists of a leucine-rich BCAA blend (2 to 4 g). I may also add 3 to 5 g of glutamine (peptides or freeform) to the BCAA strategy. Leucine is shown to stimulate protein synthesis and, therefore, muscle recovery. The other rich supply of BCAA I sometimes use immediately after a workout is a whey protein supplement, although this is likely to prompt insulin secretions that can put out thermogenic fire early.

If fat loss is your primary goal, then wait 30 minutes after exercise to eat your restorative post-workout protein/carbohydrate blend. If fat loss isn't your chief aim and muscle and/or strength enhancement is, consume your restorative protein/carbohydrate blend immediately after exercise. Glutamine supplementation is also known to reduce post-workout cortisol levels to promote anabolism. I usually consume a whey protein drink enhanced with glutamine and some carbohydrates immediately after my workout. These facts are scientifically referenced in the discussions to come.

Ageless Performance is designed to deliver results whatever the goal or ailment, simply because it heightens biological efficiency. The normal potential of the body and mind consists of health, fitness, and longevity— a potential inherent in all of us. Ageless Performance is a foundation that can be applied to combat diseases that are less understood because it empowers our natural restorative abilities, and with a better future window into the nutraceutical-gene relationships, even terminal illnesses of congenital and other origins will be eradicated.

In summary, step one of our prevention program involves dietary control of insulin as described above.

Step two for prevention is supplementation with alpha lipoic acid and chromium. Multi-vitamin/mineral supplements ensure that maximum nutrient density is maintained daily in your meals. In addition, alpha lipoic acid and GTF chromium must be added to the preventive or therapeutic program. Both supplemental alpha lipoic acid and chromium have been shown to support insulin function and even reverse insulin resistance in many cases (39, 40, 41). This mediation of insulin efficiency directs a healthy metabolic momentum. The correct chromium source must be selected, and that's not necessarily chromium picolinate, as we'll see later in this book.

In summary, step two involves nutraceutical support for insulin. Step three, which will be described later, entails a comprehensive fat-supplement program with special biochemical navigation for these fats.

AGGRESSIVE PREVENTION OF INSULIN RESISTANCE

Metformin, a common anti-diabetic drug, causes the body's cells to respond better to its own insulin production. The result is that the pancreas doesn't have to oversecrete insulin to control blood sugar. In any anti-aging program metformin can play a vital role by preventing insulin resistance from advancing at a fast rate with the passing years.

Imagine the cumulative influence insulin resistance can have over time as each meal of the day delivers a degenerative impact. The destructive hormonal cascade that ensues from each meal is further hastened by the consumption of the processed, high-glycemic-index North American diet. This type of diet can sow insulin resistance and then cultivate it.

Many research institutions, including the University of Milan, have run studies to show that metformin can reduce the incidence of insulin-related, or glucose-intolerance-related, diseases such as atherosclerosis, hypercholesterolemia, obesity, and chronic inflammation, even in non-diabetic users of the drug (42, 43). Although we face a natural decline in insulin efficiency as we age, the accelerated deterioration we're experiencing in society today is a result of our sedentary lifestyles and processed diets, not chronological time. The need for metformin administration, whether for diabetic or nondiabetic situations, is most often compensation for these poor lifestyle habits.

The age-related reduction in insulin function isn't due to chronological age. It actually has more to do with biological age and biological health. The studies that indicate the multiple health benefits of metformin administration ultimately shed more light on the fact that insulin resistance contributes to multiple diseases, demonstrating that we do have the ability to lessen the risk of developing today's common epidemics. By eliminating premature insulin resistance, Ageless Performance resets biological age.

The dietary component of Ageless Performance certainly preserves insulin efficiency to slow biological aging, but alpha lipoic acid is another factor that contributes to the same goal, as do GTF chromium, quality high-biological-value protein, curcumin (herbal extract), specific polyunsaturated fatty acids, and many other nutraceuticals. The combined effect of these factors delivers powerful prevention; however, the singular application of the aforementioned measures can limit their benefits and, in some cases, contribute to the onset of disease.

Correction of insulin resistance or diabetes involves the improvement of the diet and the elimination of environment and lifestyle factors that gave rise to the disease. Drugs used to treat Type II diabetes are usually required as compensation for a poor lifestyle. Keep on the same track that caused disease and the underlying festering will continue, even if the symptoms are relieved while on a compensatory drug like metformin.

ALPHA LIPOIC ACID IS A LIFE-SAVER

Alpha lipoic acid has been proven to deliver powerful protection against radiation (44, 45). Experiments using alpha lipoic acid on children exposed to the Chernobyl disaster in Russia revealed incredible recuperative results (46, 47). Is the Chernobyl tragedy something you have to worry about today? Not likely, but this model does serve as a good example of the powerful protection and therapy these antioxidant substances can deliver. The point is that effective health care is initiated by preventive or proactive steps and not the reactive care we're accustomed to applying. The concepts Ageless Performance is built on are preventive in nature. They represent the most powerful, most economical health-care system you can apply.

The administration of alpha lipoic acid as an adjunct to cancer irradiation is an obvious fit, as is its addition to metformin, glyburide, or other anti-diabetic drug applications. This is powerful integrative medicine that's more potent, safer, and more logical than the application of pharmaceuticals only. In fact, the primary objective of health-care professionals *must* be the application of therapies with the least side effects, and then, when absolutely required, they can use treatments that might impose a greater strain on the biological system.

In the case of diabetics, alpha lipoic acid and chromium supplementation would be the first choice of therapy, with the addition of the mineral/metal source vanadyl sulfate or sodium metavanadate as the next stage applied correctly. These vanadium compounds, as we'll see in upcoming chapters, will prove to be one of the most powerful anti-diabetic strategies available—reversing diabetes in a matter of weeks in most cases. Another step might be to use the carbohydrate blocker, phaseolamine. The last measure would be the use of glyburide, a drug that elevates insulin levels, because hyperinsulinemia (high insulin levels in the blood) is toxic. Each of these steps should be additive with each compound enhancing the effects of the other, the ultimate need for the pharmaceutical drug being minimized in dosage by the synergy, and the ultimate level of drug toxicity being minimized to nominal. Logical, isn't it? It's up to you to demand it!

Let's continue building the case for alpha lipoic acid and other antioxidants. As mentioned earlier, peroxynitrite is the dangerous free radical that's been shown to cause DNA damage, atherosclerosis, neurological disorders, and inflammation, including inflammatory bowel disease (48, 49). Alpha lipoic acid is an effective neutralizer of the scalding peroxynitrite (50, 51). In my own case, due to the onset of ulcerative colitis, alpha lipoic acid was a critical therapy and subsequently an important preventive factor in my treatment. Try it yourself in daily totals of 300 mg divided into 100 mg doses with food. Melatonin is also a powerful neutralizer of the dreaded peroxynitrite and therefore a regulator of the inflammatory process (52). Minimizing or eliminating full-blown inflammation as well as subclinical inflammation that slowly ages the body without a sign is crucial to anti-aging and disease prevention. Neutralizing peroxynitrite and preventing its occurrence is a vital anti-inflammatory strategy.

These strategies work best as *preventive* programs, keeping self-perpetuating, destructive free radicals from proliferating out of control. They empower the body, allowing it to maintain the control it was designed to wield. The problem again is that our genetic or biochemical designs weren't formulated to control the level of free-radical imposition our environment bathes us in. Free radicals of many kinds influence the reactive nitric oxide I mentioned earlier, activating it and converting it to peroxynitrite status. Therefore, an incremental nitric-oxide production that's known to occur in some tissues as we age may very well supply the reactive substance from which our environmental free radicals can produce scalding toxicity.

It's necessary to emphasize once more that inadvertent boosting of nitric-oxide levels within the free-radical-laden body isn't safe, but sports-nutrition companies still advocate the practice through oral arginine overload. The individuals likely applying these nitric-oxide boosters are athletes, who are exposed more intensely to oxidative stress to begin with because of their increased metabolic activity. Implement the Ageless Performance foundation, though, and you can boost away with arginine. Only then can you experience performance potential while protecting your body from catabolism.

Ageless Performance is a comprehensive design formulated to place controls on the production of nitric oxide as well as neutralize the exogenous and endogenous sources of free radicals that may interfere with nitric oxide. Alpha lipoic acid is at the center of this regulation, and I'm not referring to 20, 50, or even 75 mg daily. My personal program includes 900 mg of R+ alpha lipoic acid every day. You might want to start with 100 mg and work your way to 300 mg daily by age 50 or 60.

Alpha lipoic acid, sylimarin (milk thistle), and N-acetyl cysteine are now recognized as powerful protectors of the skin from the sun's rays. This protection is far more effective when it's orally administered than when it's applied topically. The point again is that supplementation is the key to longevity, and it's the most powerful health care available. Conditions such as hypertension, cholesterol anomalies, high serum (blood) fat, obesity, loss of lean muscle, insulin resistance and diabetes, and chronic inflammation are biological markers of biological age. The health status of your cardiovascular system, insulin function, inflammatory response, lean-muscle mass, and fat mass can be used to assess your biological age. You can control every one of these metabolic processes and every one of these conditions, in effect taking charge of your biological age. With the application of Ageless Performance, this control will be yours.

Alpha lipoic acid has been shown to decrease levels of fibrinogen and, as a result, reduce the risk of blood-clotting (53). As for energy, antioxidants like alpha lipoic acid are important co-factors for metabolic activity, in particular the production of ATP (54). If you're a competitive athlete, get on alpha lipoic acid or you'll lose out to someone who is. If your health is valuable to you, start the program because the alternative is a multiple-drug-popping adult life riddled with diseases that include cognitive disorders.

As we've seen, ATP is manufactured in the mitochondria of the cell. If demands for ATP increase, as is the case with athletes or less-regular exercisers, oxygen consumption goes up, mitochondrial activity increases, and the danger of free-radical generation intensifies. In particular, reactive oxygen species (ROS), a particular type of free radical, rise out of the oxygen-mitochondrial activity. These free radicals contribute to the degeneration of the mitochondria itself, and this hastens the general deterioration of tissues such as cartilage and neurons. ROS are also implicated in the conversion of nitric oxide into the destructive peroxynitrite radical.

Studies indicate that supplemental coQ10, N-acetyl cysteine, glutathione, and alpha lipoic acid, along with the drug deprenyl, protect the mitochondria from these ROS free radicals, maintaining the energy source for our cells and preventing the age-related acceleration of degeneration (55). Other studies performed with athletes confirm that alpha lipoic acid delivers performance benefits, especially in older athletes who tend to be more vulnerable to these free radicals (56).

Alpha lipoic acid is also derived in our food supply from sources such as red meat. However, to get the levels required for enhanced biological age and athletic activity we'd have to consume pounds of beef, which would have other serious consequences that I'll outline later in this book.

The need for alpha lipoic acid supplementation increases with age. As we get older, we can expect a natural decline in endogenous alpha lipoic acid production and consequently a potential reduction in energy level and tissue protection. In addition, because we tend to lose gastrointestinal efficiency with age, the food source of dietary alpha lipoic acid also becomes less readily available. The age-related deterioration in insulin efficiency can be offset somewhat with regular alpha lipoic acid supplementation.

If you're still not convinced that alpha lipoic acid is a vital health-supportive antioxidant, you'll change your mind as you read on.

6

REVOLUTIONARY SCIENTIFIC DEVELOPMENTS

HOW IT WORKS

Researchers have discovered a new level of biological activity for the free radical, a level as deep as gene expression. As I've mentioned a few times already, free radicals can influence how genetic codes are interpreted and at what rate they operate. Since environmental factors and lifestyle, including diet, have a profound effect on the oxidative status (levels of free radicals) of the body, they also significantly control how and when and to what degree genes are activated. The way we deal with emotional stress also affects genetic expression via the free radicals that stress hormones can produce.

With a simple paradigm shift of the daily events we encounter, however, a situation that can induce emotional duress can be perceived alternatively to result in another emotional outcome, a healthier hormonal cascade, a lower free-radical load and, ultimately, a different influence on genetic codes. We might think we have no control over our daily lives, our jobs, the people we encounter, and the environment we inhabit, but we do. We have total power over how we're transformed emotionally and therefore oxidatively— in short, how this free-radical stress modifies our genes. Change the perception and correct the oxidative outcome. Add antioxidants to the mix and further reduce the negative impact on genes from emotion, diet, and environment.

These recent gene-related free-radical findings add a new dimension to the understanding of emotional and environmental scripting of our cells. Free radicals can mold *how* we are at the level of genetic activity, which means antioxidants can do the same. These are the very genes we might think we're being held prisoner by, the ones that make us fat, the ones that predispose chronic inflammation, diabetes, and other diseases. We might have inherited these codes, but we still have the ability to regulate how, when, or whether they're activated. Antioxidants are the keys to the locks that imprison us, and Ageless Performance provides the precise antioxidant combination of these bindings.

Genetic expression can be significantly modified by nuclear factors that direct the rate of expression. Nuclear factors are biochemicals that are able to penetrate the nuclei of the cells where genetic material is housed. Nuclear-factor-kappa-B (NF-kappa-B) is one of these regulatory protein complexes. NF-kappa-B binds to and actually stimulates various genes to increase their rates of expression. It's been determined that our cells produce more of the complex as we age and that it adheres to more genetic material with ever-greater frequency (1, 2, 3). This simplified depiction of the research is an extremely significant finding that will transform the face of medicine and the pace of our biological clocks.

The genetic material affected seems to be highly associated with immune activity, inflammation, and even carcinogenesis (4, 5, 6). This means that as we get older the genes that control inflammation, the immune response, and the onset of cancer are compelled to function out of their normal operating ranges. We expect that with age immune-system efficiency declines, as does regulation of the inflammatory process. However, that doesn't mean that deterioration occurs with chronological aging. These new findings prove we can appreciably alter the rate of biological aging and break away from the dreadful destinies we've been brainwashed to accept. The research further indicates that we've been on the right track with many of our antioxidant compounds already but that we must fine-tune the applications to make their activity more precise.

The genetic imposition by NF-kappa-B is an important fact that must be kept in mind as we progress through the description of the Ageless Performance program. A major component of the corrective program is designed to block NF-kappa-B's negative influence, for that dreaded complex may very well be one of the more powerful accelerators of biological age and its associated diseases. NF-kappa-B has been linked to the nitric-oxide system, as well, a network we also know to be central to the development of disease and biological aging.

The startling fact is that NF-kappa-B might be one of the programmed "on" switches for the aging process and it might be possible to turn it off in the future. We now realize at least how to slow it down.

The result of NF-kappa-B-accelerated activity is an overactive immune system or autoimmune disorders and amplification or increased frequency of inflammatory activity. These two multifaceted systems, immune activity and inflammation, are intrinsically related. The development of athero-sclerosis is propagated by inflammatory-like activity.

Diseases of cognition such as Alzheimer's and multiple sclerosis are characterized by inflammation of myelin and other tissues. Colitis, Crohn's disease, and other gastrointestinal disorders are inflammatory afflictions that involve uncontrolled immune activity. Allergies are distinguished by overactivity of the immune system and inflammatory process. General subclinical symptoms of aging are typified by inflammation.

If NF-kappa-B is at the center of inflammatory activity, then it can be linked to all of the above diseases. If we can better control inflammatory activity, we can down-regulate the rate of biological aging. The prostaglandin hormones that promote inflammation and cardiovascular disease are the same ones that block thermogenesis, our built-in ability to burn fat, which means they advance obesity, as well. Many of us suffer from a relentless assault by these multiple disorders and rely on multiple drugs for symptomatic relief when the most potent treatment is correction of the common root of the diseases.

The genetic influence of NF-kappa-B causes inflammatory hormones such as prostaglandins and similar hormones (eicosanoids) to be produced at unnatural levels, creating unnatural biological results. Regulating the production and activity of NF-kappa-B will help normalize this eicosanoid hormonal activity to reduce the risk of disease and even reverse it. Imbalanced eicosanoid production is the reason many individuals struggle concurrently with diabetes, cardiovascular disease, obesity, and chronic inflammation. We're not able to eliminate this negative genetic influence completely, but we can restrict it, which suggests we can lessen the intensity of an inflammatory condition and even decrease the incidence of cardiovascular disease. In most cases these conditions can be quite easily reversed. Our recent understanding of these effects has inspired a new era in health care that's changing the way health and fitness are treated. This knowledge has only come about in the past few years and isn't likely to be part of our global mainstream health-care programs for some time to come, but we can begin to apply it now.

Our bodies try hard to take off the extra weight we may be carrying, or they attempt to rectify other biochemical anomalies we struggle with. The body strives for efficiency, so it doesn't have to overwork, and leaner measures play a big role in biological effectiveness. Correcting this common, unnatural acceleration of NF-kappa-B activity is the treatment for multiple diseases, as opposed to alleviating the symptoms of each disease exclusively with multiple drugs. Ageless Performance helps fix this root chemistry to normalize gene activity, and once adjusted the symptom-relieving drugs that might be required to keep someone alive or just tolerate life might not be needed ever again. This is likely to be the case with easy-to-correct diseases such as serum-lipid anomalies (blood fats/cholesterol), hypertension, obesity, and some forms of arthritis.

NF-kappa-B's influence on gene expression is one of the ways age-related diseases are propagated. But there are a myriad of other proteins involved in the regulation of this gene expression. Another is I-kappa-B, a protein complex that binds to the gene modifying NF-kappa-B, preventing its translocation into the nucleus of the cell where the genetic material can be affected (7, 8). In other words, I-kappa-B blocks the negative effects NF-kappa-B imposes.

Glucocorticoids (corticosteroids) are common anti-inflammatories, but their method of activity has only recently been identified. A 2002 article in the *Journal of Leukocyte Biology* indicates that glucocorticoids stimulate the production of cellular I-kappa-B, NF-kappa-B's inhibitor protein (9). A 2001 Danish study reveals that s-adenosyl-methionine (SAMe) has much the same activity as glucocorticoids, promoting I-kappa-B and blocking NF-kappa-B (10). This is one way SAMe induces its anti-inflammatory activity. SAMe is powerful stuff, and it doesn't deliver the sort of side effects corticosteroid therapy does. However, you're not likely to get a chance to use SAMe if you rely on your typical health-care practitioner for treatment advice, because few of these professionals gain any knowledge of SAMe therapy during their studies. You can, however, request that your health-care practitioner look into SAMe as an alternative to corticosteroid administration. If the powerful gluco-corticoid must be applied to penetrate the toxic cesspool that poor diet and lifestyle created for you, so be it; at least you tried a less-invasive strategy first.

Nevertheless, understand that corticosteroid therapy can't rectify the cellular chemistry causing chronic problems such as unforgiving inflammation in that nagging shoulder or knee. In fact, excessive steroid administration will actually further interfere with the chemistry of prostaglandins, the natural hormones involved in inflammatory regulation. A change in lifestyle must be applied if any sort of long-term recovery is to be accomplished, and that includes a dietary alteration. Ageless Performance promotes natural anti-inflammatory activity and long-term recovery. The nutraceutical strategy of the Ageless Performance program is geared toward correction of the NF-kappa-B chemistry, and SAMe can play an important role, especially in the case of severe diseases. I use 200 to 500 mg of SAMe each day as a preventive substance, and as much as 1,000 mg per day can be used without side effects in cases of serious pain and inflammation. Even if corticosteroid therapy is required during SAMe administration for an inflammatory condition, it might not be necessary to use such high steroid dosages, cutting down on potential harmful risks. Since SAMe stimulates NF-kappa-B's antagonist protein, I-kappa-B, to reduce NF-kappa-B's negative influence on genes, SAMe is also easy to appreciate as a powerful anti-aging substance.

NF-kappa-B is able to induce its negative effect on the genetic code *only* if it can get to the DNA, which is shielded in the nucleus of the cell. The nucleus is a highly protective storage compartment for our delicate genetic material. I-kappa-B binds to NF-kappa-B in the cell's cytosol (outside the nucleus in the cell's body), and when tightly bound the dual complex can't enter the nucleus because the former is too large to penetrate the nuclear pore. I-kappa-B is our savior, defending us against the degenerative NF-kappa-B.

FIGURE 6:

The Cell and Its Components in Relation to the Nuclear
Factors That Influence Gene Activity

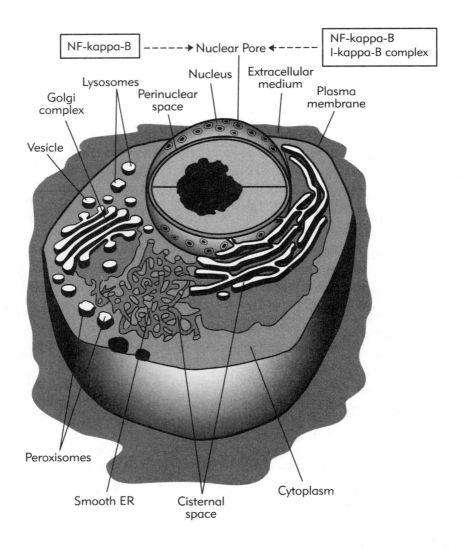

Another recently recognized cytotoxic feature of NF-kappa-B is its stimulatory influence on nitric-oxide production, an overload of which can result in cell toxicity and death (11). SAMe, of course, down-regulates nitric-oxide levels and is a fantastic preventive and therapeutic supplement that detoxifies the liver as well as the chondrocyte (cells involved in the production of cartilage) of the destructive NF-kappa-B and nitric-oxide cloud, allowing these specialized cells to perform according to their genetic programming, in other words, their potential within.

The above research is essential to our perception of genetically instigated disease. The genes involved in this assault are directly linked to eicosanoid-hormone production. An appreciation of this system allows us to understand how profound dietary, environmental, and emotional influences are on our genetic programming, cellular chemistry, and distinct potential within. Eicosanoid hormones take part in what is called the autocrine system, which differs immensely from the endocrine system. Autocrine hormones—prostaglandins, thromboxanes, prostacyclins, leukotrienes—are short-lived but very potent. The epidemics we're facing today with pharmaceutical drugs are closely connected to these autocrine hormones, and it's easy to see how regulating NF-kappa-B activity helps balance this system and maintain biological self-sufficiency. Clearly many of our nutraceuticals—SAMe, antioxidants, and essential fatty acids—fit the preventive and therapeutic program extremely well. Unlike pharmaceuticals that typically compensate for imbalance, these nutraceuticals correct the metabolic disease.

Free radicals and the byproducts of their interaction such as peroxides can impose a biochemical influence on the control factor, I-kappa-B, causing it to disassociate from NF-kappa-B (12). Consequently NF-kappa-B, free of I-kappa-B, can flow freely into the nucleus and contact genetic material to accelerate its expression. Studies demonstrate another vital link between free radicals and disease, between epidemic and lifestyle, between environmental exposure and diet, between emotional duress and disease. Essentially free radicals facilitate gene expression, and overexpression causes disease. Oxidation and its concomitant stress have a compounding degenerative influence, sparking genetic manipulation as well as the nonspecific demolition of vital molecules, cells, and tissues.

ANTIOXIDANTS EVEN THE SCORE

Many people say supplementation isn't natural and that the food we eat furnishes everything we need. Not so. We're faced with unnatural levels of free radicals and chemical poisons. Each day the degree of free-radical toxicity becomes more dire. Our only hope is to increase antioxidant potency to proportional protective levels, and food alone won't cut it.

Protecting our cells from uncontrolled free-radical ricochet will reduce the risks associated with the NF-kappa-B protein complex. Although antioxidants of all sorts are required to initiate complete protection throughout the body, alpha lipoic acid is especially effective because of its size and chemical nature, which allow it to move freely within the body and its cells.

Alpha lipoic acid and its derivatives can deliver antioxidant activity in both fat- and water-soluble mediums, in the blood, within the cell membrane, and inside the cell (13, 14, 15, 16). It can also move right into the nucleus without much obstruction, defending the NF-kappa-B/I-kappa-B complex against free radicals and preventing the protein complex from exerting its influence on genetic codes. However, any old alpha lipoic acid won't work. There are two isomers (molecular mirror images) of this wonderful stuff— the R+ and S forms. Stick to the functional R+-alpha lipoic acid, since S-alpha lipoic acid is said to be physiologically irrelevant. And ensure the form is clearly stated on the labels of products that are used. Most sources are combinations of the two, but make certain you purchase something that mostly consists of the R+ isomer.

Since alpha lipoic acid is a formidable protector of the I-kappa-B/NF-kappa-B protein complex, and SAMe assists the body in generating more I-kappa-B to bind NF-kappa-B, together they constitute a significant anti-inflammatory strategy and help prevent, down-regulate, and even eliminate other diseases. The synergy of alpha lipoic acid's activities—insulin enhancement, multi-medium antioxidant protection, ATP co-factor, gene protector, gene-activity modulator, nitric-oxide regulator, and glutathione booster—amounts to a power-packed preventive molecule that must be considered central to any supplementation program. Alpha lipoic acid is far from just an antioxidant. I rate its supplementation as essential after age 20, while SAMe supplementation is crucial for prevention after age 30.

Various bioflavonoids have protective influences similar to that of alpha lipoic acid. Curcumin, an herbal extract of turmeric, is commonly applied to combat inflammation. As such it's just as potent as many drugs, but its method of activity has remained a mystery for a long time. In 1992, through a company I once owned, I introduced a powerful natural anti-inflammatory product to the Canadian health-food marketplace. It was made up of various ingredients, including turmeric, which in turn consisted of 95% curcuminoids. The complete formulation comprised synergistic components such as bromelain, glutamine, and glucosamine. The results experienced by the application of this product were impressive, and it was awarded an industry prize in 1993. Studies indicate that these ingredients can be extremely powerful, but the variety of products in the industry aren't necessarily manufactured with the same scientific rationale or integrity.

Not soon after the industry award was granted, competitive companies released their versions of this successful formulation, but one knockoff product, in particular, was significantly less expensive, and the feedback our company received indicated why this copycat was so much less expensive. Consumers reported that the product from our company was much more powerful, yet the ingredients and label quantification for our product and the copycat's were similar. I was confident I knew what was wrong; the other company was using a 7% to 9% curcuminoid standard of turmeric instead of a 95% extract. To the untrained, the 95% extract looked and tasted the same as the 7% to 9%, but our more potent version multiplied the cost, and at that time curcuminoids were a lot more expensive than they are today.

Due to my former company's merger in 1997, I was called in to review formulation details of a third-party firm at the production plant and, lo and behold, one of the formulations presented to me was this very curcumin-containing competitive product. The formula production instructions called for turmeric (7% to 9% curcuminoids) while the label claim was turmeric (95% curcuminoids). With fraudulent label claims like that, no wonder people experience unsuccessful anti-inflammatory results! The point is that this sort of thing can happen, so choose brands carefully and don't discount the therapeutic potential of a nutraceutical that's supported by scientific evidence just because of a poor outcome with one untrustworthy brand. I no longer own this company, so my message is free of biased motivation. I simply bring this example up as a caution.

CURCUMIN—
A POWERFUL ANTI-INFLAMMATORY

Curcumin displays strong anti-inflammatory potential in the entire body, and in the near future it will be recognized as one of the vital anti-aging nutrients. It plays a core role in the Ageless Performance program. I've been using extremely high doses of curcumin (turmeric 95% curcuminoids) for various reasons, which you'll see disclosed throughout this book. Curcuminoids, extracted from turmeric, contribute a potent defense of DNA (17, 18, 19). Studies have compared its anti-inflammatory potential and anti-cancer properties against common pharmaceutical therapies to reveal, in some cases, better results and in other cases conclusive synergistic value (20, 21, 22). Have pharmaceutical companies reported on this? *No, they haven't.* The incredible facts rising out of this research reveal that curcumin, unlike a common nonsteroidal anti-inflammatory drug (NSAID), doesn't induce gastrointestinal, liver, and/or kidney toxicity (23).

Having read reports of the potential of curcuminoids to down-regulate cyclo-oxygenase-enzyme activity and eicosanoid-hormone biosynthesis, I was confident some time ago that they regulated gene expression of the enzymes involved in eicosanoid-hormone production, much like the protective NF-kappa-B gene influence of alpha lipoic acid. In this way curcuminoids prevent the overexpression of genes involved in the immune and inflammatory response.

After ongoing, relentless search, I found my answer. Curcumin had been investigated for its ability to suppress the activation of HIV to the status of AIDS. In a 1993 Harvard University study it was demonstrated that curcumin inhibited the expression of a gene in the DNA of the virus. This gene was responsible for turning on HIV to initiate the assault on the body (24). Recently, through this historical work, curcumin has been shown to block the activation of NF-kappa-B. Not only is curcumin a powerful HIV inhibitor, it can be justifiably applied as part of the anti-aging and anti-inflammatory program with scientific proof that it works powerfully alongside or independent of alpha lipoic acid.

Interestingly NF-kappa-B activation/elevation is now recognized for its involvement in the muscle-wasting associated with a sedentary lifestyle (25). This provides a window into the biochemistry/pathology of lean-tissue atrophy by disease as well as disuse. The Ageless Performance strategy maximizes lean-muscle synthesis and lean-muscle retention, and NF-kappa-B down-regulation is central to this goal. As for athletic performance and muscle building, the implications are obvious.

Curcumin also blocks tumor necrosis factor (TNF), revealing more about how it acts positively on inflammation and tissue recovery even from the damage of both rheumatoid and osteoarthritis. It's been documented that curcumin can down-regulate nitric-oxide synthase, the enzyme responsible for nitric-oxide production. And, as we've seen, nitric-oxide overload is disastrous to tissues. In this way, as well, the herbal extract delivers anti-inflammatory activity, reducing peroxynitrite accumulation (26). This nitric-oxide-synthase influence also gives us more evidence of the pharmacology of curcumin in connective-tissue regeneration, joint anti-inflammatory activity, and general biological age improvement, including brain health.

I've used this potent herbal extract as a major component of my recovery program to beat severe ulcerative colitis, and I advocate its use for all kinds of inflammatory conditions. Taken orally and/or topically for skin disease and wounds, it packs a powerful punch without side effects. In fact, if you want to talk about curcumin-related side effects, the very few are actually positive. That is, curcumin is hepatoprotective; it supports thermogenesis and cardiovascular health and delivers general antioxidant activity. In a recent 2001 British study, curcumin was shown to protect and even reverse prostate disease, including cancer, through this NF-kappa-B/nitric-oxide suppression (27).

Therapeutically curcumin is impressive. However, the preventive potential of this herbal extract is another exciting application. Furthermore, because the production and activity of NF-kappa-B accelerates with age, blocking the action of this factor is a powerful anti-aging strategy, as well, and this requires large quantities of curcumin. The gastrointestinal absorption of curcumin seems to be inhibited by food, so turmeric extracts are best taken on an empty stomach. However, people who find the extract difficult to tolerate on an empty stomach can take it with food as an alternative choice.

Supplementation with curcumin, SAMe, and alpha lipoic acid is central to the anti-aging, preventive, therapeutic, and athletic-performance nutraceutical program. Bromelain, too, must be included as part of the strategy, as it's not only synergistic to curcumin uptake but delivers its own independent anti-inflammatory potential, as well.

What sort of doses of these nutraceuticals should you be using? I'd recommend 1,500 to 2,000 mg per day of 95% turmeric/curcumin, 250 to 800 mg per day of alpha lipoic acid (R+), and 1,000 to 2,000 mg per day of bromelain 2,000 GDU. And, if you're ready to steel yourself for the costly SAMe, add about 200 mg of it daily, though as much as 500 mg per day is actually preferred. These totals are to be divided over two or three daily doses, but if you're really zealous and have the time, divide them over four daily doses.

What we know about the NF-kappa-B gene expression takes us deeper into the pathology of our common epidemics. All of this complex biochemical activity crosses into the brain to affect cognition, as well. Alpha lipoic acid supplementation has been shown to preserve brain function and, combined with acetyl l-carnitine and SAMe, the neurological benefits are profound. This dynamic trio, as I call them, has been shown to reverse damage associated with aging such as neuropathy and recall impairment (28, 29, 30). Alpha lipoic acid protects the brain from metal poisoning such as mercury neurotoxicity and defends neurons from glutamate toxicity (31, 32). Prevention of dementia and brain dysfunction with alpha lipoic acid supplementation is more than a possibility; it's a reality.

Keep in mind that the results experienced from the application of Ageless Performance will vary from individual to individual. The rate you experience changes may differ from that of your friend's simply because of the varying degrees of biochemical correction required in each of us and the different lifestyle habits as well as diverse levels of commitment to the program. In order to reverse dysfunctional chemistry that has accumulated over decades of misuse and abuse, the program must be applied for some time with diligence.

THE COMMON LINK

There's much more that links NF-kappa-B to our epidemics. Those genes that NF-kappa-B can accelerate have been connected to the production of an enzyme called cyclo oxygenase or COX (33, 34). COX is the enzyme that catalyzes the production of eicosanoids (the prostaglandin and related hormones responsible for inflammation) from arachidonic acid, the cell-membrane omega-6 fatty acid. Pharmaceutically derived COX inhibitors such as ASA are now commonly employed to block COX activity. The alpha lipoic acid/curcumin/SAMe supplement strategy is designed to correct the problem that calls for COX-inhibitor drugs; in other words, the dynamic trio modifies genetic activity that can overproduce COX and alleviates the need for symptom-relieving drugs.

Studies have unveiled that many herbal medicinals used for thousands of years are effective COX regulators. Green-tea polyphenols, for example, deliver this COX-down-regulating activity, as does reservetrol, an extract from grapes. These specialized herbal extracts or nutraceuticals can be utilized successfully to induce safe anti-inflammatory, anti-tumor, anti-cancer, anti-clotting, and general anti-aging activity (35). Their *most* powerful application today is their use as preventive nutrients to help regulate NF-kappa-B, nitric oxide, COX enzyme activity, and the hormones involved in the regulation of delicate life-support systems.

All of the above information explains the link between free radicals, gene activation for enzyme production, and essential fatty-acid metabolism. The enzymes required for the conversion of essential fatty acids to the powerful autocrine hormones, desaturase enzymes, are also largely impaired by NF-kappa-B and free radicals. Incomplete supplementation involving the common essential fats and other omega-3 oils isn't the answer to our health problems.

WHAT DOES ALL THIS MEAN?

Eicosanoid hormones are derived from a few special fats that have become popular supplements; flaxseed and fish oils deliver these fats.

These eicosanoid autocrine hormones (prostaglandins, thromboxanes, prostacyclins, et cetera) regulate biological processes that include blood pressure, inflammation, blood-clotting, neuron function, lipolysis (fat breakdown), and much more. The polyunsaturated fat, arachidonic acid, is formed from some of these often supplemented fats and then converted by cox (a special cellular enzyme) to yield various autocrine hormones. Again, these eicosanoid hormones are involved in the direction of vital biological processes that, when incorrectly managed by an imbalanced hormone system, contribute to the diseases that are now epidemics. This imbalanced system, which is founded by imbalanced nourishment, makes it next to impossible for the body to recover from basic daily wear and tear, especially when activity is extensive such as in sports.

To reiterate, the basis for Ageless Performance is a supply of the right fats for the production of the right hormones. But the program also helps control the related gene system (cox gene) so that these fats are able to achieve the necessary hormone proportions for a correct, self-regulated response to stimuli.

Insulin plays a huge role in self-regulation of health and disease, and not only of serum sugar. A December 2001 study demonstrates that insulin resistance and diabetes maintain NF-kappa-B activity in the "on" position and, as a result, this state causes an imbalanced flow of nitric oxide and eicosanoid hormones (36). In this manner, insulin resistance and diabetes give rise to associated secondary diseases. Supporting insulin efficiency is one of the ways alpha lipoic acid accomplishes general nitric-oxide control and general biological health.

All of the recent breakthroughs in how antioxidants work have taken us into a new era of athletic-performance enhancement and health care of even the most aggressive diseases. Ewing sarcoma, for example, is one of the most hostile tumors affecting people today, and despite oncological advances the prognosis is poor for the afflicted. A 2002 study published in the *International Journal of Cancer* shows that NF-kappa-B activation is a major player in the tumorigenicity of this vicious killer and that research will now focus intensely on suppression of this intracellular facilitator (37). The point again is that nutraceutical regimens that are part of Ageless Performance can help, at the very least, delay the onset of terminal diseases; reduce the

ROOT BIOCHEMISTRY IN A NUTSHELL

- NF-kappa-B stimulates the expression of genes that are associated with immune activity and inflammation.
- I-kappa-B binds to and essentially deactivates NF-kappa-B to eliminate the risk the gene modifier imposes.
- Our environment has an abundance of free-radical-producing chemicals.
- Our common processed foods and fast-paced lifestyles promote free-radical loads in our bodies.
- Free radicals cause I-kappa-B to separate from NF-kappa-B.
- Once separated, NF-kappa-B is small enough to enter the nucleus and stimulate a corresponding gene.
- As humans, and other biological systems akin to those of humans, age, they tend to produce more NF-kappa-B.
- As humans, and other biological systems akin to those of humans, age, they also tend to become less proficient in the production of intracellular antioxidants and therefore become more vulnerable to free radicals.
- Free radicals induce a greater risk of disease as humans get older, exponentially propagating the aging process, while antioxidants oppose biological aging at various levels.
- Dietary, including supplemental, antioxidants become more important to the preservation of health as we age.
- Curcuminoids can inhibit NF-kappa-B activity.
- Alpha lipoic acid will inhibit the translocation of NF-kappa-B to the nucleus where the genes are located.
- Neutralizing free radicals with a general antioxidant program reduces the risk of NF-kappa-B translocation to the genetic code.
- The gene expression that NF-kappa-B stimulates involves the production and activation of the cyclo-oxygenase (COX) enzyme.
- COX catalyzes the conversion of polyunsaturated fats like arachidonic acid to eicosanoid hormones such as prostaglandins, thromboxanes, etc.
- Prostaglandins, thromboxanes, and other similar eicosanoids have a profound influence on the body—inflammation, blood clots, pain, fever, bronchial-tube constriction, blood-vessel constriction, cancer activation, and more.
- Poor cellular regulation of these eicosanoids results in disorders that lead to the development of today's common epidemics.
- Antioxidants are critical to optimal health, evening out the free-radical score, normalizing hormone activity, reducing the risks of our current epidemics, and helping us heal their ravages.
- Supplementation with antioxidants is one of the keys to Ageless Performance and long-lived health.

intensity of the diseases' progress; aid in recovery as complements to pharmaceuticals; and even function as primary cures. The evidence is irrefutable!

VITAMIN E IS CENTRAL

A complete antioxidant system blocks the chain of interruptive activity free radicals impose on our metabolisms. We either compensate for the unnatural degree of stress or reap the consequences! But don't rely on alpha lipoic acid and curcumin alone. SAMe again is a big part of the preventive strategy, but it can be extremely expensive. Don't forget, however, to weigh the costs associated with illness against the cost of prevention. Nevertheless, you might want to save SAMe for administration when things get out of control if expense is a factor, but keep in mind that this strategy isn't much different than the reactive one we're trying to alter. Vitamin E is also crucial to prevention, and though many people are aware that it provides substantial preventive value, few understand its deep metabolic activity. The vitamin is further recognized for its influence on cellular prostaglandin synthesis (eicosanoid hormones from arachidonic acid, the cell-membrane fatty acid). In some cells and conditions vitamin E facilitates production of eicosanoids, while in others it's inhibitive (38, 39).

With the recent discovery of the NF-kappa-B gene system, perhaps more about vitamin E's precise activity will be unveiled. It's likely to be linked to NF-kappa-B or other systems similar to it, but what's known for sure is that vitamin E plays a significant part in the regulation of inflammatory hormones. In fact, studies as recent as 2000 have concluded that vitamin E supplementation can enhance the COX influence by acetylsalicylic acid or ASA (Aspirin), and that's a truly exciting revelation (40). In other words, the synergistic value of vitamin E with ASA allows for lower doses of the latter required for the prostaglandin/thromboxane inhibition (COX blockage) needed for anti-inflammatory, pro-thermogenic, and anti-clotting applications. This reduces the risk of gastrointestinal damage associated with long-term ASA use, and it may be one of the reasons vitamin E is said to be a hindrance when used in conjunction with ASA—the combination *can* promote extreme thinning of the blood or excessive bleeding times.

Frustration is what I experience when I address these issues with medical professionals. I understand their concern, including the fear of liability, but what I don't comprehend is why integrative medicines aren't considered by most of them. Vitamin E and ASA together represent a *complementary* strategy—nutraceutical and pharmaceutical synergy. A small dose of ASA daily is now known to exhibit powerful antioxidant activity, but the amount required to induce this protective effect is much less than the suggested 80 mg dose per day. High daily doses of ASA are toxic, as I've demonstrated in earlier chapters. Avoiding vitamin E supplementation to make way for higher doses of ASA doesn't make sense. It might make a lot of *cents* for pharmaceutical manufacturers, but for human health care, particularly prevention of cardiovascular disease, it makes more sense to use the pharmaceutical in 20 to 40 mg daily doses in conjunction with a healthy quantity of vitamin E and polyunsaturated fats (the latter also induces platelet-dispersing, anti-clotting properties). Magnesium, a mere mineral that we'll learn more about later in this book, is essential for healthy platelet function, as well, and a nominal deficiency can cause platelet aggregation/blood-clotting. This simple deficiency might be the reason someone needs ongoing ASA therapy in the first place.

Why would anyone choose the gut-busting, liver-toxic megadose ASA alternative after knowing these facts? For safer prevention, supplement with a multi-mineral that includes magnesium, add to the mix a little vitamin E and polyunsaturated fats such as those from salmon-oil supplementation, and throw in a small bite of an 80 mg ASA tablet each day. ASA is a great preventive *supplement*, but only if it's used correctly. The typical 360 mg per day dose isn't a healthy daily application; it's more like a sudden metabolic brake for a chemistry raging out of control. The common 80 mg dose might not be tolerable for all people who administer it on an ongoing basis, either. It, too, is understood to be compensation for metabolic impairment. What I do is take just a quarter to a half of an 80 mg tablet each day (20 to 40 mg of Aspirin), and what I get in return are no side effects and a facilitative, fat-burning, healthy result. However, we must apply Ageless Performance to synergize the positive influence of the smaller ASA dose. If we don't, we'll need megadoses of ASA, but only because our metabolic chemistries need massive correction.

Vitamin E has a major influence on our hormone systems because it protects the integrity of the polyunsaturated fats in our cells. We know that vitamin E is fat-soluble. When the vitamin's status in the body is at healthy levels, it's imbedded in the cell membrane's lipid bilayer (two fatty layers making up the cell membrane), protecting phospholipids (building blocks of the membranes that are made with fats) from free-radical damage, essentially reinforcing membrane integrity (41). This protective activity alone promotes a healthier intracellular and membrane phosphatide and fatty-acid balance, which translates into a better eicosanoid-hormone balance.

Vitamin E supplementation reduces the neuron-membrane-degeneration rate associated with age. Put another way, it slows the pace of age-related brain degradation, and this, too, is connected to phospholipid preservation of brain cells (42). Even if the aforementioned were vitamin E's only role, it would be vital to the balance of the eicosanoid- or autocrine-hormone system and essential to cellular health. Studies show that the main source of polyunsaturated fat for the production of autocrine hormones is the phospholipid of the cell membrane, the building block that vitamin E protects (43).

Hormone balance is a function of many nutritional factors that Ageless Performance is accurately designed to optimize.

CELL-MEMBRANE PHOSPHOLIPID BILAYER

To increase the efficiency of vitamin E as well as reduce its oxidative potential, vitamin C must be supplied in quantities proportional to the former's intake. Alpha lipoic acid, as we've seen, plays a role in this system of co-dependent synergy, as well, and so, too, do selenium and glutathione.

Vitamin E exists in several forms in nature—various tocotrienols and multiple tocopherols. They're all found in different plant oils, with wheat germ oil being one of the densest natural sources and safflower a far second. Vitamin E is also found abundantly in leafy greens.

The *activity* of vitamin E is measured in alpha tocopherol equivalents. Alpha tocopherol is used as a standard to rate other vitamin E sources. However, this doesn't mean the other forms of E that rate many times lower than alpha tocopherol for tocopherol activity aren't as beneficial as alpha tocopherol to the complex human biochemistry.

If we measure the activity of alpha tocopherol on the biological influence that a tocotrienol has, it might not deliver as effectively as the tocotrienol would for its specific biochemical function. Vitamin E doesn't work alone; it requires all of the factors we've been discussing in order to deliver its full potential, and that includes tocotrienols. Natural, undenatured food provides this complementary balance; processing desecrates it. As we've seen, vitamin E depends on selenium, which has been shown to enhance significantly the immunoregulatory properties of the human leukocyte (immune cell) by promoting a more rapid lympocyte response to foreign intruders or antigens (44). Ageless Performance is formulated in consideration of this and many similar synergies and nutrient co-dependencies.

Nature and science aren't necessarily the way we interpret them; they're what they are for reasons we might never know. Because of this, supplements can't replace good eating habits. A diet consisting of whole foods in balanced proportions is critical to optimal health; it's the solid foundation from which our nutraceutical supplementation can work. Ageless Performance incorporates the supplement program into a solid, undenatured dietary foundation. Without the foundation, supplementation has little ground to stand on.

Don't get discouraged about the complexity and vastness of these nutrient relationships. The science sounds convoluted, but it will eventually be boiled down into a simple application that turned my life around from life-threatening disease to Ageless Performance. Remember, this proven formula took me from physical breakdown and near-death to above-average health and championship bodybuilding form. Today Ageless Performance persists as the cornerstone of my prevention strategy, preserving optimal physical and mental function.

VITAMIN A AND CAROTENOIDS

As with vitamin E, there are different types of vitamin A. It's a fat-soluble vitamin, but typically we recognize two categories for this essential: the fat-soluble retinol and retinal and the water-soluble carotenoids of which there are many more than just beta-carotene. In fact, there are more than 600 carotenoids in nature and 10% actually have vitamin E activity. We only know a lot about a handful of these carotenoids. The fat-soluble vitamin A is generally found abundantly in foods of animal origin such as liver, dairy products, and fish. Vivid reds, yellows, and oranges characterize carotenoid-rich plants.

Beta-carotene is converted to retinal by the mucosal cells of the intestines upon being absorbed. Studies show that diabetics experience a reduced ability to metabolize beta-carotene and that vitamin A bioavailability is reduced. This is caused either by the increased oxidative stress induced by the diabetic state, which turns the antioxidant over at a faster rate, or the poor metabolism of the vitamin due to insulin impairment. Supplementation is shown to reverse the deficiency (45). These facts shed light on the possibility that vitamin A deficiency can begin to advance with the onset of insulin resistance long before diagnosis, and this factor alone can propel free-radical proliferation, degeneration, and aging. Since we all face varying degrees of insulin resistance as we get older, regardless of lifestyle, supplementation is a logical preventive solution. Vitamin A deficiency results in LDL cholesterol exposure to free radicals, contributing to the progression of cardiovascular disease that can be reversed or proactively avoided by vitamin A supplementation (46).

Like vitamin E, carotenoids are important protectors of the special fats that make up cell membranes and hormone precursors. In fact, studies reveal an intimate interaction between vitamins E and A at the site of the cell membrane. This interaction is critical for the maintenance of phospholipid and membrane integrity—the very membranes that essentially hold our forms. The synergy of these two fat-solubles has been shown to inhibit general lipid peroxidation and cholesterol oxidation, more evidence that vitamin A is vital for membrane integrity and therefore hormone health. Not only are the fats of these membranes employed as building blocks for autocrine hormones, the membranes incorporate the receptors that endocrine hormones such as insulin, estrogen, testosterone, thyroxine, and others must trigger for healthy activity. Membrane integrity is critical for endocrine activity to ensue with precision, as well.

Some carotenoids display tissue-specific activity. Lycopene, a carotenoid found in red tomatoes, has a more powerful effect than most carotenoids. Lycopene defends against cardiovascular disease and prostate cancer (47, 48, 49); tomatoes, a great source of lycopene, deliver potent cardiovascular protection. However, recent studies have revealed that the tomato's lycopene content is only one component of this protective activity. The yellowish fluid around the seeds of the tomato contain the active protective compounds adenosine and cytidine, which promote anti-thrombin activity (50). In many food preparations this nutrient-loaded fluid is discarded. Whole food holds the complementary keys to good health. Supplement with powerful preventive nutrients like lycopene but not as a replacement for whole foods like tomatoes. Rely on whole foods only, however, and the concentration of key antioxidants required to combat our unnatural concentration of free radicals won't be obtained.

Lutein, another protective carotenoid, has a high affinity for the tissues of the eye (51, 52). The incidence of age-related macular degeneration, or eye disease, can be reduced with lutein supplementation. There's no reason to accept eye disease as a function of chronological age. You can prevent it! Has your health-care professional mentioned these significant preventive and therapeutic nutrients? Likely not, and that's because most medical practitioners haven't been exposed to this scientific research in their education.

Vitamin A also plays an important role in the metabolism of protein (53). With more dietary protein, more vitamin A is required for efficient metabolism and utilization. Athletes who shovel in protein supplementation without considering the rest of their needs are wasting their time and money, not to mention their health. A lack of vitamin A can result in impaired growth, not to mention the well-known fact that this vitamin is essential for optimal eyesight (54, 55, 56, 57). Vitamin A metabolism is also closely linked with coenzyme Q10 (coQ10) metabolism, vitamin D, and squalene biosynthesis (58). Synergy is the key!

coQ10 is a nutrient the body produces in the liver from ubiquitous, or abundant, dietary supplies of ubiquinone. Do we need to consider supplementing with coQ10? Yes, unless you want to bet against your health! coQ10 is an important fat-soluble antioxidant that guards against cardiovascular disease, but it's also required as a backup co-factor for the production of ATP, especially when the body is pushed to extremes (59, 60).

As in the case of alpha lipoic acid, coQ10 production can be impaired with age (61). Also, as with alpha lipoic acid, a lack of coQ10 can, *in part*, cause the limitations in performance potential we may experience in our later years. Heart-muscle performance tends to decline with age, and coQ10 supplementation clearly enhances myocardial aerobic performance when under stress (62).

How much coQ10 do we need daily? Since our bodies are able to manufacture it even if the production capacity is meager, it's not considered essential by government regulatory bodies, so there is no recommended daily intake. As we reach our forties, coQ10 *is* essential as part of a *comprehensive* antioxidant plan, and if you're actively pursuing elite levels of athletic performance, you might not reach your full potential without it (63, 64). I'd say with confidence that coQ10 is ergogenic, especially for older athletes!

Athletes carry higher levels of stored coQ10 than less-active individuals (65, 66). The body will adapt to produce more coQ10 if regular activity is incorporated into the lifestyle. Oral supplementation can also elevate cellular levels of coQ10, but it must be supplied concurrently with complementary antioxidants so that its full potential can be experienced. In fact, without the simultaneous supply of the correct proportions of glutathione, alpha lipoic acid, and vitamin E, supplemental coQ10 can deliver an oxidative (negative) result (67, 68).

coQ10 protects "free-flowing" serum cholesterol from oxidation (69, 70). Understand that serum cholesterol is most harmful or contributory to cardiovascular disease after it's been oxidized. Upon being oxidized, LDL cholesterol becomes the dreaded blood-vessel choker we all fear so much. Before then it doesn't pose the same danger. Therefore, antioxidant protection is just as important as reducing serum LDL levels for optimal cardiovascular health.

Also recognized as an important factor in protecting us from photoaging or skin damage due to ultraviolet irradiation (71), coQ10 has just recently been identified as an obligatory constituent in thermogenesis or fat loss (72). However, coQ10 isn't exactly a fat-loss substance; more to the point, a deficiency of it results in general metabolic impairment, which induces less-efficient thermogenesis—reduced incineration capacity

(73). If you're using statin drugs for cholesterol regulation, coQ10 supplementation is essential as these drugs—pravastatin (Pravachol) and simvastatin (Zocor)—will deplete coQ10 in the heart muscle and bring it to cardiac arrest.

GLUTATHIONE BLASTS THE BAD GUYS

Glutathione is "nonessential"—the body can manufacture it, too. However, if demands are extreme, normal rates of production of glutathione might not be able to fulfill the body's needs, and believe me, you don't want to be caught one molecule short of this antioxidant. Glutathione is found virtually everywhere in the body, displaying a variety of functions: a powerful free-radical scavenger, a neutralizer of carcinogenic compounds, a crucial agent for the immune system, a protector of cell membranes, and a supporter of insulin efficiency.

It's present in high amounts in the liver as a detoxifier, and it's concentrated in lymphocytes and other immune cells responsible for the elimination of invading microbes (74, 75). When the immune system fights off instigators of disease, demands for glutathione increase dramatically, leaving body tissues in a state of competition. A recent study performed by the National Institute of Occupational Safety and Health demonstrated that exposure to diesel exhaust caused inflammation of the delicate lung alveoli, boosting cellular demands for cysteine and glutathione as detoxifiers. Limitations of these antioxidants result in progressive cellular damage, while preestablished saturation of these potent detoxifiers in the cells of the body through supplementation protects the cells from diesel fumes. We're all exposed to these carcinogens daily! An immune system performing at above-average levels requires a greater-than-average supply of glutathione and other antioxidants (76).

Exposing the body to excess free radicals whether from environmental toxins, radiation, or physical activity taxes glutathione stores. Restrict its availability and we're doomed. Again, the more active we are, the more free radicals we produce and the more glutathione we require. Although glutathione displays impressive antioxidant protection, its function is limited to the availability of other synergistic antioxidants and co-factors mentioned earlier—in other words, vitamins E and C, selenium, and alpha lipoic acid.

Glutathione also works alongside vitamin E to protect the fatty bilayers of every cell membrane in the body, and this makes it a vital component of Ageless Performance (77, 78). Oral supplementation with glutathione can raise plasma and cellular levels, but the result is nominal compared to the enhancement a good-quality whey protein isolate can deliver (79, 80).

Cysteine availability seems to be the limiting factor in intracellular glutathione biosynthesis. Whey protein isolates that have been prepared or processed correctly will supply an abundance of active peptides (glutamylcysteine) that contain the important building blocks for glutathione (81). For this reason whey peptide supplements have become advocated therapeutic staples for individuals recovering from surgery, trauma, immune dysfunctions, and extreme physical work, which includes exercise. Not only do these special protein sources contribute the building blocks for glutathione (which is made up of three amino acids—glutamine, or glutamic acid, cysteine, and glycine), they deliver an abundant supply of essential building blocks for general tissue maintenance. Despite the whey/casein controversy, studies comparing casein supplements versus whey supplements show that whey boosts antioxidant capacity of the body *way* better than casein (82). N-acetyl cysteine (NAC) also works closely with alpha lipoic acid to boost cellular glutathione levels and defend our genes from NF-kappa-B's negative influence (83).

NAC is an effective and safe way to drive cysteine intracellularly for glutathione synthesis (84, 85). The supplementation of NAC has become recognized by more conventional medical practitioners as essential in the battle against liver toxicity as well as a powerful anti-rheumatic therapy. (86). In fact, this natural power-packed nutrient is known to be the mightiest hepatodetoxifier, clearing toxicity from the liver induced by man-made chemicals such as acetaminophen (87, 88). That's right, acetaminophen, found in Tylenol, can be extremely toxic to the liver and kidneys, especially if combined with alcohol. Manufacturers of ASA and acetaminophen-containing drugs should take responsible action to include an efficacious, glutathione-boosting dose (100 mg) of NAC in their formulations for your protection. In fact, this inclusion should be mandatory. For now, though, this means we have to take the initiative and supplement NAC in higher doses than average (more than 150 mg per day) when we use acetaminophen or high levels of ASA. However, I can't see how these over-the-counter drugs will be sold without the inclusion of NAC in the near future; not to add NAC is plain ignorance.

Can you guess which nutrient has recently proven to be one of the most powerful boosters of cellular glutathione? Alpha lipoic acid is the answer (89). In a Japanese study in 2001, gingko biloba was also shown to increase cellular glutathione levels (90). If you're looking to create or sustain better health and longevity, build and maintain saturated glutathione status at all costs by employing as many of these complementary boosters. Ageless Performance is designed to develop extraordinary levels of glutathione and ensure this protective state.

PROTEIN SUPPLEMENTS SUPPORT AGELESS PERFORMANCE

As we age, the common problem of reduced gastric secretions and general gastrointestinal wear can cause limited digestion and absorption of protein and amino-acid building blocks. This includes impaired absorption of NAC and other cysteine sources. Cysteine and other sulfur-supplying amino acids like SAMe play a major part in alpha lipoic acid biosynthesis and insulin production by the body (91, 92). We've already touched upon the gastrointestinal pH problem and the related digestive and absorptive impairment of nutrients. Protein malabsorption is another profound result of insufficient gastric acid secretions, and you'll read about others later.

For this reason high-quality protein supplements have been shown to provide tremendous promise as longevity supporters. Protein supplementation is becoming more and more common, and not just for athletes. So mainstream, in fact, that most people who use protein supplements don't even really understand how they enhance good health, only that they do and that they must be part of the daily nutrient intake.

Whey supplements are now acknowledged as important factors in geriatric health for the very reason that geriatrics experience, with high frequency, altered gastrointestinal acidity and whey is assimilated by our cells without requiring significant digestion. Without these building blocks and co-factors, cellular glutathione levels diminish, lean-muscle levels decline more rapidly as we age and, as a result, biological aging advances exponentially. Studies performed on mice comparing casein-based chow with whey-based chow revealed the latter significantly enhanced longevity, possibly due to the measured increase in liver and heart glutathione (93).

Glutathione is vital to chromium's role, which in turn is crucial to insulin's function in the body's chemistry. Therefore, glutathione depletion may also contribute to insulin resistance much like chromium deficiency does, and from this standpoint alone the antioxidant's deficiency promotes biological aging. The highly dependent relationship of alpha lipoic acid, glutathione, chromium, and insulin hasn't yet been clarified conclusively by science, but I'm betting that one explanation for the insulin support that alpha lipoic acid delivers is the intracellular glutathione enhancement it promotes. In this way alpha lipoic acid sustains chromium in its job as an insulin activator. Again the synergy of nutrient supplementation is critical.

If correctly processed, these whey protein supplements don't need significant acid hydrolysis (digestion by acid) and can be absorbed rather effortlessly by the gut to build glutathione levels throughout the body. Another fundamental factor that protein delivers to the health equation is a positive influence on the fatty-acid biochemistry and hormone production discussed earlier. Additionally protein sources high in leucine, such as whey, contribute to anabolism, helping to maintain healthy lean-body mass for all walks of life from the athlete to the sedentary elderly (94, 95).

The hormone cascade that dietary protein initiates combats the negative inflammatory influence that excessive insulin secretions can impose on fat metabolism and eisosanoid-hormone production (such as prostaglandins). High-glycemic-index foods trigger insulin secretions, which accelerate the conversion of essential fats (such as those from flaxseed oil) to eicosanoid hormones that are characteristic of disease, while protein tends to induce the secretion of glucagon, which inhibits this activity (96, 97, 98). In other words, if you supplement with flaxseed oil to deliver hormone precursors (the essential fats) and you haven't considered all of the elements that guide these fats in the cell to balanced hormone status, essential-fat supplementation is futile. The activity of dietary protein includes metabolic guidance for these fats; the result of this guidance is better thermogenic regulation, anti-inflammatory activity, anti-diabetic influence, and cardiovascular protection. But don't start inadvertently shoveling in the protein; it's just one component of Ageless Performance.

The program is intricate and very involved, but you don't have to memorize all of the information we've covered so far. Just know that each facet of the strategy is carefully crafted to play a vital part in the symphony of efficient cellular chemistry. In the end, Ageless Performance in its entirety will be available through summarized instructions. Along the way, I'll present updated summaries of the strategy. The first up-to-date version of these summaries will be presented at the end of this chapter.

The miracle of life comes with the miracle of prevention and therapy built right into our genetic instruction. It's not our duty, nor is it within our capabilities, to manipulate this programming. What we must do, however, is allow this miracle to function according to design, and that requires our active participation. It's up to us to apply these proven strategies; block the unnatural state of toxicity, and deliver the substrates our cells depend on.

BREAKING THE CYCLE

Later on in this book you'll be exposed to groundbreaking research that involves an amazing substance that may be a powerful *cure* for Type II diabetes and a possible adjunctive therapy to insulin administration for Type I diabetics. It's been shown to reduce the quantity of required exogenous insulin for Type Is and to reverse completely the condition of Type II diabetes. The recovered state is maintained in many cases even after oral administration of this special substance is terminated.

This incredible substance may become one of the more popular insulin enhancers in the near future as the battle against insulin resistance or Syndrome X escalates out of control. Synthetically derived metformin, a common diabetic drug, is a fantastic insulin enhancer, but it can't reverse the anomaly that causes insulin resistance or diabetes.

Dependence on metformin is indefinite for the majority who resort to applying this strategy alone. Metformin is compensation to lean on much as a crutch is for a broken leg. The formidable substance you'll read about in Chapter 8 is different. It's been shown to be corrective. As soon as more trials are done with humans, I'm confident this substance will be the insulin-efficiency restorer of choice, and yes, you do have a *choice* in the matter of your health.

Even with the administration of this possible cure for diabetes, however, the habits and impositions that contributed to the development of diabetes and the rest of our mushrooming epidemics must be removed from the equation for a recovered state to be maintained. Without this change the factors that created the first round of disease will slowly reverse the correction this special substance can induce.

A change in diet alone can reverse many instances of Type II diabetes. In the case of extremely advanced states of disease the administration of Ageless Performance on its own might not be enough to prime the system toward expeditious recovery. In these cases a little more augmentation, a sturdier crutch to lean on, might be required to get things rolling in the right direction. That might involve buttressing insulin's role with metformin or orthomolecular levels (extremely high levels exceeding even those that are preventive) of alpha lipoic acid, chromium, or other specialty ingredients I've referred to but not yet specified.

With this support, *with this crutch*, your body will be better able to utilize the essentials required to rescue your cells from imbalance and distress. The special substance I'll introduce you to soon must be used in this way—as a primer for proper insulin function and general metabolic health. But the main objective of therapy must always be recovery and recuperation, not mere compensation.

If you broke a leg, for example, and required a crutch, your aim would be to heal to the point where the crutch was no longer needed. If your dietary habits were sound and rest time sufficient, healing would be whole so that you could run, hop, skip, and jump as you did before your injury. If your recovery program was less than optimal, you might have to limp along, functioning at less than your maximum potential. You might have to rely on that crutch for the rest of your life.

As a consequence of this impediment, secondary problems would inevitably arise. Your hips would develop imbalance and joint disease. Your good leg would wear faster, and an accelerated rate of degeneration would set in throughout your body due to lack of physical activity. Your spine would incur a newly developed stress. Your neck and back muscles would strain, bringing you more discomfort and pain. The pressures of pain and discomfort would result in hormone imbalances and stress-hormone secretions, more free radicals, increased oxidative stress, and greater general biological damage. Drugs such as metformin, prednisone, NSAIDs, antibiotics, and antidepressants are themselves crutches to lean on until the body has had the opportunity to recover and proceed normally. Rely on them indefinitely and secondary metabolic strains—diseases—are sure to arise.

We've learned to accept long-term pharmaceutical drug use as a coping mechanism for disease, which means we've surrendered to the inevitability of secondary diseases. However, the goal must be recovery and the role of pharmaceuticals has to be temporary. A prolonged battle against disease establishes a state of metabolic imbalance of extreme proportion; the recovery period for such conditions if employing nutraceutical strategies might take as much as six months or more. In fact, if metabolic disarray is severe, it could take longer than a year. Patience and perseverance will serve well.

If corrective strategies are applied, eventually insulin support from the pharmaceutical drugs can be alleviated and orthomolecular levels of nutraceuticals reduced to typical preventive levels, just as a healed leg would eventually not need a crutch any longer. Again, in order to get off the crutch, you have to get off the drugs! You can't get off the drugs unless you promote healing with natural chemistry. Your diet and supplementation must provide the right quality and quantity of building blocks and hormone precursors and facilitators that support recovery and correction. The result of this approach is biological self-sufficiency, the potential within we were all born with.

Could you imagine running a marathon with a broken leg and then not being able to understand why it's more broken than before the event? No, not likely. The situation is no different when you've developed insulin resistance or diabetes and you place stress on your body with sustenance that it can't tolerate such as refined, processed, high-glycemic-index foods—the typical North American diet.

Can you eat cake, candy, white pasta, processed bread, raisins, and pastries frequently and abundantly while battling diabetes? No, of course you can't. These are the high-glycemic-index foods that strain an already struggling system—the foods that caused the original problem. If you do indulge in these foods and are battling diabetes, the outcome is disease with greater severity, just as a marathon could pulverize to an unrecoverable state a previously broken leg. However, the pounding the body takes from the inside isn't apparent the way the damage a leg receives from a marathon run is. It's up to you to recognize the subtle signs that come from within and change the course you're on so that you're moving along a healthier path.

Rest in the case of diabetes, insulin resistance, cardiovascular illness, and inflammatory disease requires that the compromised biochemical system be released from its strain. The stress is caused by poor diet and lifestyle, which includes emotional, mental, and physical activity. Persisting with a poor diet just because you can lean on a crutch like metformin (in the case of diabetes) only makes the disease worse in the end. The underlying festering that's been allowed to accumulate will surface as a worse case of the primary condition or as other diseases. That's inevitable.

It won't be long before irreversible damage results and the need for amputation develops. But how do you amputate the immune system or the insulin/glucagon axis? You can't, and don't think that more drugs are the answer to this advanced problem, either, because they're merely the solution for the suspension of death.

Allow me to highlight a common problem. As diabetes progresses beyond the help metformin can deliver, glyburide is often prescribed as an additional or alternative drug. Metformin enhances the response of cells to insulin, but if a Type II diabetic state is severe, the drug can't stimulate the cellular response enough and more insulin must be secreted by the pancreas as compensation to clear glucose from the blood. This is precisely what glyburide does. It instructs the pancreas to pump out more insulin to bombard those desensitized cells. However, hyperinsulinemia (high blood insulin) is a problem; it contributes to the propagation of disease, as well. Insulin-responsive cells will also eventually resist this higher dose of endogenously produced insulin, and one day it might become necessary to inject an exogenous insulin source to force the cells to take up blood sugar, provided the subject survives the glyburide-metformin combo. More insulin propagates more disease as high insulin levels distort eicosanoid and other hormone systems.

I'm continually frustrated by the fact that alternatives can be used long before glyburide is applied. If these alternative strategies work, this excessive flow of insulin might not be required and the body will be spared damage. Doctors can try using the drugs miglitol and acarbose in conjunction with metformin instead of glyburide. These drugs block or slow intestinal digestion and absorption of dietary sugar to reduce the glycemic impact of a meal and decrease dependence on insulin.

A natural bean extract called phaseolamine that impedes the digestive enzyme amylase, reducing dietary sugar digestion, absorption, glycemic impact, and insulin requirement, can also be employed. Phaseolamine is a common ingredient in health-food industry "carbohydrate-cheater" products that are designed to allow the consumption of carbohydrates without the same insulinogenic impact (99). Green-tea extract also obstructs salivary amylase, an enzyme responsible for carbohydrate digestion (100). Black and green tea are great accompaniments to any meal.

Why the concern about glyburide? Long-term studies have finally confirmed that the combined treatment of metformin with glyburide increases mortality rates (101, 102). But those plagued by a diabetic condition can choose to be in control and nutraceuticals can play a huge role in possibly reversing diabetes completely.

I've seen many people eat the wrong foods while battling diabetes. They say, "Oh, the doctor said I can tolerate some of this cake since I absolutely can't live without it, but I can do so only if I time my medication correctly." That's insanity! You can live without cake. In fact, you'll die because of it!

This cake-eating diabetic is no different from someone wanting to run a marathon with a broken leg and relying on a crutch to carry him along. He might make the journey, but not without secondary damage and not without the danger of amputation.

Yet with the proper program it might not be long before a disorder such as Type II diabetes is completely healed. Once efficiency is instilled, those afflicted with the disease can go back to an occasional treat because their bodies will tolerate the strain but not before their metabolisms have reached a state of self-sufficiency.

Ageless Performance is a facilitator of maximum potential and optimal biological performance that drives elite-level immune function, saturation of antioxidant systems, efficient neural function, undisturbed hormone communication, and superior cellular operations. Most of us accept a general decline in our ability to enjoy life as we age. It doesn't have to be that way, though. We can enjoy life to its fullest until our last days. Ageless Performance will make that possible.

⚖️

Before moving on to the next chapter, you'll find a summary chart of what you've learned so far. If the strategies outlined on the next page are applied, your body will be prepared with a protective biological foundation. With this foundation in place you'll be ready for your subsequent introduction to polyunsaturated-fat and mineral supplementation, the central components of the program.

The relatively aggressive *preventive* doses in the following chapter are for most individuals and can be used for *therapy*. For more expeditious therapeutic results, however, the levels of some nutraceuticals may be increased to intensify the genetic influence on the body and promote a healthier outcome faster. These intensified levels of nutraceuticals will exceed those listed in the chart on the next page and will be discussed in "Getting with the Program," the last section of this book. In addition to these enhanced programs, adjunctive ingredients conducive to highly specific therapy will be discussed in the final chapter, "Condition-Specific Therapies."

You can start right away on Ageless Performance with what you know now and apply adjunctive components as you proceed through this book. With every addition your health and athletic potential will improve beyond your wildest dreams as you extract more and more of the miracle that's waiting to surface.

To your health!

Prioritized Summary Table for the Ageless Performance Program

Priority #1: Instill or ensure insulin efficiency

	All Ages	Age 5 yrs+	Age 12 yrs+	Age 18 yrs+	Age 25 yrs+	Age 30 yrs+	Age 40 yrs+	Age 50 yrs+	Age 60 yrs+
Minimize consumption of processed food in the diet.	✓	✓	✓	✓	✓	✓	✓	✓	✓
Consume whole fresh foods as much as possible.	✓	✓	✓	✓	✓	✓	✓	✓	✓
Consume quality complete protein with every meal. (See Appendix C for the list of preferred protein sources.)	✓	✓	✓	✓	✓	✓	✓	✓	✓
Consume carbohydrate sources that rate below 55 on the glycemic-index scale. (See Appendix A for the glycemic-index table.) Higher glycemic-index meals/foods are allowed after activity/exercise only.	✓	✓	✓	✓	✓	✓	✓	✓	✓
Supplement every day with a quality multi-dosed multiple vitamin/mineral formulation to set a foundation for nutrient density of nourishment. (See Appendix B for guidelines for choosing a multiple.)	children's formula	children's formula	✓	✓	✓	✓	✓	✓	✓
Supplement with additional vitamin C to reach these maximums.			✓ Max per day 250 mg	✓ Max per day 750 mg	✓ Max per day 3,000 mg	✓ Max per day 4,000 mg	✓ Max per day 4,000 mg	✓ Max per day 4,000 mg	✓ Max per day 4,000 mg
Supplement with additional alpha lipoic acid (R+) to reach these maximums.				✓ Max per day 100 mg	✓ Max per day 100 mg	✓ Max per day 150 mg	✓ Max per day 150 mg	✓ Max per day 250 mg	✓ Max per day 300 mg
Supplement with additional curcumin—turmeric (standardized to 95% curcuminoids).					✓ Max per day 350 mg	✓ Max per day 550 mg	✓ Max per day 1,000 mg	✓ Max per day 2,000 mg	✓ Max per day 2,000 mg
Supplement with additional GTF chromium.				✓ Max per day 100 mg	✓ Max per day 200 mg	✓ Max per day 500 mg	✓ Max per day 500 mg	✓ Max per day 600 mg	✓ Max per day 600 mg

7

MINERALS: STITCHES IN THE BIOLOGICAL FABRIC

MINERALS VIBRATE WITH LIFE

Our bodies are essentially atomic entities, embodiments of earthly minerals. We can't complement or be part of the cosmic order if the universal design isn't allowed to materialize. The human and other biological designs of the *animate* kingdom require a complete array of minerals without limitation. The demand for all nutrients, including minerals, increases significantly when assailed by the chemical scalding our environmental toxicity imposes.

If we can't meet today's higher demand for minerals, we'll be as vulnerable as the perforated sail of a sailboat in a windstorm; we'll seem to move at a progressive pace in life but at a rate that's far short of our potential. Like the sail pummeled by roaring gusts, the living material that embodies our essences will rip at our points of vulnerability when a storm hits. Ageless Performance is designed to knit an impermeable fabric that can withstand bad weather and propel us forward through life's exigencies. An adequate supply of minerals is crucial to the Ageless Performance program, and whole foods alone won't meet the need if self-sufficient health is the goal.

The prevalence of insulin-related disease today is a global concern. The reason for this worldwide impact is the adoption of processed foods that are stripped of important fibers, phyto-antioxidants, special fats, vitamins and, of course, minerals. Today diabetes, inflammation, and obesity are prevalent among the young, and mineral deficiencies and imbalances play a huge role in this pathology. Minerals or elements are the foundation of all matter; they make up every molecule, every essential or nonessential nutrient in the body. A deficiency of just one interrupts life.

MEET THE MACROMINERALS

Studies show that excess dietary sodium chloride, or table salt, can cause hypertension, but equimolar (sodium equivalent) amounts of sodium citrate, sodium bicarbonate, and sodium phosphate induce no change in blood pressure (1, 2). Is chloride the culprit? It's possible, but you'll see in a moment that the issue involves much more than just one mineral.

One thing we do know is that dietary sodium has an influence on calcium status in the body. Excess dietary sodium increases calcium excretion, and calcium *deficiency* has also been linked to hypertension (3, 4). Studies demonstrate that communities drinking sources of hard water (calcium- and magnesium-rich water) have lower incidences of cardiovascular and associated diseases than those consuming soft water (less calcium and magnesium in relation to hard water). This represents a clear example of environmentally linked epidemics that aren't at all connected to a toxicant (5, 6, 7).

Highly processed foods tend to be depleted of these health-supportive minerals, but to compound the problem these same foods are typically loaded with added sodium from sodium chloride, sodium benzoate, and sodium bicarbonate to enhance palatability as well as shelf life. The natural balance of the altered food is thrown offline by this *man*ipulation, and the biochemical balance within our bodies becomes a direct reflection of this alteration.

If you're like most North Americans, this processed diet and the sedentary lifestyle that often goes with it probably seeded and cultivated disease. And if disease hasn't struck you yet, it might not be too long before it does. The pharmaceutical industry profits as few industries can in today's compromised global market, and it's at your expense and with your complicity. Calcium channel blocker drugs such as Procardia have become popular new-age pharmaceuticals that may only be required to battle the epidemic proportions of high blood pressure because of our global malnutrition—the sort of malnutrition that rises out of mineral imbalances. These calcium channel blocker drugs are a new wave of anti-hypertensive medications designed, as the drug companies might say, to work better than common diuretics to combat high blood pressure.

Let me emphasize, however, that diuretics work well for most people as blood-pressure-reducing agents when required. The mad dash by pharmaceutical companies to produce new, patentable, and *more expensive* drugs has given rise to this new fashion—anti-hypertensive drugs the manufacturers market with millions of dollars as the latest and greatest. Millions of unsuspecting, naive health-care professionals buy into the claims to sell these heart busters to us on an experimental basis.

That's right. These new drugs may deliver nominal anti-hypertensive activity, but they also increase the risk of heart failure due to their capacity to interrupt calcium activity in almost every cell of the body, in particular the cells of the heart and central nervous and respiratory systems where calcium balance is critical. Such drugs are also known to influence the intestinal cells significantly. You've likely never heard about this negative effect and you'd be surprised to hear that your health-care professional may have very well placed the same blind trust in the pharmaceutical company that designed the profit-generating product. The irony of this specific model is that anti-hypertensive drugs are supposed to diminish myocardial strain and the risk of heart failure, which hypertension increases, but these new drugs can make things worse (8, 9). Typical diuretics deliver results without the same danger, but the saddest fact of all is that the problem in most people's cases is a sedentary lifestyle coupled with a processed diet, and drugs aren't at all required to alleviate the condition if the correct lifestyle and nutraceutical strategies are applied.

The processed diet is stripped of most minerals essential to metabolic health, potassium included, and potassium status influences biological calcium condition significantly, as well. Calcium deficiency will lead to metabolic havoc that permeates beyond cardiovascular disorder if, and only if, the body can survive, limping through the impairment. Osteoporosis and hypertension, for example, develop after metabolic havoc has festered for a long time, but they're merely symptoms of the pervasive disarray.

Potassium supplementation is known to *oppose* hypertension (10, 11). The intake of potassium has a tremendous influence on calcium status by decreasing the rate of excretion to the point where it reduces the recurrence of calcium oxalate (urinary-tract stones) crystallization in the urinary tract (12, 13). In essence, potassium fights the negative effects of sodium on calcium status, and if you're physically active, particularly if you indulge in endurance training, you should know that exercise also boosts the rate of calcium excretion. Potassium supplementation, specifically with potassium citrate, defends against urinary-stone development even in postmenopausal women who tend to be predisposed to excessive calcium loss (14). In my opinion, citrate (citric acid) as much as potassium is the anti-calcium oxalate factor. It inhibits urinary-stone development, since it tends to lower the pH of urinary-tract contents, which in turn increases the solubility of urinary calcium, reducing the crystallization potential to help dissolve existing stones and prevent new ones.

Why all of these seemingly unrelated examples of natural prevention? The point is quite relative: healthy lifestyle, healthy diet, and nutraceutical supplementation constitute a formidable preventive strategy that outperforms our accepted reactive health-care protocols. Prevention is the key to powerful health care. You're the administrator of prevention; you're in complete control of your health.

As much as each mineral is recognized for its distinct function or requirement by a unique system of the body, minerals display a great deal of interaction, co-dependence, and synergy. These interactions occur at various levels in the body from absorption, transport, and incorporation into tissues and enzymes, as well as simultaneous independent activity on a common system.

The case of bone mineralization is a well-known example of this multi-mineral requirement. Most people understand that the bone matrix consists of a myriad of minerals, but the influence of multiple minerals on hypertension isn't so commonly comprehended. Magnesium profoundly affects cellular potassium and calcium status, as well. The supplementation of magnesium promotes relaxation of smooth muscles to help *reduce* hypertension (15). The point again is synergy and complementary function—supplementation with magnesium, potassium, and calcium together with a sodium-limited diet can reverse hypertension and maintain healthy blood pressure without the need for drugs. It's that simple! It's your choice to use drugs to combat a nutrient imbalance, and it's just as easy to choose the more logical solution—nutrient-dense, whole food and supplementation.

Is a daily multi-vitamin/mineral supplement essential today? I'm betting on it. If you're an athlete, healthy potassium, calcium, and magnesium status are even more difficult to maintain. Supplementation is important and for much more than prevention of cardiovascular risks. Furthermore, high-sodium diets, like those that include processed and preserved foods, will result in an imbalance. In fact, excessive sodium intake has an ergolytic (performance-impeding) rather than ergogenic (performance-enhancing) effect, decreasing pulmonary efficiency, especially in the case of endurance sports (16).

MINERALS CATALYZE LIFE AT ALL LEVELS

Calcium is most usually associated with bone health, but it has many other notable roles in the body, which in essence accounts for its limited availability for bone maintenance when inadequate dietary supply persists for prolonged periods. Critical to the clotting process, enzyme regulation, and cell-membrane integrity, calcium, like sodium and potassium, is also an important factor in muscle contraction and nerve-impulse generation and propagation.

Cyclic AMP (cAMP) is a molecule that relays the hormone's message from the exterior to the interior of the cell through the membrane. cAMP is a secondary messenger whose function is dependent on cellular calcium availability (17). Studies as recent as 2002 confirm our historical notion that cAMP is highly dependent on calcium for maximum activity and that calcium itself is a secondary messenger inside the cell acting like a delegate, so to speak, from the cell surface inward for some of our regulating hormones. Limit calcium availability and hormone activity is impaired.

Oddly enough, our first line of therapeutic action in these cases is to bombard the cell with high levels of hormones from exogenous (oral or injectable) sources before ever determining whether this mineral limitation is the cause of hormone insensitivity. These are uninformed, drastic measures, especially when the diets of the majority of North Americans are calcium-deficient, which makes hormone dysfunction common, mineral deficiency the most likely cause, and supplementation the more reasonable solution.

Hormones, neurotransmitters, prostaglandins, and other communicators transmit their influence to target cells by stimulating production of intracellular cAMP and the influx of calcium, usually concurrently. Calcium is critical to hormone communication and vital to general biological harmony. In order to maintain cell life, tissues that aren't directly involved in critical life support, such as bone, will sacrifice calcium if dietary calcium is in short supply. A diminished calcium status in the cells of the heart or liver, say, is quickly compensated for by bone resorption—calcium extraction from bone. Osteoporosis, then, is more a symptom of a deeper problem than the disease we think.

Ginseng has been shown to induce its adaptogenic or biological-regulating influence through cellular calcium regulation. In a 2002 in vitro study a particular gensenoside (active constituent of ginseng) was found to modulate the activity of calcium channels in neurons (18). Ginseng helps convey the correct hormone message in the right proportion from the outside of the cell to its interior. Furthermore, this facilitation of calcium influx promotes cellular resensitization, causing cells to function according to design and at more youthful levels.

Coleus forskohlii is another common herbal application used to boost cell responsiveness to hormones. It primes cells by inducing cAMP production inside them, initiating the appropriate cellular response to hormones more expeditiously. Recent studies also show that forskolin, the active compound of coleus forskohlii, induces nitric-oxide production (19).

Biological aging results in the "numbing" of cells to the stimulus of communication molecules such as endocrine hormones and the autocrine's prostaglandins, thromboxanes, and other eicosanoid hormones produced from our essential fats. The result of this resistance is obvious: cells don't function in synchronicity and the body may compensate by raising secretions of communication molecules, leading to possible health risks.

General metabolic inefficiency develops because of this cellular sluggishness and perpetuates a series of problems that experts believe can contribute to poor weight management, slow immune reactivity, and more. A lack of energy and strength are often consequences of this metabolic lethargy. These energy deficiencies represent subtle signals we can heed if we're perceptive about our internalized messages. If we're receptive to the signs our bodies give us, we can make changes in our diets and lifestyles before diseases are pronounced.

Calcium deficits are a likely underlying cause for these hard-to-detect symptoms, and the resulting bone resorption usually goes unnoticed until a fracture sheds light on the problem. Coleus forskohlii administration may prove successful in priming cAMP, regulating nitric oxide, and enhancing cellular response to our bodies' communication systems. In other words, this herb can improve biological efficiency, strength, and energy.

However, raising efficiency in this way doesn't change cAMP's dependency on calcium. In fact, if the rate of cAMP production increases, so does the requirement for calcium. If cellular desensitization is caused by limitations of calcium, whether by poor diet or inadequate gastrointestinal absorption of the mineral, the result of this priming by coleus forskohlii is an accelerated resorption of bone minerals as calcium is used up in cells to support cAMP and other cell activities.

Herbs like coleus forskohlii and ginseng can only elicit long-term benefits if a functional nutritional foundation is in place. Our cells can't perform without adequate calcium, and so our bodies will always fulfill this primary requirement to keep us alive even at the expense of bone mass.

Caffeine has an effect similar to coleus in that the former blocks an enzyme called phosphodiesterase. Phosphodiesterase enzymes have various functions in the cells, one of which is to "chomp" on cAMP, reducing the "excited" status of the cell. Caffeine interferes with phosphodiesterase activity and raises the cellular response rate and intensity to signals (20). With higher cAMP levels, cells respond more quickly to hormone and other signals characterized by the hypersensitization caffeine promotes. Calcium is vital to this process, which means chronic caffeine use or abuse can result in the depletion of this valuable mineral.

Colon cancer, too, is associated with inadequate dietary calcium (21, 22). Excess dietary sodium, poor dietary protein *quality*, and abundant caffeine consumption can inhibit calcium absorption and status and indirectly magnify the risk of cancer. Supplementation with calcium will thwart this danger as will the elimination of the factors inhibiting positive calcium status in the body.

Caffeine has a compounding negative influence on biological calcium status. It promotes urinary excretion of calcium and induces its expulsion from the intestinal tract, resulting in fecal loss of the mineral. Moderate alcohol consumption further exacerbates poor calcium status as well as magnesium excretion (23). An individual consuming alcohol and caffeine abundantly, relying on the typical processed, mineral-stripped, sodium-enriched diet, is at tremendous risk for calcium deficiency and its associated physical fallout. Again, osteoporosis is only one of the clinical risks. The underlying mess that occurs concurrently festers until other metabolic disasters are developed.

Studies today show that calcium status in the cells may also play a significant role in the synthesis of glucose-transport proteins, with calcium deficiencies resulting in impaired serum-glucose regulation (24). This relates or even contributes to the onset of insulin resistance and diabetes.

The bone-density-status relationship of dietary calcium can serve as a model to describe the development of disease from the dietary shortfall of any essential nutrient. The biological manifestation of disease as a consequence of deficiency isn't a sudden occurrence that arrives without warning. The calcium model conveys the body's extreme level of tolerance to depletion; the fact that one system is robbed to maintain an immediate need is a message we all must heed.

The debt must eventually be paid back, even though, on the surface, health seems apparent. Similarly a diet consisting of limited or incomplete protein can sustain a healthy metabolism, as well, but at the expense of systems that have less-immediate requirements. If the liability isn't paid back to the body, the robbed systems suffer until they can steal from one another. Persist with the dietary limitation and levels of intolerance will creep from one biological system to another and eventually one of them will fail and allow disease to surface. Long before diagnosis, disease will fester. During that state, the signs will be clear, but most people will ignore the smoldering until it flares into the wildfire we call disease. We can stomp out the early flames, but we'll need a lot more help if the fire blazes out of control.

When it comes to protein and essential amino acids, this failing system is likely to be the immune system and/or gastrointestinal tract. However, the immune system relies on vitamins, minerals, and fats just as the rest of the body does. The answer to dysfunction or disease isn't vitamin C, NAC, protein, or glutathione supplementation to support immune function. These specialty nutrients can only deliver expected results when a functional foundation is already in operation. They all depend on one another; they all rely on minerals.

Food intake must be densely packed with a complete array of minerals in order to meet the body's needs and, if met, the intrinsic protective system will ward off disease with ease. A diet abundant in whole grains, fruits, and vegetables is essential for optimal health from this standpoint alone. However, bioavailability of minerals in our food supply is a critical issue that must be considered. Vegetarian diets are loaded with minerals, but the form in which these elements are delivered isn't always the most bioavailable.

That's why animal protein sources are strongly recommended adjuncts to a mostly vegetarian diet. Minerals such as iron, zinc, selenium, and even calcium are much better absorbed when consumed either in conjunction with animal protein or as constituents of it. Vegans, studies show, are vulnerable to iron, zinc, and selenium deficiencies that can cause grave consequences that may never be linked, especially if they're marginal.

Iron supplementation has become intensely controversial, but don't be caught one atom short! The body has devised a method of closely regulating absorption of iron—the greater the need the faster the absorption rate. The only way we can dispose of iron is through damaged tissue, which means we have little control over it. However, various factors influence how well iron is absorbed, especially in the case of deficiency.

The form of dietary iron consumed is crucial; vegetarian, nonheme-iron sources display a significantly lower rate of absorption (25, 26). Animal meats are loaded with heme-iron (iron incorporated into hemoglobin), delivering it in a state more easy utilized by the gut. In addition, dietary protein enhances iron absorption, so take iron supplementation with dietary protein (27, 28). One cautionary warning, though: phytate-rich soy proteins can reduce mineral bioavailability, while phytate-free soy proteins can enhance supplemental mineral bioavailability even better than most animal protein sources. This includes calcium, iron, zinc, magnesium, and phosphorus absorption (29).

In other words, strict vegans and even vegetarians such as lacto and ovo can be susceptible to iron deficiency, especially amid disease, trauma, surgery, or the rigors of sport. Athletes are more vulnerable to iron deficiency due to plasma expansions during exercise, loss through sweat, and foot-strike heamolysis (30). When endurance activity is involved, even tiny depletions of iron can result in significant shortcomings in athletic and immune-system performance (31, 32, 33). Protein and iron supplementation for athletes is critical if optimal performance is desired, despite the controversy regarding the potential toxicity of iron supplementation.

The reason dietary protein enhances iron absorption isn't completely understood, but I'm willing to guess that the increased acidity (lowered pH) of the gut encouraged by dietary protein has something to do with the improved iron bioavailability. Vitamin C and other pH-lowering foods are suggested adjuncts to iron supplements as they, too, promote absorption potential.

There are some experts who claim that ascorbic acid, an acidic form of vitamin C, will react with iron to propagate free-radical generation from iron (known as the Fenton reaction generating the hydroxyl radical). Other forms of vitamin C such as ascorbyl palmitate, a fat-soluble C source, won't advance the same risk. However, my investigation of the research reveals that this isn't entirely so; there's much more to this issue than merely ascorbic acid. Cysteine and other thiols (sulfur-containing compounds), for example, are also implicated reducers of iron, turning it into its dangerously reactive state, yet we know them as powerful antioxidants for the body (34). The problem isn't ascorbic acid or cysteine; the trouble is more or less caused by a pro-oxidative system, a biological system that lacks the co-dependent antioxidant mix referred to in previous chapters. If the system has all of the antioxidants required in the complex *antioxidant chain of events*, iron and the entire body are more likely to be protected.

In fact, there is more documented research pointing to the exact opposite of the above claim; co-supplementation of ascorbic acid and iron reduce the incidence of iron-induced lipid peroxidation (fat/membrane destruction) and DNA damage in comparison to iron-loading only (35, 36, 37). I prefer to use blends of different vitamin C sources (magnesium ascorbate, ascorbyl palmitate, calcium ascorbate, and ascorbic acid), and you might want to consider the same. Ageless Performance is balanced and complete with all of the antioxidants required by the antioxidant chain of events.

The iron controversy is justified, and we've seen examples of why that's so. It's a double-edged sword: too little iron causes disease and just a bit too much promotes the same. Excessively accumulated iron can increase the risk for proliferation of pathogens and free radicals (38, 39). The solution is to use safe iron supplements in moderation and in conjunction with a complete antioxidant program.

Iron accumulation in the body increases the oxidative potential of the organs and promotes free-radical generation from catecholamine (stress hormones and neurotransmitters) secretions (40, 41). Therefore, the iron-loaded, stressed individual faces an intensified free-radical load. Take away iron and the oxidative potential is reduced, but so is the oxygen-transport and oxygen-utilization mechanism throughout the body. So it's more logical not to limit iron intake, but to take better control of internal oxidative stress with an effective antioxidant program and healthier lifestyle.

The source of iron I prefer is lactoferrin, an important fraction of the whey protein supplement. Regular consumption of whey supplementation delivers this safe source abundantly. In addition, lactoferrin (the iron source itself) imparts anti-microbial activity by inhibiting microbe adherence to the gut wall (42). Lactoferrin provides iron in a form that the intestinal cells can absorb actively and more rapidly. A good-quality whey protein isolate (better than a whey concentrate) supplies iron safely but only if the label of the product specifically indicates that lactoferrin is present. Some whey protein supplements, such as ion-exchanged variations, don't contain lactoferrin. Cold, cross-flow membrane extractions tend to contain the lactoferrin fraction.

Iron is essential in the body for numerous activities that extend beyond oxygen transport and transfer. The substance is involved in the metabolism of sulfur and sulfur-containing compounds, including the endogenous synthesis of biotin and possibly alpha lipoic acid (43). This ushers the potentially oxidative iron into an important antioxidant role, demonstrating how delicate its balance is to the body. Iron is also an important component of other antioxidant systems such as that found in the catalase molecule, and without catalase function you're doomed.

Animal protein sources are loaded with a great many important minerals, not just iron. They supply calcium, phosphorous, magnesium, zinc, sulfur, chromium, and others incorporated in the tissue and closely related to the proportions required by human flesh.

Lately we've seen a lot of hype about zinc in muscle magazines. In fact, both magnesium and zinc are getting a lot of media time, but all is not what it seems. The claims surrounding zinc and magnesium as testosterone and growth-hormone boosters are a little stretched. In fact, I'd have to say the situation has left the realm of reality. This issue is another example of sports-nutrition companies taking authentic nutritional research and reporting it with a twist to cloud the facts.

The boasts of products containing varieties of zinc and magnesium aspartates (mineral chelates) are partially valid. It's not so much that zinc and magnesium supplementation can enhance testosterone production and anabolic potential as much as a deficiency in the minerals can cause severe metabolic impediments that result in compromised hormone production and activity (44, 45). Studies show that zinc- and magnesium-deficient *males* will produce healthier testosterone levels and more lean-muscle mass with the administration of these minerals as long as all other dietary requirements are met. However, contrary to the cleverly worded implications of advertisements, megadoses of these minerals don't create testosterone levels that are above normal. You might have seen the ads for ZMA- and ZMASS-type (zinc/magnesium supplement) products that supposedly improve testosterone and muscle mass; the supplements might work for you, but only if you're deficient in the first place. This is an example of how vital mineral status in the body is to healthy metabolic activity. Even the smallest deficiencies can result in severe hormonal impediments.

As we get older, gastrointestinal problems can evoke mineral malabsorption, and it's easy to see how this trivialized difficulty can result in severe hormonal deficiencies that are attributed to old age. Lack of testosterone response is an age-related disorder affecting libido, strength, and muscle mass, but so is the malabsorption of nutrients such as zinc and magnesium. Instead of trying to treat these disorders nutraceutically, however, we tend to use drug therapy first. Is it possible that we in our modern Western world are deficient in zinc or magnesium? Today's processing of our food supply, accompanied by the higher demand created by our stressful environments, surely makes shortfalls likely.

Impotence is definitely on the rise these days and is fast becoming a widespread epidemic. And it's a good bet that nutrient deficiencies as outlined above are the primary culprits. Abuse of pharmaceuticals is another reason for the epidemic proportions of impotence. Ironically pharmaceutical companies capitalize on the situation by promoting hormone therapy to rectify drug-induced impotence when all along we just need the raw materials to be supplied sufficiently by our diets—not drugs.

The solution you've been searching for may be as simple as taking a potent mineral supplement. But don't expect an improvement overnight. Rectifying nutrient status takes time and often requires more than one synergistic nutrient. That's why the entire Ageless Performance program is important; it's hard to determine how many factors are deficient. If you're like Mr. and Mrs. Average North America, you're lacking a lot. Supplement your mineral intake or you'll suffer the wrath of multiple drug requirements to compensate for nutrient deficiency.

Sports-nutrition companies also claim that zinc promotes growth-hormone production, so athletes race to megaload the mineral, hoping to secrete more growth hormone. Again the scientific fact is that zinc deficiency results in compromised insulinlike growth factor (IGF-1) activity, severely impairing general growth, fat incineration, immune function, and more. Supplement the deficient individual and growth ensues, but not beyond the healthy norm (46, 47, 48).

Based on these facts, zinc deficiency also instigates the accumulation of body fat! But don't take this to mean that zinc supplementation is a fat-loss strategy; it only demonstrates that nutrient deficiency impairs efficient metabolic function. Ageless Performance ensures maximum nutrient saturation and maximum biological efficiency.

Our bodies have the ability to self-regulate body fat and ward off diabetes, inflammation, cognitive disorders, and endocrine diseases. Very simply put, we require the tools and fuels to accomplish our preprogrammed efficiencies. So when are we going to accept the fact that nourishment is the key to health, and malnourishment is the primary cause of disease? If you're not supplementing amid today's nutrient-scant nourishment, free-radical-loaded environment, and stressful lifestyles, you're malnourished, and disease is a high probability in your future.

MICROMINERALS DO MATTER

Microminerals such as selenium are just as important as any other essential nutrient, even though they're required in minute amounts. Selenium concentration varies drastically in the soils of different regions around the world to result in a related geographical variability of selenium status for people. Seafood is generally a good source of selenium as are organ meats. The diverse forms of selenium have various characteristics. Inorganic selenium from plant sources (selenite and selenate) aren't as well absorbed as organic-delivery types (selenomethionine and selenocystiene) from animal meats (49). Strict vegans living in regions where deficiency in the soil exists are at risk for selenium deficits; deficiency is a serious matter that can instigate disease without apparent cause.

Interestingly the organic forms of selenium are versions of sulfur-containing amino acids, with the sulfur component of the amino acid replaced by selenium. Selenium and sulfur display similar properties. The former is required as a vital component of our antioxidant systems, working closely with vitamin E and glutathione. Selenium is essential for the function of glutathione peroxidase enzymes, the catalysts that provide exceptional antioxidant protection in almost every cell of the body (50).

There are five different glutathione peroxidase enzymes in our cells, four of which are completely selenium-dependent. A shortfall in selenium can result in a lack of glutathione peroxidase activity in the liver (51).

Since the liver is a detoxification site for the body, this deficiency presents grave danger. You can't afford to be a single atom short of selenium; one of the most critical antioxidant systems in the body, the glutathione, depends on it. Studies demonstrate irrefutably that supplementation with vitamin E and selenium concurrently supply considerable protection against liver and other cancers (52). Research concludes that selenium shortages result in a general increased risk of disease (53, 54). Deficiencies are characterized by poor thyroid hormone metabolism; impaired growth; weakness and muscle tenderness; cardiac, myopathic, and pancreatic degeneration; whitening of the nail beds, and a loss of pigmentation in the hair and skin (55).

Chromium is an important nutrient that Ageless Performance accounts for with serious consideration. Still, some experts insist chromium isn't crucial to human health. Some of the minerals previously discussed can be supplied in sufficient quantities by combining a healthy diet with a multi-dosed multi-vitamin/mineral supplement; that is, a multiple vitamin/mineral augmentation consumed over two or three single doses to make up the daily total. You'll find that the requisite levels of dietary chromium I recommend will be impossible to achieve even with a multi-vitamin/mineral supplement complementing a healthy diet.

Health Canada doesn't allow a supplement to deliver more than 500 mcg of elemental chromium daily. However, I consume between 500 and 800 mcg per day from supplemental sources. For individuals who exhibit signs of insulin resistance or have been diagnosed with diabetes, some experts suggest as much as 1,500 mcg daily in divided doses.

As much as chromium supplementation is shown to improve insulin function in many cases, it's not the fat-buster most claim it is. In fact, people in the health-food retail or consultation business know very well that the response from chromium supplementation from client to client isn't at all consistent. It doesn't deliver better energy, strength, fat loss, and lean-muscle gain to all who administer it. Those who experience the expected metabolic improvements from supplemental chromium were probably deficient in chromium prior to supplementation. In other words, if you're getting enough dietary chromium, supplemental chromium won't likely enhance insulin's function above baseline values.

Another factor determining the efficacy of chromium supplementation is co-dependence on other nutrients to complete the chemistry it partakes in. Once more the synergy of nutrient supplementation, as employed by Ageless Performance, is critical to achieve a positive outcome.

CHROMIUM—GOLD OR GUNK?

As we know, insulin resistance results in the oversecretion of the hormone to compensate for a lack of efficiency in it. In this compromised state every time a meal is eaten the pancreas is instructed to pump more insulin into the bloodstream. One of insulin's roles is to activate the glucose-transport sites that clear glucose from the blood and into the cells of the insulin-responsive tissues. Once in the cells, glucose can be used for mitochondrial energy production. Without insulin tissues starve and death becomes imminent. Higher levels of insulin promote storage of substrates like fat and carbohydrate to keep the former from being oxidized as a source of energy efficiently.

Try exercising in this insulin-resistant, hyperinsulinemic (high levels of insulin in the blood) state and you're less likely to burn fat or even build muscle. In fact, since we all face a certain degree of insulin resistance as we age, this is one of the main reasons athletic performance and lean measures are more difficult to maintain as we get older. The elevated insulin and glucose levels that arise out of this inefficiency are toxic, too. The liver comes to the rescue by converting high levels of insulin and glucose into fat, which contributes to increased serum lipids (fat in the blood) and an uncontrollable accumulation around the waist and hips. The excessively loaded fat cells further interfere with insulin's role by secreting hormones that impede insulin activity. Even mild states of insulin resistance can quickly progress to a worse condition and induce metabolic havoc and diabetes, a situation that must be corrected before it gains momentum.

Ageless Performance is the solution to this epidemic condition, and chromium supplementation is an integral part of the *comprehensive* strategy. Studies confirm that chromium supplementation can boost insulin's capacity to regulate serum glucose. An improvement in insulin's potential means fat can be burned more efficiently as an energy source, especially during exercise. As I've previously indicated, research irrefutably demonstrates that chromium status in the body tends to decline with age (56, 57, 58) and this, in part, contributes to the acceleration of biological aging.

Supplementation with chromium by Type II diabetics improves glucose control and serum-lipid variables and at the very least reduces the drug dosage required to regulate the condition (59). In fact, more recent studies indicate that chromium helps down-regulate corticosteroid production, which decreases the catabolic damage caused by mental, emotional, and physical stress, including that induced by intense exercise (60). This is likely due to chromium's ability to enhance glucose control and therefore reduce glucose-stress hormone reactivity in the blood, which we now know gives rise to excessive free radicals. Supplementation with chromium is mandatory for optimal health, but let's get something straight: the mineral isn't a miraculous substance. It's not a pharmacological chemical with symptom-relieving, healing properties. It's a minuscule element required in the grand scheme of biological complexity, and just a slight limitation throws the entire works into disarray. This serves as a model for all of the factors Ageless Performance incorporates. Deficiency results in disease.

Insulin promotes the movement of amino acids into the cells for protein synthesis, further stimulating cellular protein synthesis. This is a highly important step for cell maintenance, lean-muscle restoration, and general life support. By instilling insulin efficiency, muscle is sustained better and fat is more readily used for fuel. There's a kind of exponential dynamic that develops with chromium supplementation when the mineral's status is deficient. The new level of chromium promotes healthier lean-muscle mass, which is able to burn more calories throughout the day while enhanced insulin efficiency allows for proper fat oxidation by muscles during exercise. Second, insulin efficiency supports optimal thermogenic activity. All in all, the healthier dynamic promotes leaner measures with much less physical effort and a lot less dietary sacrifice.

Studies show that chromium, through its activity with insulin, improves the secretion of glucagon, a hormone that slows insulin secretion to inhibit hyperinsulinemia (extraordinarily high insulin secretions). Keep in mind that hyperinsulinemia triggers an imbalanced cascade of other hormones that are responsible for inflammation, fat accumulation, blood-clotting, asthma, and even cancer. This is the basis for the broad preventive and therapeutic activity of Ageless Performance—the reversal of multiple diseases by addressing a few of their common roots such as insulin resistance and nitric-oxide deregulation. The process involves biological regulation of insulin and nitric oxide—the central activity of Ageless Performance. Ageless Performance is about regulation that achieves balanced hormone cascades and mineral systems.

Again chromium is a critically important co-factor for insulin function. Once dietary needs are met, additional chromium won't advance additional fat loss or above-normal insulin activity. That's probably why chromium supplementation works for some but not others as a weight-loss supplement or anti-diabetic agent. Diabetics who experience no improvement from chromium supplementation likely already have healthy chromium stores, and the disease may be caused by other factors, which Ageless Performance also accounts for.

There are different forms of chromium supplements available in the marketplace, and one of the more common, chromium picolinate, might not be the best source. There are many studies that demonstrate picolinate's positive effect on insulin and glucose metabolism, but there's an equal amount of research to show that it doesn't work as well as most experts once thought (61, 62, 63). In fact, studies like the one performed at the University of Alabama and reported in April 2000 prove that the picolinate of chromium can be quite toxic (64). The toxicity stems from the method in which the picolinate version of chromium is used in the body. It enters the cells via a mechanism that's different from the common protein-transport-mediated chromium. This study reveals that the metabolic problem arises when chromium is released from the picolinate carrier. This reaction instigates the extremely toxic hydroxyl radical, a potent free radical that can scald the cells and tax the body's protective antioxidant status.

Other forms of chromium don't manifest this hydroxyl radical. The more likely individuals to use chromium supplementation are those who are in a diabetic state, those who want to lose weight, and athletes who are trying to enhance performance. All of these individuals will experience relatively higher free-radical impositions as a consequence of their condition or lifestyle. This extra picolinate-induced hydroxyl activity only contributes to the free-radical toxicity in the body and most likely causes an incremental depletion of glutathione, creating greater susceptibility to disease.

Some studies indicate that elemental chromium (chromium only) might not be the active factor that facilitates insulin at the cell-membrane receptor sites. In fact, in the 1960s and 1970s at the U.S. Department of Agriculture, observations made by Walter Mertz and colleagues led to the discovery of a category of active molecule called a glucose-tolerance factor (GTF). The interesting finding was that nicotinic acid *plus* chromium or niacin-bound chromium was an active constituent in the cell membrane with regard to insulin activity. When Mertz replaced this niacin component of the molecule with picolinic acid, the activity was significantly reduced (65).

Further studies performed at the University of California resulted in similar outcomes. In 1992 the findings were announced at the American College of Nutrition Symposium on Advances in Clinical Nutrition: the complex of chromium nicotinate resulted in retention of 311% more chromium than with chromium picolinate and 672% more than chromium chloride.

Chromium is naturally complexed in the cell membrane with nicotinic and amino acids. At the cellular-membrane level this complex lends activity to insulin-receptor kinase, an enzyme involved in the signal communication from insulin to the insulin-responsive cell (66, 67, 68). This phosphorylation is the chemistry that triggers insulin activity, hence, the role of chromium in the comprehensive scheme—it facilitates phosphorylation to activate insulin. Other studies that don't specify the structure of this chromium complex and refer to it as a naturally occurring low-molecular-weight oligopeptide form of chromium have also confirmed its critical role, showing it can improve efficiency of insulin-receptor kinase by as much as seven times (69). Of course, I'm *assuming* these studies refer to the same or a related chromium complex and the same underlying chemistry—the GTF (chromium + multi-amino acid + multi-nicotinic acid).

Vanadium, a substance we'll learn more about in the next chapter, delivers tremendous insulin enhancement in a similar fashion, including the stimulation of insulin-receptor-kinase activity, providing a powerful anti-diabetic remedy, even more powerful than that of chromium's (70). Nevertheless, chromium is central to this vanadium function, as well, disproving the historical controversy that vanadium and chromium are antagonistic and demonstrating that these two minerals are synergistic when used supplementally.

Complexes similar to the chromium-nicotinate-amino-acid one have been synthesized using various amino acids with nicotinic acid to emulate the natural GTF, but these synthetic forms have proven less efficiently absorbed than the natural GTFS. Interestingly the GTF is formed using the three amino acids that make up glutathione whose availability in the cell is therefore an important factor influencing insulin efficiency. Glutathione is involved in glucose transport! It may very well be that this is one of the ways alpha lipoic acid supplementation contributes to insulin efficiency, since the nutraceutical is one of the more powerful protectors and boosters of intracellular glutathione.

In fact, alpha lipoic acid could be *the* most powerful booster of intracellular glutathione (71, 72, 73). Independent studies, discussed earlier, show that it combats insulin resistance and even facilitates normalization of glucose metabolism in some diabetics on its own. Based on the scientific literature, I'm convinced that alpha lipoic acid's insulin support is due to its ability to bolster glutathione status, maintaining glutathione availability for the insulin receptor's GTF complex. In the true spirit of Ageless Performance, alpha lipoic acid, GTF chromium, and glutathione boosters like whey protein and N-acetyl cysteine, or NAC, are able to deliver tremendous synergistic value as combined supplements. The benefit of the combination is as powerfully therapeutic as it is preventive of many of our common ailments, even those as severe as cancer and diabetes.

Glutathione functions throughout the body at various vital points in cells. It neutralizes carcinogens in the liver and the rest of the body, protects the integrity of cell membranes, and is intricately involved in the active transport systems of cell membranes. That means it's required for the absorption of nutrients by our cells, and not just the cells of our internal works.

Actively involved in the digestive tract's mucosal cell membranes as a critical part of absorption, glutathione initiates nutrient transport, such as that of selenium, from our digestive lumen into the mucosa and onward to the blood (74). The gut is exposed to food-borne oxidants that tend to deplete mucosal glutathione significantly. Rat studies have revealed that the mucosal cells secrete significant levels of cysteine and glutathione right into the gut lumen to deliver protective antioxidant activity to the food bolus. This activity is thought to support nutrient transport across the mucosal membranes, as well, with cysteine playing a role in iron absorption (75). To maintain mucosal-lining functionality, glutathione is quickly robbed from the rest of the body if it becomes depleted in the intestinal mucosa (76).

Since alpha lipoic acid is a powerful booster of glutathione, it's as vital in a supplemental program as other more conventional glutathione boosters such as whey protein. And because selenium is essential to glutathione's role, it, too, is crucial. Furthermore, vitamin E works with glutathione, as do vitamin C and chromium. And the interdependence doesn't terminate there. It's as though this indispensable synergy never ends, and the only factor that can supply a version of this synergy as close to the one that's functional is our *supplemented whole food.*

And that brings us back to chromium and the fact that brewer's yeast provides a reasonable level of the mineral in the most bioavailable, most bioeffective form—the natural GTF complex.

THE GTF COMPLEX

Generally our food supply seems to lack chromium, but to compound the problem absorption of this mineral is typically poor, as well. Supplementation with niacin-bound chromium, or chromium nicotinate, has been proven in various independent studies to lower serum-lipid levels in humans (77, 78). Of course, the indication is that chromium deficiency results in the lipid anomaly and supplementation corrects the deficiency status. It's obvious that this lipid correction is probably due to insulin correction.

The rise in inflammatory conditions, cardiovascular disease, cognitive disorders, and adult-onset diabetes may be caused by several factors, and perhaps chromium deficiency plays a small part overall. But they all stem from a common chemistry gone awry—insulin biochemistry. For some individuals, though, this chromium deficit might be the problem that gives rise to insulin resistance and all of its associated secondary diseases. Since insulin resistance, or Syndrome X, is now an epidemic raging out of control, chromium research and the results of these studies have been accepted with open arms. GTF supplementation can help restore insulin efficiency, enhance lean body mass, reduce fat, decrease the risk of today's common epidemics, and boost energy.

The biochemical influences that take place every time we eat food are profound. Food is much more than a source of fuel, building blocks, vitamins, minerals, and antioxidants. Our diet triggers an immense hormonal cascade, and the profile of this cascade is a function of insulin efficiency and the food we eat. The cascade permeates the body, influencing every biological system in one way or another. Poor insulin efficiency instigates an unhealthy cascade of hormones, and the trouble is exacerbated by the high-glycemic-index sustenance common in North America. Supporting insulin efficiency with multiple nutraceutical strategies promotes a healthier hormone cascade, biological harmony, and self-sufficiency.

Insulin efficiency determines how the body uses various dietary nutrients, including essential fats such as those from flaxseed-oil supplements. Supplemental chromium polynicotinate and GTF chromium help accomplish correct fatty-acid metabolism and healthy hormone balance. Raising the efficiency of insulin improves serum-glucose regulation to reduce the chance of free-radical generation. Better insulin direction allows for better nutrient incorporation into tissues and biochemical systems. Obviously without chromium our bodies can't do what they were designed to achieve. Our genetic potential depends on chromium's availability, and our food can only supply the mineral as follows: one cup of whole milk has 2.4 mcg; one tablespoon of brewer's yeast yields 3.3 mcg; one cup of whole brown rice furnishes 12 mcg; three ounces of raw oysters provide 12.6 mcg; eight ounces of beer contain 2 mcg; one raw apple delivers 7.5 mcg; and one cup of white mushrooms contributes 33 mcg.

Whole grains and meats are excellent sources of chromium, but the milling of the former removes the mineral. Organically complexed chromium, which meats have a lot of, is far more bioavailable than inorganic sources of the mineral. In addition, as we saw previously, the pH of the gastrointestinal tract influences how well chromium is soaked up. Acidity improves absorption, which might be how concurrent vitamin C administration enhances chromium utilization. In fact, dietary protein also advances chromium absorption, probably because it, too, lowers stomach pH.

Some studies indicate that concurrent vitamin C and chromium supplementation can be toxic, since ascorbate can act as a reducing agent—similar to the case of iron—to convert chromium into genotoxic and carcinogenic forms of the metal. Other reducing agents such as glutathione and cysteine are said to impose the same toxic outcome. The reality is that we can't live healthily lacking any of these compounds. However, it isn't any specific mineral that causes toxicity; rather, it's an imbalance of them that leads to a free-radical-loaded system (79). A healthy antioxidant status prevents toxicity from developing from any one of these nutrients; Ageless Performance instills the correct nutrient balance and a dense, protective antioxidant status.

Chromium supplementation can ameliorate dysthimic depression disorder. Dysthimic depression is a mild illness that persists for decades, starting early in life. It's characterized by a gloomy, pessimistic, humorless personality. The individual is usually an introvert displaying extreme skepticism, self-reproach, and significant lack of libido. One could say these are common traits in any normal individual from time to time, but in the long run these emotional disturbances impair personal growth and often develop into deeper depressive states and impaired social integration. Chromium is now known to potentiate the effects of common pharmaceutical drugs such as sertraline, which is used to treat this condition. The result of the integrated approach for treatment is a remarkably lower dose requirement of the drug and consequently reduced side effects (80). In my consultation experience, chromium supplementation has delivered significant emotional enhancement on its own and with even better results with the right dietary program. Ageless Performance can be more potent than drug therapy for disorders such as dysthimic depression. The program corrects the metabolic damage that gives rise to the need for drugs.

The absorption of chromium is often disrupted in the elderly since hydrochloric-acid secretions in the gut are frequently limited. I've mentioned this impairment a few times. It must be taken seriously, because even minute absorption deficiencies could result in considerable metabolic consequences that lead to physical and psychological impediments that are usually treated with drugs unnecessarily.

It's clear these mild gastrointestinal deficiencies can propagate insulin resistance, since multiple factors that support insulin are undermined by pH anomolies. Regular use of antacids will also contribute to the same dysfunctional nutrient absorption. Alkaline is opposite to acidic. An acid-poor gut impairs the absorption of glutathione, glutathione-supportive protein, cysteine, NAC, chromium, and the B vitamins, all of which support insulin efficiency. Concurrently an acid-poor gut *promotes* carbohydrate digestion, which enhances the glycemic impact of a meal. Carbohydrates require alkaline environments for optimal digestion. If this acid-deficiency condition persists, food induces a higher glycemic impact on the body than expected and a multiple-disease state is the unfortunate outcome.

This acid impairment of the gut coupled with a processed diet that strips chromium and other vital elements from foods can spur the development of diseases associated with old age, diseases that proliferate at an exponential rate with the mere induction of hydrochloric-acid deficiency. Studies demonstrate that chromium status in the body declines steadily as we age.

Yet if the diet is healthy and supplementation complete, these age-related deteriorations don't occur and symptoms of disease may never be experienced because biological age will have progressed slower than the actual passage of time. It's scientific fact, and supplementation is an easy choice to make and apply instead of accepting disease passively. One dose of supplemental chromium polynicotinate or GTF each day in addition to your multi-vitamin/mineral's content may suffice as insurance. I take about 500 to 800 mcg of supplemental chromium per day.

Methylsulfonylmethane (MSM) can be an important addition to the foundation of a therapeutic or prevention program. Our food supply is naturally rich in sulfur, particularly MSM, as is our body. In breast milk sulfur is usually the sixth most abundant mineral, and in the body it's the third most common mineral by weight. Studies of MSM go as far back as a quarter century ago at the Oregon Health Sciences University where it was concluded that supplementation with MSM could produce various health benefits, ranging from anti-inflammatory to improvement of glucose tolerance.

Sulfur is another substance influenced by food processing. The mineral is a critical component of specialized amino acids such as methionine, taurine, and cysteine. It's important to note that these sulfur-containing amino acids are essential to the maintenance of protein structure in the body. Sulfur is crucial to protein cross-linking, which is necessary for connective-tissue integrity. It's responsible for the rubbery, cushiony characteristic of cartilage, hence the tremendous value of glucosamine sulfate over that of glucosamine hydrochloride. Tertiary and quarternary structures of the protein strand provide the three-dimensional structure that enzymes, hormones, cell receptors, and transporters rely on for specific communication. Without this structure the special keys or communication systems of the body are inoperative. Sulfur plays an important role in the body's communication system.

Taurine is integral to cardiovascular well-being, including the maintenance of healthy blood pressure. It down-regulates the ill effects of homocysteine. In fact, according to a study performed in 2001 at the University of Kobe in Japan, the pathology associated with homocysteine elevation was shown to be another example of dietary- and lifestyle-induced modulation of gene expression (81). Homocysteine is a toxic metabolite that can be escalated if the diet is low in B vitamins and folate and is disproportionately high in methionine-rich foods such as red meat. Eat red meat abundantly without sufficient vegetables or multi-vitamin supplementation and you'll likely succumb to the ravages of homocysteine in the long run. According to the Japanese report, homocysteine induces its deadly assault by interfering with the genes responsible for superoxide dismutase (SOD) expression and secretion by the vascular smooth-muscle cells or blood vessels. SOD is an antioxidant that protects the vessels from free-radical damage and ultimately from atherosclerosis. While homocysteine impairs SOD production and secretion, taurine prevents homocysteine's negative activity by improving SOD gene activity. In fact, taurine, a sulphonyl amino acid, delivers exceptional cardiovascular protection.

In 1994 an epidemiological study revealed that the people of Hakka, a Chinese sub-ethnicity, retained their old lifestyle practices and as a result enjoyed longer-lived health than the rest of us (82). A field survey on the Hakka's diet, blood work, and urine samples showed lower sodium and higher potassium intakes than the average, and taurine levels in men were as high as those found in Mediterranean cultures. In Hakka and Mediterranean communities cardiovascular disease is nominal. The serum levels for taurine discovered in the Hakka's women were even higher, approximating those existing in the heart-healthy Japanese villages of Okinawa. It's been demonstrated that Okinawans experience the greatest longevity and lowest mortality rate in the world.

The mystery of these youthful people isn't a secret at all; the answer lies in their relaxed lifestyle and abundant consumption of fresh fish, whole fruits, soybeans, and visceral organs. All of these foods are packed with the goodness that Ageless Performance delivers—a balanced array of essential nutrients that are easy for the body to absorb and use.

Taurine seems to play a part in glucose transport (83). But is it essential? Taurine is synthesized in our bodies using methionine and cysteine and is thought to be a dietary necessity for infants and the elderly. In my opinion it's critical at all stages, simply because it's a powerful thiol (sulfur-containing compound with antioxidant properties) compound much like cysteine. The bottom line is that taurine is essential for good health. It can be considered nonessential if suboptimal health is acceptable. I choose to supplement it.

Cysteine, a sulfur-containing amino acid, is an important component of insulin, as well. A deficiency of cysteine can cause impaired insulin function and glucose tolerance, which is likely due to the compromised glutathione status that can occur due to the same lack of cysteine. The amino acid is significant in the manufacture of endogenous alpha lipoic acid, glutathione, and other biological enzymes, all of which rely on sulfur for their special activity. The value of MSM supplementation is profound, since this sulfur is also a central component for endogenous production of SAMe, glucosamine, chondroitin sulfate, and other important regulatory and structural molecules we've mentioned, including cysteine (84).

Studies indicate that cysteine is a valuable antioxidant independent of the antioxidants it constitutes, and this activity again is highly attributable to the sulfur in its structure (85). NAC down-regulates the gene and the protein conversion responsible for the acceleration of Alzheimer's disease (86). A 2001 study proves irrefutably that Alzheimer's is associated with neuro-impairing amyloid plaques, which themselves are derivatives of a protein (amyloid precursor protein or APP) produced by the overexpression of a gene in specialized neurons. Oxidative stress, once again in this model, acts in a genomodulatory fashion, accelerating this toxic gene and the detrimental plaque formation manifesting disease. The model shows that a natural sulfur-containing antioxidant such as NAC plays a genetically specific role, down-regulating this overactivity. This study also demonstrated that the disease-inducing rate of gene activity was returned to the dysfunctional state when cells reverted to a NAC-free medium.

The potential for disease is in all of us, so what keeps it from being triggered in everybody? The answer is our biochemical uniqueness, which influences the activity of genes in a singular way in every human, promoting distinct outcomes. Diet looms large in this phenotypic (physical outcome from genes) distinctness, just as a nutraceutical strategy can protect and facilitate a healthy gene activity from the same genetic profile that can manifest disease. Sulfur figures considerably in this properly operating gene activity, and that's why MSM supplementation delivers a variety of health benefits amid the processed, sulfur-deficient North American diet.

The activity of glutathione is highly dependent on the sulfur in its structure, and is vital due to its multiple roles in the body, including the support of immune function. A shortage of sulfur can influence many systems, resulting in a number of conditions such as glucose intolerance, cardiovascular disorders, inflammation, cartilage damage, and dementia. The claims made for MSM supplementation have been so broad and profound that it's difficult to believe its advocates at first. One would almost think MSM is a miracle cure for every ailment under the sun. Although a placebo effect might be a possible explanation for many of these testimonials, I'm betting on the few scientific reports and the understanding of sulfur's crucial biological role, including that of genomodulation, that MSM is integral to prevention and therapy.

A variety of rat studies show that MSM supplementation can decrease inflammation, allergenic response, the onset of tumerogenesis, cancer, and rheumatoid arthritis. The findings reported in a 2002 publication of the *Journal of Alternative and Complementary Medicine* detail a study performed by the GENESIS Center for Integrative Medicine in Graham, Washington. The findings conclude that "2,600 mg/day for 30 days of MSM supplementation may be efficacious in the reduction of symptoms associated with seasonal allergic rhinitis (SAR). Furthermore, few, if any, side effects are associated with the use of this compound." SAR afflicts in excess of 23 million Americans (87).

As is the case with many other important nutrients, MSM isn't a miracle cure-all. It's the absence or limitation of sulfur in the diet that instigates disarray and disease. Supplementation with MSM simply reverses a state of deficiency. The fact that sulfur-containing antioxidants such as alpha lipoic acid, cysteine, glutathione, and chondroitin display genomodulation and nitric-oxide regulation activity doesn't necessarily imply that these substances are pharmacological agents as our health authorities want us to believe. Our health-protection or federal-regulatory agencies may lead some of us to think these substances should only be made available by prescription because of their powerful biomodulatory activity. But that belief system is the sort of reasoning that keeps humans, as well as many of our companion animals, in a state of disease and a mode of reactive health care, which is absolutely absurd.

Dimethylsulfoxide (DMSO) is a common topical agent used abundantly to treat equine and canine leg strains and sprains. Oral MSM shows similar promise, and many experts prefer it due to the controversy surrounding DMSO. Some say that DMSO forms deposits in the body and is difficult to metabolize, but I disagree. In fact, many studies demonstrate DMSO's therapeutic effect with tremendous safety, protecting immune activity, reversing autoimmune disease, and contributing to experimental cell preservation in cryogenics (88, 89, 90, 91).

MSM supplementation *must* be considered part of your essential nutritional foundation if you insist on consuming processed foods abundantly. Ingestion of a whole-food diet will reduce the necessity for large daily doses of supplemental MSM. However, the 250 to 500 mg capsule doses of MSM that are common in the marketplace might not be appropriate unless you're ready to swallow handfuls of capsules for each dose, since 2.5 to 5 g could be required each day.

I add a heaping teaspoonful of MSM to a protein drink three or four times per week. That equals about 10 to 16 g of supplemental MSM per week, and even that might not be considered enough by some experts' standards, except that my diet consists mainly of whole foods and lots of fresh, lightly cooked vegetables—all good sources of MSM. Fish, milk, and milk products are also excellent sources of MSM, though conventional pasteurization techniques can destroy it. Just like other special nutrients, MSM is highly susceptible to degradation by heat and can be removed or destroyed by food processing.

Manganese, zinc, and copper are important co-factors for the powerful SOD. Without these minerals SOD can't do its job to neutralize free radicals, and without SOD activity we'd burn from the inside out in a matter of minutes. Despite what many people think, orally supplemented SOD can't increase cellular SOD levels. The alternative strategy for escalating the levels of cellular SOD is to make certain that all of the body's nutritional needs are met, which includes abundant supplies of the minerals necessary for SOD's role.

Copper, like chromium, zinc, and other minerals, is involved in far more than just SOD activity. It figures in hemoglobin manufacture, connective-tissue synthesis, and bone-matrix construction. Copper is also involved in hormone production and thyroid, epinephrine, and dopamine regulation. Minerals are critical to general hormone balance, and their status can decline significantly with age and become the root of age-related metabolic deterioration.

However, few health-care professionals identify mineral deficiencies as a cause when their patients are faced with thyroid, adrenaline, testosterone, IGF-1, or dopamine anomalies. Drugs instead are the first line of treatment, which is a shame, because they're poor compensation for a simple mineral deficiency. The consequence of just drug therapy can be more disease as the original problem persists and the new medications induce unnecessary biological interference, including scientifically documented additional nutrient depletion.

Minerals constitute the matrix of interconnected molecules that make up our tissues. They're essential to the body's ability to maintain pH balance. Some minerals contribute to acidity, while most of those available from whole grains, fruits, and vegetables are required in order to buffer acidosis. The absence of one or multiples of these sparks of life results in the development of disease or disorders that over time degrade our bodies to the point of no return. A related death is then attributed to disease and rarely, if ever, to the deeper cause—the limitation of these critical building blocks and co-factors.

Conventional health professionals treat mineral deficiencies with pharmaceutical drugs simply because they have no education regarding these implications. After being exposed to this science, you have to agree that the maintenance of insulin efficiency is critical in the prevention of disease. The very strategy of life extension takes this achievement as a primary initiative, and the goal requires that all of these vital minerals be supplemented to make sure we don't fall one atom short.

CHELATED MINERALS

There are many forms of elemental mineral sources, but they definitely don't deliver the same potential. Let's delve a little into the chelation of minerals. Chelated minerals have become widely accepted sources of bioavailable supplementation. However, not all chelates are equal.

We'll start with the controversial iron supplementation, since it really is a confusing issue for consumers. Iron bisglycinate chelates, manufactured by mineral specialist Albion Laboratories, deliver iron in a protective chelate made up of two amino acids. The Albion chelate is better protected from oxidation (alteration by free radicals and reducing agents) and isn't as likely to propagate free radicals in the gut as most other sources of supplemental iron will. Ferrochel and ferrous bisglycinate, Albion chelates, were both deemed safe even at extreme doses of 500 mg/kg tested on rats, with no short-term toxicity (92, 93)! That's an equivalent dose of 75 g of each of these iron sources for a 150-pound human. This form is actively absorbed the way a peptide (protein) is sucked up in the gut, it has a higher absorption rate, and it's much less likely to induce gastric upset than less bioavailable sources such as iron sulfate (94, 95).

Albion Laboratories produces a series of extremely effective mineral chelates. The technology the company delivers truly provides a difference you can feel. In fact, as I've mentioned before, the mineral *in* this ligand (molecule that binds to the mineral acting like a carrier) is enveloped— sandwiched—by two amino acids.

Intralumen chelation occurs when two minerals come together and form an insoluble complex in the gut that can't be absorbed. Both minerals can be lost due to this process. The loss is common with multiple-mineral formulations in which abundant calcium joins with phosphates and magnesium to create the insoluble, unabsorbable calcium-phosphate-magnesium complex (96). Special chelates like those of Albion Laboratories reduce the risk of this development. Many other minerals are antagonistic to one another and, as a result, absorption from a mineral supplement is highly compromised unless this special chelate system is used.

FIGURE 7:

Amino Acid
Albion Chelate

Iron Bisglycinate

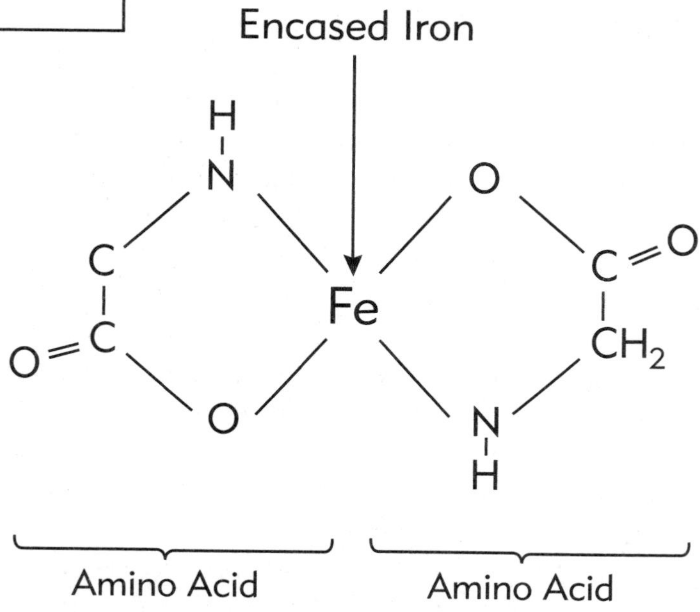

Encased Iron

Amino Acid   Amino Acid

Ironically calcium is often combined with magnesium in typical cal/mag formulations, and this in itself presents an antagonism most manufacturers are oblivious to. It actually reduces the absorption potential of both the calcium and the magnesium. Recent studies have shown that supplementation with calcium and magnesium concurrently can help lower serum cholesterol levels by somehow blocking cholesterol reabsorption by the gut (97). Calcium and magnesium are important for many functions, only one of which is bone-mass maintenance, but the mineral source that's used is just as significant.

A minute shortfall of calcium and magnesium will result in profound metabolic disarray that can be quickly rectified with a multiple-mineral supplement. Calcium incorporation into bone requires proportional magnesium availability. Bone mineralization necessitates phosphorous, zinc, and many more minerals, as well, but getting all of these into the body at the same time is tricky. However, one of the few ways the antagonism is avoided is through the administration of chelates that protect the mineral in the way the Albion bisglycinate is designed to do. These special chelates guard the minerals they carry against mineral-mineral antagonism, but they also defend against nonmineral antagonists that exist in our food such as phytates and oxalates from fibrous plants, coffee, and tea.

Recently I formulated an incredible lineup of supplemental minerals for a Canadian manufacturer of sports and other nutritional products. The products have an innovative but commonsense strategy. In the formulation, among the Albion chelates, I included phytase, the enzyme that digests phytates. By concurrently administering phytase with mineral supplementation, antagonism from food- and drink-derived phytates is reduced. Synergy in supplementation is crucial.

Minerals are central to enzyme function throughout the body. Magnesium is important for bone integrity, neuron health, testosterone activity, and muscle contraction, and it's crucial to the enzymes involved in platelet adhesion (platelet collection in clot formation). Oral doses of magnesium can be assessed for retention potential by measuring platelet-adhesive changes. Studies indicate that the bisglycinate chelates of magnesium are much better absorbed and *retained* than magnesium salts like magnesium oxide, especially amid gastrointestinal impediments (98). The measure of a nutrient's potential is highly related to its retention possibilities, and absoption doesn't necessarily translate into retention.

The role of magnesium in reducing platelet adhesion is significant (99, 100). Research comparing this potential to EPA/DHA (salmon-oil) supplementation has been quite remarkable, with platelet-adhesion reduction quite similar. Obviously the subjects in the study were deficient in magnesium, otherwise their natural chemistry would have maintained healthy platelet function. In this case, EPA and DHA worked to ensure enhanced platelet activity when magnesium was missing from the supplement mix, but the fats might very well be the factors that compensated for the root problem—magnesium deficiency—by correcting the symptom in this case.

Magnesium deficiency contributes to cardiovascular disease. Supplementation to guarantee an adequate supply of the mineral is the best cure for this problem—much smarter than ongoing ASA administration as compensation for a nutritional deficiency that could be the cause of increased clotting risk. It's ridiculous that the magnesium status of the body isn't determined before something like ASA megadosing is recommended for life!

Albion has recently produced a magnesium-bound creatine. This chelate has superb potential for sports and general prevention, since magnesium and creatine have synergistic value for muscle function and other biological activity. However, it's a bit pricey, and until the cost comes down, taking a different Albion magnesium chelate such as a bisglycinate in conjunction with creatine monohydrate will be more economical. That's probably why we haven't seen this innovation explode into the market-place yet.

There are different types of mineral chelates available, some of which don't involve amino acids. The kreb cycle intermediate chelates are common as are other proteinate chelates, but unless the mineral is tightly bound, enveloped, and actively absorbed like the sandwiched bisglycinates are, they won't deliver the same potential. Calcium citrate, for example, is also considered a chelate, though it's a mediocre source of calcium compared to the preferred bisglycinate chelate. Calcium-citrate-malate sources of calcium, however, are better than the citrate type.

Despite these wonderful advances in supplementation, the whole, fresh, unprocessed diet must constitute the solid foundation within which supplements operate. The whole, fresh, color-rich diet is a critical component of Ageless Performance, but it does deliver an abundance of antagonistic phytates and oxalates, and because of that the Albion chelate will serve best as a supplemental form of precious minerals.

Let me remind you that you're not what you eat but you are what you're able to digest and absorb. The bioavailability of your nourishment is a major factor influencing how proficiently your biological health develops.

Calcium carbonate, for instance, delivers more calcium per gram than a calcium bisglycinate form might. However, calcium carbonate is less efficiently utilized; higher levels of calcium from calcium carbonate aren't necessarily better than lower levels of the more readily absorbed form, since the better absorbed bisglycinate is less likely to antagonize other minerals. Take large quantities of calcium carbonate and you'll interfere with the bioavailability of other essential minerals in the diet. Mineral bioavailability is crucial for optimal health and maximized athletic performance. Albion chelates are my preferred choice, and I suggest you look carefully at product labels for this type of mineral supplement.

NORTH AMERICANS ARE MINERAL-DEFICIENT

The West is by no means free of mineral deficiency. An estimated 75% of the U.S. population doesn't meet the government-recommended daily allowance of magnesium, 68% are short of their requisite calcium, 58% are deficient in iron, 50% aren't getting their required manganese, and 40% fail to consume enough zinc. Mineral and other nutrient deficiencies are especially likely with gastrointestinal disease (101).

Furthermore, these statistics are based on recommended daily intakes that are on the low side to begin with. As disease proliferates, we look to new technology for treatment, but the efficacious treatment most often lies in the correction of mineral deficiency. Symptomatic relief with drugs like ASA and Coumadin (Warfarin) only mask the problem and allow more disease to develop from the underlying festering. If drugs such as these are absolutely needed to reduce the risk of clotting, use a magnesium-repletion supplement at the same time. Then, with your doctor's approval and monitoring, try to come off the drug after a few months of mineral supplementation and don't terminate the supplement afterward. Salmon-oil and magnesium supplementation in combination will probably do the job better and more safely than any drug, but again only apply these strategies with your medical professional's approval and assistance when dealing with health problems. Ageless Performance is designed to deliver health benefits as a normal biological function to prevent such conditions from ever developing. That's the ultimate goal of the program—self-sufficiency.

Mineral supplementation is an important part of the Ageless Performance plan. Still, supplementation isn't compensation for poor diet. It might help overcome deficiency and dysfunction that poor dietary habits are responsible for, but for the full preventive potential of supplementation to be realized a natural whole-food underpinning must be in place to maintain optimal metabolic momentum.

Anti-aging or life extension isn't something mystical or magical; very simply, it's an extremely aggressive prevention program. Death is inevitable, but we're born to live. You can decide to enjoy a life with long-lived vigor by employing these basic principles, or live a slow death by depending on human-made compensation for the human-created nutritional inadequacies and excessive toxic imposition that we see in our technological age.

Since insulin efficiency is integral to prevention, therapy, athletic performance, and anti-aging, in the next chapter we'll examine in more detail the miraculous, insulin-potentiating substance I alluded to earlier—vanadium. The potential of this remarkable *metallonutrient* has been kept from us by authorities who have been and continue to try to limit our access to disease-preventing, disease-reversing substances unless prescribed by health-care professionals after illness has been diagnosed. But this is a reactive health-care strategy, and we know that prevention is a lot more effective. The relatively inexpensive vanadium can be taken in short cycles by individuals predisposed to the multibillion-dollar, profit-generating, life-suffocating Type II diabetes. The result can be complete reversal and prevention of diabetes—a disease that's become the bread and butter of the pharmaceutical industry.

8

MINERALS: METABOLIC MIRACLES

DIABETES: THE SHORT AND SWEET

Within the membranes of insulin-responsive cells, insulin-receptor sites can diminish and glucose-transport sites can decrease in number. Age, diet, lifestyle, and genetic predisposition have all been implicated as causes for this occurrence. As a consequence of this membrane interruption, the cellular response to insulin is impaired. If the number of glucose-transport sites, referred to by researchers as GLUT4, falls by 65% or so, a diabetic state is imminent.

In this condition, with the consumption of each meal, the body signals the pancreas to secrete more insulin than normal as compensation for the glucose blockade and metabolic *numbing*. This is the very premise for Type II, or adult-onset, diabetes. In this situation the cells that are normally responsive to insulin become desensitized. Type II diabetes is quite different from Type I.

In Type I, insulin isn't produced in sufficient quantities, or at all, and the clearance of glucose from blood can't proceed efficiently. After eating a meal, a Type I or Type II diabetic person's blood sugar can rise to toxic levels as a result of poor insulin response. Diabetic neuropathy, glycation of protein, circulatory impairment, organ damage, and many other disorders soon follow.

Since blood glucose can be highly reactive, this condition promotes the generation of free radicals and premature aging of the body, making antioxidant supplementation unequivocally vital to the diabetic condition—both Types I and II. Ageless Performance meets the antioxidant needs. Of the 20-plus million diabetics in North America, 5% or so are Type I. Therefore, about 95% of today's diabetic population can potentially reverse the disease—the Type II condition—unless the damage has progressed beyond repair.

As I've mentioned previously, we all face a degree of insulin resistance as we get older, but this degeneration can be down-regulated or slowed down. Our processed lifestyles accelerate the development of insulin resistance to a diabetic state. Today age-related insulin anomalies are common among adolescents. Experts blame a genetic predisposition for this migration of disease. I'm not convinced the human genome has changed in the past 10 years, resulting in a greater frequency for these diseases in our young. Evolution just doesn't work that way.

It can take thousands of years to create genotypic change significant enough to make such a difference in a species as evolved and as intrusive in the natural selection process as human beings are. Many people with whom I've consulted have completely reversed this condition with relative ease. In fact, almost every case can be turned around or at least reduced to a mild condition despite what we've all heard from conventional health-care professionals.

As we've seen, the glycemic index of our diets is a major player in the cause as well as the reversal of this metabolic problem as is supplementation with key nutrients such as alpha lipoic acid, chromium, glutathione, whey protein, and even MSM. Keep in mind that these aren't miraculous nutrient cures for disease; they're simply essential to normal human biochemistry. Supplementation amid deficiency gives rise to healing and the perception that these substances are curatives. The preventive activity of these common supplements is also indicative of how essential these nutrients are to our well-being. Even our whole food can't provide the level of compensation we require because of our plastic lifestyles and environments. Supplementation is essential!

Prevention involves avoiding unnecessary toxicity when possible. The implications of metals on biological function are profound, which prompted me to investigate their use in dental restoration. Most of us are aware that mercury from typical dental amalgams imposes serious toxicity throughout the body, especially the neurological system. I uncovered some evidence that reveals that some forms of ceramic, gold, and copper dental restoration materials significantly increase insulin secretions, while one type of material, Vita vmk 95, radically reduced the release of the hormone (1). Both influences are potentially poisonous over the long term, promoting oxidative stress and inflammatory hormone cascades—inflammation that can instigate multiple diseases, including diabetes. The point is that preventive strategies will reduce the risk of disease, and that includes taking proper care of teeth.

The powerful protective substance I've been teasing you about is also a metal and has been a topic of controversy, as well. Vanadium is a *metallo-mineral* found abundantly in Earth's crust. Whether or not vanadium is essential to human life has been an ongoing debate, but studies have conclusively shown that in its vanadyl sulfate (vs) form and other similar biochemical types it has tremendous medicinal or pharmacological value. This suggests, in my opinion, that vanadium *might* also be critical to our well-being and that deficiency in it *might* give rise to the need for the orthomolecular doses required for resolution of the problem deficiency creates.

vs has considerable insulin-potentiating properties; in effect, it enhances the function of the hormone. Experts point to the insulin-mimicking qualities of vs as the method of activity, but that isn't a correct description of its performance, because it doesn't deliver insulin potential unless the hormone, insulin, is concurrently present in circulation with it. vs boosts the potential of circulating insulin, promoting its efficiency and reversing the body's resistance to the hormone.

Taken in short bursts, vs can provide amazing preventive potential, but it's also effective therapeutically for Type II diabetics and can even reverse their condition! Consumed in conjunction with exogenous insulin by Type I diabetics, vs can improve the hormone's efficiency, dramatically reducing the amount required in some cases. In fact, studies have disclosed that vanadium works through a biochemical pathway that's different than insulin's, which can add to the value of injections of the hormone required by Type I diabetics (2). And if you decrease insulin requirement, you cut down on insulin-related risks. These studies show that vanadium won't advance the development of hypoglycemia, either. Amazing results, but what's even more unbelievable is how vs has been kept from the over-the-counter market in some countries.

These exceptional results were originally discovered in tests with rats, where it was found that when the administration of vanadium ceases, the newly established insulin efficiency remains in place—again, it corrects the membrane damage that causes Type II diabetes! Human tests have yet to be performed to confirm this persistence after vanadium administration stops, but the anecdotal evidence I've seen suggests it does occur. Tests on humans have, however, demonstrated decisively that vanadium sources such as vanadyl sulfate, sodium metavanadate, and others have powerful anti-diabetic activity and excellent potential to block the progress of insulin resistance. Studies also indicate that results are experienced within 72 hours of commencing therapy and, most important, without significant side effects.

One of the obvious applications of vanadium supplementation is the promotion of insulin efficiency for fat loss. As is the case for many other nutraceutical substances already discussed, vanadium isn't a fat-loss substance; it merely helps correct the metabolic problem that contributes to body-fat accumulation and many other diseases. I employed this corrective or metabolic reset strategy to prepare for bodybuilding shows as far back as 1988, reaching leaner measures than most, if not all, participants I competed against. The other easily apparent use is the maintenance of insulin efficiency for anti-aging purposes, therapy for insulin-related diseases, and athletic-performance enhancement. Truly insulin health is the crux of the conceptual fountain of youth!

Despite positive scientific findings by credible researchers from respected institutions, the Canadian government hasn't allowed vs to become an over-the-counter supplement in the doses required to induce corrective results; in fact, its sale is totally prohibited, while in other countries such as the United States it can be purchased legally in any health-food store as easily as one would buy a multi-vitamin. There are a few studies that point to the potential toxicity of vs, but they were poorly executed and were followed by multiple studies that demonstrated a nontoxic nature. The benefits of vs far outweigh minor side effects such as stomach upset and mild diarrhea, which are only experienced in some cases. Pharmaceutical drugs make it to the market all the time displaying horrific side effects like internal bleeding, bone degradation/osteoporosis, impotence, lost libido, hair loss, nausea, stunted growth, irritability, psychosis, depression, hyperactivity, suicidal and homicidal tendencies, gum bleeding, friendly bacterial imbalance, ulcers, anemia, edema, heart palpitations, blood-pressure anomalies, sleep disturbances, inability to focus mentally, optic impairment, kidney strain, and liver toxicity. Public introductions of these foreign chemicals are examples of global experimentation where profit is the primary aim.

The only real side effect that's been experienced with large, orally administered doses of vs is gastrointestinal disturbances—a bit of gas, gurgling and, in some cases, diarrhea, a far cry from gum bleeding, homicidal tendencies, stunted growth, and osteoporosis. In most cases, by slowly working up to functional doses, this stomach upset can be avoided. Researchers are now attempting to develop a different chelate, or version, of this substance to eliminate the gastrointestinal disruptions associated with it. Metformin is also known to induce mild gastrointestinal difficulties, which makes it not much different from this newcomer. However, metformin can't do what vs does! Why are metformin and lethal substances like acetaminophen (Tylenol) approved and marketed to become household items, and vs, a relatively safe substance, banned?

I imagine the reluctance to legalize vs and other related vanadium sources in Canada is based on the volumes of research that show metals to be toxic to humans in various ways, including genetoxicity. However, many of these studies have also revealed that the toxic activity is caused by reactive oxygen species (ros) generation by the metals (3). These metals tend to act as catalysts to produce harmful oxidants, and ros is a powerful free radical that damages metabolic activity, including mitochondrial and genetic. But what about iron? It's a metal and it's as essential as chromium. This takes us back to two of the central points of Ageless Performance: that free radicals are dangerous disease instigators and antioxidant systems are critical synergists in all forms of disease prevention and therapy, including vanadium administration. However, in opposition to this disease-instigating case a study in June 2002 identified novel anti-carcinogenic and anti-tumor applications for vanadium (4).

VANADYL SULFATE SUPPORTS INSULIN SAFELY

Experts have claimed for some time that vs can assist insulin in its physiological role, but only if a condition of insulin resistance or glucose intolerance previously exists. Research has revealed that insulin function isn't raised above baseline levels and, as a result, an individual with normal insulin function isn't affected negatively by the administration of vanadium in the orthomolecular doses I recommend. That is, hypoglycemia isn't a common occurrence with vs administration.

Type II diabetes and insulin resistance often go undetected until they reach advanced states. Long before diagnosis, the secondary damage insulin resistance elicits will induce severe metabolic havoc. Avoiding early stages of insulin resistance and diabetes is critical to general disease prevention and anti-aging. Using vs supplementation as an occasional membrane reset, as we'll see, is a great preventive strategy.

vs has been shown to undo completely the damage in the cell membrane that results in insulin resistance and Type II diabetes. However, vs doesn't compensate for poor insulin function by simply raising the body's sensitivity to insulin the way metformin might. The metallo-mineral actually promotes reconstruction of the functional system that might have broken down. A 2002 study from the Faculty of Pharmaceutical Sciences at the University of British Columbia indicates just how this pharmacology unfolds. The report demonstrates that vanadium stimulates the transcription and translocation of the glucose transporter GLUT4. Concentrations of GLUT4 on the cell membranes increases toward normal levels with supplementation of vs or Bis (maltolato) oxovanadium, an organic type of vanadium. The metallo-mineral actually fuels or activates gene activity to normalize cell sensitivity to insulin—another example of nutraceuticals reviving the genetic potential within.

Reincorporation of these transporters into the insulin-responsive cell membranes reestablishes normal insulin responsiveness. Its activity isn't stimulatory but more like a reconstruction of the normal regulatory system. This also explains how the normalized activity stays in place after administration of the vanadium source is terminated. These studies clearly illustrate that a healthy metabolic state in the nondiabetic or insulin-normal individual isn't affected by vanadium administration. Normal levels of GLUT4 can't be further enhanced. In fact, research demonstrates that metabolic homeostasis or glucose control is maintained with lower plasma insulin levels after vanadium supplementation (5). That's the ultimate goal of the anti-aging strategy!

By instilling insulin efficiency, vs can reduce the risk for the discussed secondary diseases associated with insulin resistance: cardiovascular disease, inflammatory afflictions, obesity, asthma, cognitive disorders, and more. Research commencing in 1984 at the University of British Columbia by Dr. John H. McNeill, et al, showed that oral vs could eliminate diabetes in rats, seemingly reversing the condition and "normalizing" insulin sensitivity. Multiple studies that followed this early report clearly confirmed these findings. Many human trials conducted in the mid-1990s confirmed the results found in rats, with human daily doses of vanadyl sulfate and/or sodium metavanadate ranging from 100 mg to 300 mg daily and, most important, with indications of *no* toxic effects (6, 7, 8, 9, 10)! The preceding references are documents generated at Harvard University, Albert Einstein College of Medicine, Temple University, and the University of British Columbia, a wide array of credible independent work. It's as though vs resets the biological clock and, in a sense, it does. These studies also disclose that vanadium enhances glucose uptake by the heart.

Dr. Julian Whitaker wrote about the therapeutic potential of vs in his November 1994 newsletter. He advocated the use of vs in daily quantities of 150 mg, and his very statements conveyed that this was "without adverse effects other than some gastrointestinal disturbances" for some. He, too, referred to an early McNeill University of British Columbia study to support his claims for vs.

I've worked closely with other medical and research professionals in the field of sports nutrition, anti-aging, and therapeutic and general preventive nutrition and have lectured nationwide on these topics. The positive feedback from individuals who have applied these strategies is heart-warming.

A few experts still insist, however, that vs can be toxic, but there are just as many who feel that the metallo-mineral is safe. One concern in a recent debate I was involved in pointed to studies performed on rats that ended in multiple deaths of the animals which, of course, is something to worry about. In fact, I was already using vs when the studies demonstrating it could be toxic became public. However, the results many people had experienced with vs were just too amazing to discount the supplement out of hand, so I dug deeper to find more evidence to support its safety. Besides, those who were using vs on my recommendation, including myself, didn't experience side effects, and I'd been taking it on and off for several years.

However, in order to appreciate how safe vanadium is we must remember that, like other metals or minerals, it exists in different forms. In addition, certain factors—such as oxidative status of the body—can contribute to toxicity of an otherwise nontoxic substance. In fact, many factors would be involved in the metabolism of this substance just as the case is with all of our common nutraceuticals. The right synergy is the key to its correct application.

Studies have shown that vanadium as vanadate can compete with phosphate transport at the specialized carrier proteins in cell membranes responsible for the movement of phosphates into the cells. One particular study revealed that when taken in high doses—in excess of 10 mg orally daily—vanadate can inhibit amino-acid transport across the intestinal mucosa (11). The result can be severe immune depression, lean-mass catabolism, and even death in extreme cases. However, subsequent studies indicate that vanadium doesn't affect amino-acid transport (12). This contradictory evidence was quite frustrating for me. There are so many positive health benefits for vanadium administration, including the ability to reduce elevated serum-free fatty acids (13). My intense research eventually paid off.

Interestingly studies also show that in minute doses, vanadate stimulates the same phosphate-transport protein system instead of inhibiting it, in turn promoting alanine (an important amino acid) dispersal and increasing cAMP production intracellularly. As described earlier, this incremental cAMP helps prime cells much as the cell-rejuvenating herb coleus forskohlii does.

The vs doses we're talking about for therapy for insulin resistance or diabetes, though, far exceed 10 mg daily, but the important fact is that I'm not advocating supplementation of vanadate, the form the studies show to be toxic. The source of vanadium to use is the reduced form, vanadyl sulfate (vs). Vanadium is reduced by glutathione into the vs state in the gastrointestinal lumen before absorption (14). This reduction also takes place via glutathione mediation in the plasma and other body fluids as well as within cells.

Why is all of this biochemistry relevant to vanadium's safety? If vanadium does interfere with amino-acid absorption, it's the vanadate form we should be concerned about. Studies demonstrate that surrounding cellular conditions predispose the cell to the potential toxicity of the metal. The factor promoting toxicity is oxidative stress—free radicals. The vs form has been shown *not* to compete with the phosphate-transport proteins or amino-acid dispersal, but when oxidized to its vanadate form by free radicals, it can be toxic. vs isn't catabolic as many previous studies have concluded.

The trick to supplementing vs safely and more effectively for insulin control is to use it concurrently with glutathione boosters such as NAC and alpha lipoic acid—500 mg of the former and 300 to 400 mg daily of the latter in divided doses. This extra cellular augmentation of glutathione will support the reduced, less-invasive state of vs in the body while the enhanced glutathione and alpha lipoic acid levels will bolster the previously outlined cell membrane's GTF complex for better insulin function. It might be a good idea to supplement vs concurrently with glutathione itself to help maintain the reduced state of the former in the gut. In our cells vs exists as a complex of protein or peptides such as the glutathione-vanadium type.

This strategy has worked wonders for me and for those who have applied it. My 225-pound, massively muscled physique during my competitive bodybuilding years was definitely not a picture of an individual facing protein or amino-acid deficiency. Besides, even if vs did present some level of toxicity, it might not be the sort insulin resistance or diabetes blasts the body with. Second, since vs only has to be employed in short bursts, if there are any toxic effects, they can be eliminated with proper strategy.

To discuss my own findings and results, I spoke directly with Dr. John McNeill at his University of British Columbia office, and he enlightened me about several facts. His research on vs began back in 1984. It was his work that prompted me to begin using vs in 1988. He disclosed that the animal deaths my colleagues justifiably heeded were finally attributed to a lack of water consumption, which for diabetic subjects imposes grave danger. McNeill said that vs saturation of the drinking water seemed to cause the animals to refrain from drinking. Eventually the researchers overcame the problem and the studies progressed with success.

Not drinking water might also account for the catabolic effects on lean mass that some scientists attribute to vs administration. Dehydration could cause measures that infer lean-muscle catabolism. Dr. McNeill claims that vs affects amino-acid transport nominally, if at all, and catabolism caused by amino-acid-starved tissue isn't likely, which confirms my findings.

Until recently the method in which vs induces insulin efficiency wasn't known. Today we understand that vs actually enters the cell to facilitate the incorporation of more glucose-transport sites at the membrane surface by modifying gene activity—kick-starting the healthy potential in all of us. In addition to this remarkable finding, even more recently, resistin has been shown to be inhibited by vs. Resistin is a newly discovered hormone that adipocytes, or fat cells, produce. If you carry more body fat, you tend to produce a greater amount of resistin, which is somehow involved in cytokine production and insulin function. Both cytokines and insulin are involved in and significantly influence inflammatory and immune-system activity.

At first the conclusions from these groundbreaking studies were that resistin interfered with insulin to induce insulin resistance, but apparently that's only partially true. It's now known that resistin does somehow interact with insulin, but the precise activity hasn't been determined. Resistin also facilitates tumor necrosis factor (TNF) production, which is implicated in inflammatory conditions such as arthritis and other common diseases (15).

Carry more body fat and you carry a higher risk for disease. vs blocks resistin activity to prevent this disease-promoting factor. It also decreases the risk of hypercholesterolemia, hypertension, and atherosclerosis (16, 17). Based on the newly found resistin hormone chemistry, vs administration should also have a positive influence on chronic inflammatory conditions. However, I must stress that the anti-inflammatory activity is anecdotal and even theoretical at this point.

Since gut absorption isn't very efficient, one of the problems with vs supplementation is the volume—30 to 150 mg daily—required to achieve results. I tolerate the high doses well when I administer a cycle, say, over a three- to five-week period. Once or twice each year I use vs in bursts to upgrade my insulin function in case operating efficiency has dropped. If you feel you could benefit from vs, you might want to try small doses, starting with 10 mg daily, then working up to a daily total of 45 to 70 mg. For cases of progressed Type II diabetes, 150 mg daily might be necessary. (See the detailed application instructions for vs displayed in this book's final section, "Getting with the Program.")

vs supplementation is a great way to initiate the Ageless Performance program to ensure that any state of insulin resistance is rectified while the essential and other omega-3 fatty acids of the regimen are introduced. It isn't necessary to use vs, but if you do, begin with the small doses (10 mg per day) and work up by 10 mg increments each week.

Insulin-receptor sites depend on the right fats for correct and secure anchoring, and the co-dependence of these nutrients is remarkable. While vs can enhance insulin efficiency, insulin efficiency will allow essential fats to be converted into the right structural components of cell membranes and the proper precursors for autocrine hormones.

Subsequently the new membrane fat balance can result in improved insulin response by cells—exponential amelioration of cell membranes and exponential improvement of insulin function simultaneously. It's this dependent dynamic that requires the assistance of substances such as vs to get the cycle moving in the right direction—a priming of metabolic correction.

HOW I USE VS FOR COMPETITION

First of all, avoid vs if you're allergic to sulfur-containing drugs. I start with 5 mg two times per day or 10 mg at a time, each dose with a meal. After one week, I increase to 10 mg two times daily—again, each dose with a meal—and go from there. vs is better absorbed on an empty stomach, but it's also more likely to induce gastrointestinal disturbance this way. If you're battling diabetes and are using pharmaceuticals of any kind, consult with and request monitoring by your physician while taking vs. It's safe and doesn't interfere with common diabetic drugs. In fact, it's likely to enhance their results. You and your health-care professional will be astounded with the results!

The need for other insulin-supportive drugs might be alleviated with vs use, but not indefinitely unless you change the dietary habits that caused your original problem. If you use vs to reinstate healthy cell function and don't alter the lifestyle habits that pummeled your cells in the first place, you'll lose out to the toxic bombardment, and insulin resistance and/or diabetes will reappear.

Now let's dive into the subject of fats—the core of our program.

9

GENERAL FAT FACTS

DIETARY FAT IS ESSENTIAL FOR HEALTH

Many of us spend our adult lives avoiding dietary fats. However, as we get better at eliminating fatty foods, controlling our diets becomes more difficult. Eliminate fat and we'll crave more!

Do away with fat and more than likely carbohydrate intake will increase significantly to accommodate for the caloric restriction. As we become addicted to the carbohydrate-consumption cycle, which I discussed earlier, appetite and eating habits begin to veer out of control and it isn't long before a calorie-restriction plan doesn't work anymore if it worked at all in the first place. Familiar?

If you're like many people, the next step you'll take while on your failing low-fat diet will be to step up your exercise program a notch. Eventually more and more exercise is required to fight the fat-deficient, dysfunctional metabolism until one day you may resign yourself to the misconception that your aging metabolism is the cause of your weight-mismanagement issues. Finally you'll surrender to what you think is a genetic influence you can't control.

If the above is your experience, you've given in to a phenomenon you can overcome. In fact, you've likely caused the struggle. The solution is a lot less straining than the emotional anguish and hard physical work you've employed. These same fat-deficient dietary habits promote cardiovascular problems, diabetes, and other diseases you may battle and eventually lose out to. Too much of the wrong fats and too little of the right fats instigate disease. It sounds complicated, but the program I've created is quite simple.

One of the most powerful forces driving your metabolism against your objective is the low-fat diet. Your dietary-fat demands are partly driven by a highly addictive opiatelike substance your body produces in response to the high-fat meal; in other words, an endorphin rush is the likely culprit and addiction to this rush propels you into a feeding frenzy (1, 2). Most of us attempt to fulfill this desire with the wrong fats. Failing to get what it asked for, the body keeps the "craving button" in the on position, turning up the heat until it gets what it needs. If you don't know how to satisfy that need, the struggle persists with ever-increasing intensity. You eat more of the wrong fats and the cycle is perpetuated. If you think you can beat this magnetic attraction to food, you're wrong; you'll lose every time until you address the underlying chemistry that keeps the addiction alive. Ageless Performance obliterates the craving naturally.

Your body will fight you to the grave for its requisite levels of essential fats, and when you consume the wrong fats as a consequence of an uncontrolled binge, you only get one step closer to disease. Fat calories are very dense and deliver more than twice the amount of energy per gram than carbohydrates and protein. Once fat is eliminated from the diet, the calories required to fuel the body may be severely limited, and this factor can heighten the desire to feed. This calorie-restriction-induced desire to eat is independent of the cravings caused by the addiction to the endorphin rush, compounding the hypnotic surrender to food.

Since some of the fats that have been eliminated from your diet are essential for hormone function and cell construction, your body will yearn for these building blocks with an unforgiving relentlessness. These desires stem from a need for essential building blocks that when limited give rise to a nutrient-deficiency craving (NDC). Again the body initiates these NDCS in an attempt to get the nourishment it needs to survive (3).

The NDC phenomenon is real, it's documented, and it's powerful. Keep in mind that this is only one of three things driving your uncontrollable eating habits. Endorphin addiction, calorie deprivation, and NDCS will team up, bringing the typical dieter to breakdown. However, breakdown in this case only means more of the same—the rampant consumption of food devoid of essential fats and other necessary nutrients because the common, uncontrolled binging involves processed junk food.

Consequently this binge further exacerbates the uncontrollable appetite and continued consumption of empty foods. Caloric intake might be sufficient and even excessive, but nutrient ingestion is rarely met by these valueless foods and, as a result, satiety levels are seldom sufficient. Processed foods don't deliver essential nutrition in requisite quantities. They usually provide more than enough dietary carbohydrates, some damaged protein, and the wrong fats, but these largely worthless foods are typically short of vitamins, minerals, and other micronutrients crucial to the metabolism or cellular processing of carbohydrates, protein, and fats. This shortfall prompts the body to rob metabolically necessary micronutrients such as vitamins and minerals from other systems until it gets you to eat more food.

The body's objective is to collect more nourishment, but as you fulfill this whim with unsuitable food again and again, more calories are consumed than required to satisfy the need. The craving is simply a desperate attempt to make these specialized micronutrients and scarce essential fats available. That's not much different than the gasping for oxygen when your supply is cut off, except you can survive a little longer with nutrient scarcity than you will with oxygen deprivation.

The nutrient-deficient diet is driven by panic, except that the food still carries calories that have to be stored as the body attempts to extract every bit it can from the inadequate food, depositing unnecessary calories around your waist in the process. It's easy to see how supplementation can help alleviate needless cravings.

By supplying the right fats from whole, fresh foods, you can soothe uncontrollable cravings without contributing to your midsection or your bottom end. These fats fire up the "furnaces" that burn the unnecessary dietary and body-deposited fats. Essential fats and the multitude of special polyunsaturated fats that our cells manufacture make up the delicate membrane and communication systems that unify our cells. These fats are key components of complex hormone systems, neurotransmission, and healthy cognition.

We might have many facts about the motivators of appetite. As much as all of the above is scientifically documented, the interactive dynamics of this intricate network render a reliance on any one of the concepts for relief from uncontrollable cravings extremely useless. In fact, many studies demonstrate that food yearnings are powered by mood or emotion and are completely independent of these previously cited aspects (4, 5, 6). The consumption of carbohydrate-rich foods is associated with incremental serotonin secretions in the brain, and a lack of this neurotransmitter is implicated in depression (7, 8). Depressed? Eat carbohydrates and maybe you'll feel a little better. Food is, in fact, a drug.

So the controversy is whether or not mood is the primary engine of food cravings, or is it the reverse? My position is that the mood disorders that are so prevalent today are provoked by poor diet and environmental toxicity, which brings us right back to a healthy lifestyle as the solution to the appetite problem. This mood dynamic involves a much greater complexity that comprises stored chemistry stemming from emotional experiences in our lives. Addressing these issues is critical if absolute maximum physical, mental, and emotional health are desired. Still, the healthy cleansing of this toxic chemistry relies on a nutritional status that supports detoxification. With regard to diet, essential fats are known to be crucial to a healthy cognitive and emotional state. Limit dietary fats and the mood factor sets in to drive a feeding frenzy. Antioxidants consequently are critical in the preservation of these mood-supportive fats, since they're extremely vulnerable to destruction by free radicals—synergy is the point!

This debate presents a classic chicken/egg scenario: are food cravings caused by poor diet/lifestyle, or are they sparked by mood disorders? Since the focus here is more on the nutritional influences, we'll stick closer to this dynamic, but don't underestimate the power of stored emotional chemistry and spiritual status. Ageless Performance is formulated to take in all the facts about fats, carbohydrates, and other nutrient factors that might prompt uncontrollable appetite responses. The program improves state of mind and emotion as well as state of body.

The common dietary restrictions we impose for weight management actually add to the development of mental, mood, and physical disease. They amplify the conditions of our toxic environment and nutrient-deficient foods by further limiting nutrients that would otherwise protect us from the environmental assault. They can also increase the free-radical load on the body, especially when noradrenergic drugs like ephedrine and abundant caffeine intake enter the picture. With a little conscious effort to increase the essential nutrient density of the diet, the body will become self-sufficient and appetite will automatically become controllable.

Fat isn't the bad guy we've been led to believe it is. It's true the wrong dietary fats will promote misery and disease, but it's equally correct that the right ones will make prevention and therapy easier goals to achieve. As for athletic performance, these proper fats will deliver performance potential that will propel us beyond the levels we're at today as long as the other nutrient co-factors, the ones we've discussed up to this point, are supplied with them.

The specialized polyunsaturated fats provided by the Ageless Performance program instigate enhanced neural function, muscle innervation, oxygen transport, blood flow, and cardiac output. All of these features are crucial to optimal health and biological age. They're also important for maximum athletic performance.

POLYUNSATURATED FATS

Metabolism is simply the compilation of the chemical processes that occur within a living organism. This involves the breakdown or digestion, absorption, chemical alteration, and use of a nutrient for energy and for tissue, hormone, or other biochemical synthesis. Animal meats are rich in many of the polyunsaturated fats required for healthy metabolic function. However, animal protein sources also deliver many of the fats we must avoid. These include saturated fats and a few less-preferred polyunsaturated fats, as well.

The body is preprogrammed to manufacture all of the fatty acids it requires except two: linoleic acid (omega-6) and alpha linolenic acid (omega-3), the only fats our diets must provide. In effect, these are the essential fats, often referred to as EFAS or omega fats. Limit them in the diet and biological life is proportionately constricted. The healthier, *cleaner* sources of our essential polyunsaturated fats are the oils of various seeds.

Flaxseed oil delivers a healthy proportion of omega-3 to omega-6 fats. Hempseed and pumpkinseed oils are also good, and next on the list in my descending order of favorites are soybeans and walnuts or their oils. Polyunsaturated fats give our foods as well as our tissues, once they've been incorporated, a fluidlike nature.

The term *polyunsaturated* refers to having many sites within the structure of the fat molecule that are unsaturated or, as a chemist might say, having multiple double bonds. These double bonds give the polyunsaturated-fat molecule a curvelike tendency, allowing the long chain of carbons that make up its backbone to flow in a wavelike formation. This snaky nature imparts the liquid character to polyunsaturated oil so that molecules can flow freely.

The saturated-fat molecule, on the other hand, is straight and rigid and doesn't wave, curve, or flow freely the way its polyunsaturated cousin does.

FIGURE 8:

Comparison of Fats with Different Levels of Saturation

Oleic Acid, C18:1—Monounsaturated Fat

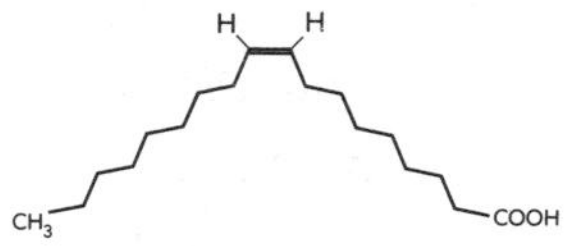

Linoleic Acid, C18:2—Polyunsaturated Fat (Essential)

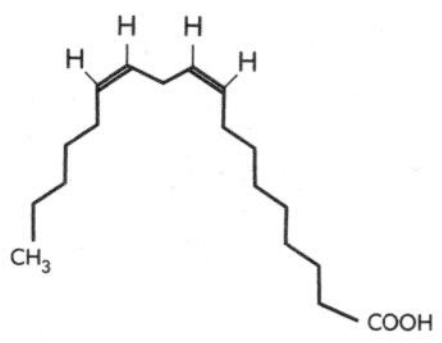

Alpha Linolenic Acid, C18:3—Polyunsaturated Fat (Essential)

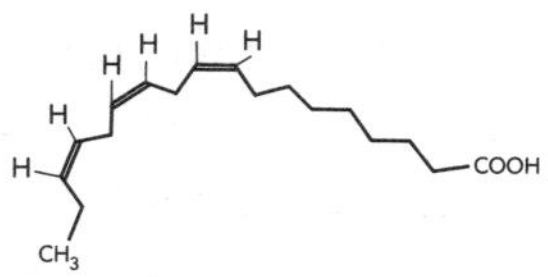

Palmitic Acid, C16:0—Saturated Fat

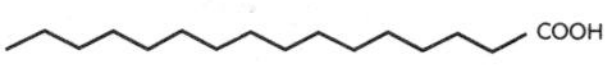

At room temperature saturated fat tends to be solid, its molecules clumping together, while polyunsaturated fat is liquid, which is why most of the healthier sources of fat come from oils.

Grapeseed, safflower, and sunflower oils are often included in the list of essential fat sources; however, they're not that good since they don't provide the critically important omega-3 linolenic acid. Grapeseed oil isn't the same as grapeseed extract, the powerful antioxidant. Omega-3 is the fat most often limited in diets and the one we have to supplement in order to bring balance to our food intake and to our cells. To consciously consume more omega-6 fat can and usually does aggravate the imbalance our diets already deliver.

Olive oil is one of the safest vegetable oils to cook with, and it's one of the more stable fats among unsaturated oils. Over and above this cooking application, olive oil delivers numerous health benefits. It helps to lower serum LDL or bad cholesterol and serum fats, reduce abnormally high blood pressure, diminish the risk of platelet aggregation (clotting), and generally decrease the danger of cardiovascular disease (9, 10, 11, 12). Regular consumption of olive oil is now recognized as so powerful for prevention and recovery from cholesterol elevation that health professionals often advocate its aggressive introduction into the diet instead of pharmaceutical administration. However, today's typically stale olive oil falls far short of its wholesome potential.

Studies indicate that olive oil provides antioxidant activity and combats inflammation, as well (13). Interestingly most experts point to oleic acid, a fatty acid in olive oil, as the element that accounts for the majority of its activity. The monounsaturated omega-9 fatty acid in olive oil, however, is only one of the factors that contributes to its health benefits. Research comparing oleic acid to whole extra virgin olive oil confirms that the latter is far more effective against cardiovascular and inflammatory disease than the former alone (14, 15). This implies that there's much more to olive oil than merely the omega-9 monounsaturated fatty acid.

Olive oil is loaded with polyphenolic compounds. Phenolic compounds are natural chemicals that demonstrate potent antioxidant activity. These antioxidant compounds contribute largely to the benefits olive oil delivers, and they've been shown to increase LDL cholesterol's tolerance to oxidative stress (free radicals), reducing cardiovascular disease associated with LDL oxidation (16, 17). However, cooking with olive oil at high temperatures oxidizes the delicate antioxidants, diminishing the beneficial activity.

Although processing and heating can destroy antioxidant activity, oleic acid can survive the strain to deliver some of olive oil's benefits. Uncooked, fresh extra-extra virgin olive oil still contains the most potent protective activity, but the stuff available in clear containers that display the oil's rich color aren't the best choice. Heat, light, oxygen, and other forms of energy can obliterate precious antioxidants. The clear plastic or glass bottles of olive oil sitting on intensely lit supermarket shelves have had their antioxidant activity significantly compromised. Oleic acid will survive, but its activity constitutes only a fraction of the oil's potential.

Buy your olive oil in opaque, oxygen-tight containers and purchase enough to last only a couple of weeks in order to limit exposure to the air. Every time you pop the lid to pour your requirements, precious antioxidants are assaulted by the elements. I use olive oil on every serving of a mixed, colorful salad and that means about one salad each day. This same light- and oxygen-limiting strategy must be considered for flaxseed-oil use, too. However, flaxseed oil, which contains a high level of polyunsaturated fats, is much more delicate and should be refrigerated, as well.

THE TERROR OF TRANS FAT

Unlike the relatively heat-stable monounsaturated fat of olive oil, polyun-saturated-fat-rich oils such as flaxseed shouldn't be used in cooking, since heat can destroy the fat component of flax, rendering it somewhat toxic to the body. That's how foods deep-fried in so-called light polyunsaturated vegetable oils can deliver deadly consequences.

Just because your deep-fried french fries are cooked in vegetable oil doesn't mean they're a healthier choice. On the contrary, the repeated and prolonged heating or boiling of these oils oxidizes their polyunsaturated fats to produce free radicals and the dreaded trans fats.

By now most people understand they should stay away from trans-fat-loaded foods, but too many don't really know why. Trans fats are hidden in many of our foods *except* those that are whole, fresh, and unscathed by human hand. This isn't entirely true, since small amounts of trans fat do exist in nature. However, the level of healthy polyunsaturated fats is so high in nature that the naturally low levels of trans fats can't compete successfully against the healthy fat in our body unless processing increases the odds in favor of trans fats.

Polyunsaturated fats exist primarily in cis form in nature. This cis form is the fluttering, free-flowing fat molecule I previously described. The curved, flickering characteristics of natural cis polyunsaturated fats differ greatly from the straight, rigid, lifeless configuration of their nemesis, the trans fats.

Trans fat has the same inflexible structure of saturated fat. As we've seen, saturated fats don't have the double bonds unsaturated fats possess. As a chemist would say, saturated fats are drenched with hydrogen atoms to create tight, unbendable molecules. cis and trans fats might be only slightly different in their structure, but their chemical properties are quite dissimilar. Food processing gives rise to trans fats, which are abundant in hydrogenated vegetable spreads (margarine), dressings, and candy coatings. Trans fat is often employed to make candy coatings because it forms a hard or stiff complex, unlike natural polyunsaturated oils.

The rigid property of trans fat, however, is passed on to the cell membranes of the body after consumption. Trans fat competes in the body with cis fat as a building block for cells and tissues. cis polyunsaturated fats provide a healthy foundation for our cell membranes and are used to form the elements of their lipid bilayers. If your diet supplies an abundance of trans fats from processed foods and a scarcity of cis fats, trans fats will beat the good fats to your cells, making their way to your cell membranes as imposter building blocks. The result is an unyielding, unforgiving element in the membranes, making them extremely dysfunctional.

Imagine the membranes of your cells packed with linear trans fats. Picture many decks of playing cards squeezed together to form a barrier so tightly crowded that slipping between two cards is impossible. Nutrients and waste can't move in and out through this rigid medium. That's what happens when trans fats are used as the building blocks for cell membranes. However, with curved cis fats in place, cell membranes

FIGURE 9:

Three Different Portrayals of a Phospholipid

Our cell membranes are built using phospholipids as building blocks.
The phospholipid is made using the described fatty acids.

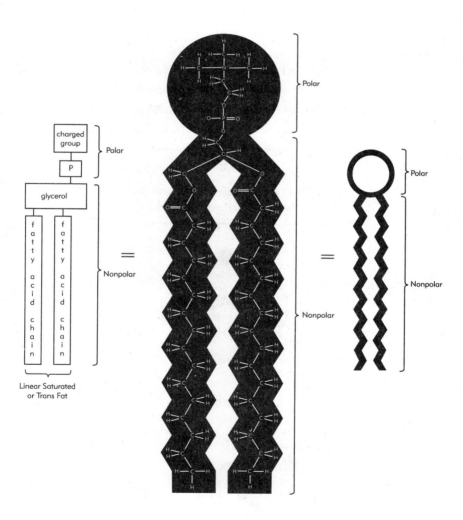

are fluid, flexible, and functional, and nutrients move in easily and toxins move out without interference. Figure 10 shows the placement of the correctly manufactured phospholipid in the cell membrane. With a trans-fat-built structure your brittle body will crumble under stress. Maintain your processed-food diet and you'll build a processed body that will lack both physical elasticity, resilience and immune defense.

Even before reaching your cell membranes these fats impose a negative influence on blood chemistry. Most fats that are hard or solid at room temperature will flow slowly in the blood. This characteristic makes our blood more viscous and sludgy and a lot more difficult for the heart to pump. The combination of more brittle membranes and a strained heart leads to disaster, namely, cardiovascular breaches that result in death without

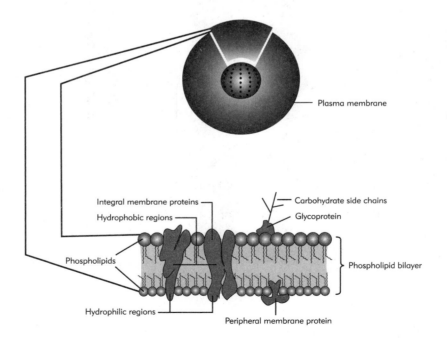

FIGURE 10:

Cross-Section of Cell Membrane Built Correctly with Polyunsaturated Fats

Plasma membrane

Integral membrane proteins

Hydrophobic regions

Carbohydrate side chains

Glycoprotein

Phospholipids

Phospholipid bilayer

Hydrophilic regions

Peripheral membrane protein

prior warning. The American Heart Association reports that "57% of men and 64% of women who died suddenly of cardiovascular disease had no previous symptom of this disease." Proactivity is a logical measure.

It's safer to fry with animal fats than it is with trans-producing *light* vegetable fats. We view the *light* property of oil as a healthy thing. We think light oil is less likely to clog arteries. It appears to be free-flowing, the way we want our blood to circulate in our body. However, the lighter the cooking oil, the greater the chance for trans-fat-associated toxicity when cooking is involved. Containing fewer polyunsaturated fatty acids and more of the saturated fatty acids, animal fats are generally safer for cooking at higher temperatures than vegetable oils. But abundantly consumed saturated fats turn blood into a slurry, as well, stressing the heart and contributing to insulin resistance (18, 19). So, you ask, just what fats are safe to eat?

Butter is a healthier bread spread than hydrogenated vegetable oil such as margarine. No matter what your health professional tells you about elevated serum cholesterol levels, replacing butter with margarine isn't the answer. Margarine and mayonnaise, like common hard-candy coatings, are usually loaded with trans fats, products of our artificial hydrogenation process.

Today some of these hardened fats are produced through an alternative processing method called fractionation. If the label reads "Does not contain hydrogenated oils; contains fractionated polyunsaturated oils only," the product still contains hydrogenated trans fats, though less than an oil that's been hydrogenated. Hydrogenation is now getting such a bad *rap* in the candy and health-bar market that new applications are being used but often with similar toxic results. So-called fractionated fats can still contain hydrogenated fats; if your health bar has a hardened chocolate or other candy coating, trans fats set the coating.

A trans-fat-built nervous system can't operate normally, and a common result is depressed and/or manic states, attention-deficit hyperactivity disorder, and other cognitive and mood disorders. A 2002 study performed at Bastyr University in Seattle, Washington, demonstrates that trans fat can decrease mitochondrial function, and multiple studies today reveal that a deterioration in this is central to many of our epidemics, including dementia

(20). The mitochondria produces the fuel of life (ATP), and impairment leads to an increased rate of biological aging and a rapid decline in health.

We're tricked into accepting trans fats in our foods and then misled again to use drugs as compensation for the metabolic damage trans fats produce. Trans fats are known to promote hyperlipidemia (high blood-fat levels), increasing bad cholesterol (LDL), but most alarming is the fact that dietary trans fats also reduce the amount of circulating good cholesterol (HDL)—a double whammy (21, 22)! Yet we're still directed by uninformed health-care practitioners to use trans-fat-loaded spreads freely as alternatives to cholesterol-rich butter when cardiovascular disease is a risk. Trans fats have been known to increase cardiovascular risks for some time, but research today has confirmed our fears. A 2002 study at the University of Washington's Cardiovascular Health Research Unit (Department of Medicine) verifies that trans fats amplify the risk of cardiac arrest (23). In a 2001 report by the Family and Preventive Medical Unit of the University of Utah, trans fats are shown to escalate the risk of colon cancer, yet we're *still* directed by media and health-care professionals to move from consuming a high-fat diet, substituting natural fat with trans-loaded artificial fats such as hydrogenated and fractionated spreads (24). It's still a high-fat diet, but now with an added risk. Our mainstream health-care choices are mind-boggling!

Our bodies rely on natural chemistry, and a limitation of natural essentials amid a bombardment of disease-instigating, man-made products results in disaster. Obviously federal regulatory agencies aren't going to act on behalf of consumers positively; their focus has been on delisting supplements that can help prevent disease, making them available only by prescription. Drugs aren't the cures for these diseases, nor is reactive nutraceutical administration. This strategy only promotes the failing *reactive* health care we're employing. Strict regulations should be imposed on the manufacturers of poisonous processed foods, and just as with cigarette manufacturers, the labels of these foods should clearly display powerful health warnings.

Imagine a warning on your Twinkie or hydrogenated margarine: "This package contains harmful chemicals that, over long-term use, can induce cancer, cardiovascular disease, diabetes, cognitive disorders, and immune-system failure." That's not so farfetched, and you might very well experience this labeling transition in the next 10 years. More likely, however, manufacturers will stop using these chemicals to avoid the labeling imposition when the laws are passed. Just remember how tobacco smoking was perceived only 20 years ago compared to today before you dismiss what I'm saying as absurd.

The studies are conclusive: these foods maim, impair, and kill! They maim because they induce insulin resistance and diabetes, and diabetes is a major cause of amputation. The American Diabetes Association reports that in the United States "each year 56,000 amputations are performed among people with diabetes."

The processed diet seeds our epidemic of diseases. Trans fats aren't acceptable dietary inclusions if you care about your health. The Ageless Performance program is designed to limit trans-fat consumption. On days when toxic exposure is greater due to consumption of processed foods, the combative strategy is to increase the amount of health-promoting omega-3 fats, in supplemental form, to compete more successfully in the body against the incidental increment of trans fats from deviations in the diet.

That makes sense, doesn't it? If you provide more of the right fats, there's a better chance for the correct fats to reach your cell membranes to build a flexible, resilient body. Ageless Performance incorporates all the requirements to prevent negative factors from interfering with your natural healing and health-maintenance programming. If healthy eating makes up the major portion of your food intake, the occasional minor lapses that deliver trans fats and other harmful dietary factors can't undermine your solid foundation.

The following table displays the constituent fats of a few different vegetable oils. Make a special note of the omega-3 and omega-6 contents for each of these sources. The objective of supplementation is to offset the typical dietary imbalance. Remember, the common diet is abundant in omega-6 fats. The objective is to supplement with omega-3-rich fats and avoid the omega-6 variety. The oils have been placed in order of preference as essential-fat supplements. The oil at the top of the table represents my preferred source.

Proportion of Unsaturated Fats in Common Vegetable Oils

Fat/Oil	Linolenic Acid (Omega-3 Essential)	Linoleic Acid (Omega-6 Essential)	Monounsaturated Fat	Order of Preference
Flaxseed	54	14	23	1
Pumpkinseed	15	45	32	2
Soybean	11	44	30	3
Walnut	5	50	29	4
Canola	8	26	57	5
Almond		17	68	6
Extra Virgin Olive		12	77	7
Safflower		70	18	
Sunflower		66	22	
Corn		59	25	

Flax contains the highest percentage of omega-3 and among the lowest contribution for the omega-6 fats in the above list of fat sources—a perfect offset for the typical omega-6-rich North American diet. Oils that contribute to the omega-6 load without delivering the commonly limited omega-3 fats abundantly should be avoided unless you're confident you're operating with a functional cellular balance. Most of us lean toward an unhealthy balance in our eating habits and consequently must consciously try to supplement the omega-3-rich fat sources.

However, even if your dietary habits are healthy, limiting the omega-6 payload from supplemental fats is still a good idea. Omega-6 fats such as linoleic have been recently implicated as contributors to insulin resistance, as has trans fat (25, 26, 27). These fat factors compound the influence our high-glycemic-index, processed dietary carbohydrates impose. The North American diet promotes insulin resistance and diabetes in multiple ways. Flaxseed oil as supplementation or as a condiment is the better of the above seed-oil choices.

On the other hand, studies demonstrate that the omega-3 fat, in particular the DHA (docosahexaenoic acid) found in fish oils such as salmon and tuna, combats insulin resistance and diabetes—omega-3 fish fats help clear blood sugar (28, 29, 30, 31). Just for the record, keep in mind that the clearance of glucose through insulin-efficiency enhancement is a lot different than better glucose control caused by an induced insulin secretion by the pancreas. Enhanced insulin efficiency results in lower insulin levels required to do the job while the incremental secretion, such as that caused by diabetic drugs like glyburide, gets the job accomplished with higher levels. Hyperinsulinemia—high insulin levels in the blood—isn't a healthy state. Fish-oil supplementation supports normal metabolic function of the body with lower levels of insulin and therefore a reduced risk of secondary diseases associated with excessive insulin.

Studies also show that the content of neuromembrane DHA declines significantly with age, contributing to neurological dysfunction (32). Therefore, supplementation with omega-3/linolenic acid and DHA makes perfect sense. Fish fats lower serum triglycerides (blood fats) and raise the levels of good cholesterol (HDL) in the blood (33). This influence on circulating HDL is a critically important activity that differentiates salmon and other cold-water marine oils from any other cholesterol therapy. I'm big on salmon-oil supplementation, but not just any type.

Fish oils can contain many fat-soluble toxins such as PCBS, heavy metals, and other common industrial poisons that enter our waterways. So you should supplement with molecular-distilled versions of fish oils to eliminate the risk of this toxicity. The Biologic Nutritional Research Inc. Web site (*www.biologicnr.com*) presents an unbiased display of recommendations approved by our in-house research program. It lists a few brands that use marine oils sourced from clean waterways and cleared of such toxins by way of guaranteed analysis. The synergy that DHA delivers to insulin function, whether as an insulin transporter or general biological efficiency promoter or both, is now recognized as a powerful pharmacological recovery potentiator for diabetics. DHA is being assessed as a pharmacological agent for insulin delivery and is likely to become a regular adjunctive therapy in mainstream medical insulin formulations in the near future (34).

But you don't have to wait for disease to come your way before you apply these powerful strategies—reactive health care has proven to be dysfunctional. The most powerful application is prevention—proactive health care. I strongly recommend that you mix the bounty of extra-extra virgin olive oil with fresh organic flaxseed oil and use these fats when condiments are desired. In conjunction with these plant-oil sources, the inclusion of salmon-oil supplementation is critical to the production of the right omega-3-to-omega-6 ratio in the body. The salmon supplementation is best consumed in gel-capsule form; including fish fat in salad dressings just doesn't quite work in terms of palatability. I make a fantastic salad dressing by combining flaxseed oil, extra virgin olive oil, balsamic vinegar, low-sodium soy sauce, a few freshly crushed/chopped garlic cloves, and a couple of tablespoons of finely chopped onions. This dressing is easy to make, it tastes great, it's free of trans fats and sugar, and it's full of healthy fats and antioxidants.

HEART HEALTHY SALAD DRESSING

1 oz of organic, cold-pressed flaxseed oil
1 oz of extra virgin olive oil
1 oz of balsamic vinegar
1 oz of soy sauce

Finely chop one to two garlic cloves, then finely chop one to two table-spoons of onion. Mix the chopped garlic and onion into the combined liquids and shake. A teaspoonful of lemon juice is another optional addition. Add vitamin E to the mixture to protect the fatty acids from oxidation. Take a gel capsule of your supplemental alpha tocopherol (vitamin E) and squeeze a few drops into the mix. Use the remainder of your vitamin E supplement as your daily supply. It's important to store this blend in an opaque, airtight container in the refrigerator to keep light and oxygen from oxidizing the delicate fats and maintain the tem-perature low (refrigerate) to protect the biological activity of the fats. Make enough to last a few days to keep your batches fresh.

This dressing is incredibly tasty on salads or as a bread dip and is a great addition to canned tuna, giving it the zest it needs. Even though a multiple green salad is the best accompaniment to a serving of tuna, I find myself making an alternative snack for a change. Slice a couple of tomatoes in a bowl and add some onion. Put in a can of tuna and pour a little of the well-shaken Heart Healthy Salad Dressing over the snack/meal. Pour as much as you need to satisfy your taste buds. Better yet, use fresh, lightly seared tuna to get an even healthier array of natural, nondenatured fats and protein. Don't be afraid to employ this dressing in abundance. The omega-3 fats provided by this mix stimulate the genes involved in the inhibition of fat-cell hypertrophy, which means they impose a genetic influence that blocks excessive body-fat deposition (35). Dietary fats that burn body fat!

MARGARINE ISN'T A HEALTHY ALTERNATIVE

The objective of the hydrogenation process is to take away the fluid nature of the oil, improving resistance to oxidation or rancidity and making the substance more viscous and even solid at room temperature while enhancing its shelf life. This viscosity induces the same rigidity in the membranes. One of the marketable advantages of the hydrogenated plastic fat you've likely been bombarded with in advertisements is that it *appears* to be a lot like butter but without the cholesterol component.

By using trans fats in their foods, manufacturers can still claim they're using polyunsaturated fats because, actually, the former *are* polyunsaturated. But they don't have to tell consumers that trans fats act much like saturated fats in the body. Even worse, as I eluded to earlier, trans fats deceive the body into accepting them as membrane components in the positions where flexible cis fats are supposed to be placed.

One such trans fat is elaidic acid, the product of hydrogenating linoleic acid, a cis essential fatty acid. Unfortunately elaidic acid can't be used in our bodies the way essential fat is programmed for use. Worse, this pernicious trans fat competes for biological activity or, more accurately, cell-membrane placement with healthy linoleic acid. In effect, elaidic acid fails to activate the proper cellular activity and even blocks the entrance of the correct fat. This trans fat can be incorporated right into the cell membranes of neurons partaking in substandard brain activity, thus making the body vulnerable to cognitive disease (36, 37).

In Figure 11 we can see what these fats actually look like. Notice that the hydrogen atoms (H) sit on either side of the double bond in trans fat while they reside on the same side in the cis double bond. This equal distribution in trans fat is the unnatural force that makes the fat resemble the linear structure of saturated fat.

FIGURE 11:

CIS Fat Versus Trans Fat

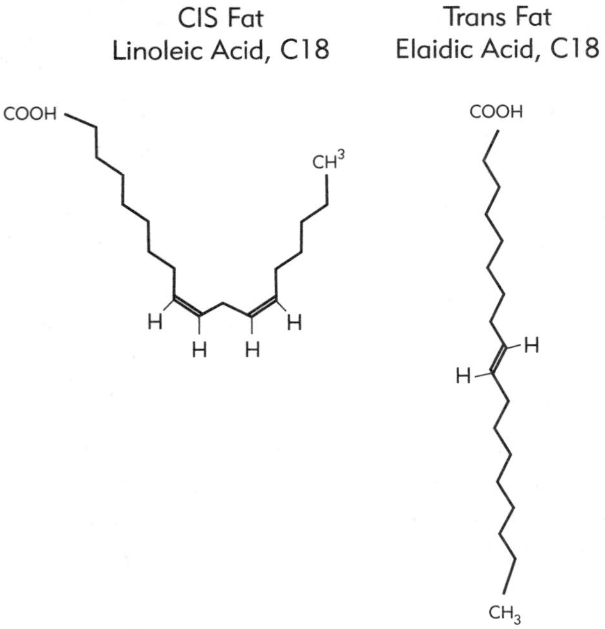

CIS Fat
Linoleic Acid, C18

Trans Fat
Elaidic Acid, C18

A diet that delivers an abundance of trans fats is typically limited in the right essential fats, allowing the former to make their way into the body without competition. Neurons depend immensely on omega-3 polyunsaturated fats. As much as dementia may be propagated by limitations in these fats, neurological performance can be severely impaired at a subclinical level to result in suboptimal cognition that may be accepted as a normal genetically programmed level of intelligence quotient (IQ). Add the compounding negative effect of the processed trans-fat-rich diet, and cognitive performance can decline even further. IQ is a function of many things, and diet is unequivocally a factor that can be controlled. Omega-3 fatty-acid supplementation is advocated in multiple sclerosis nutraceutical therapy. Fish-oil and plant-seed omega-3 fat supplementation in tandem with aggressive vitamin augmentation has been shown to ameliorate the condition (38, 39, 40).

Ageless Performance is a perfect therapeutic fit for such neurological disease, delivering multiple anti-inflammatory benefits, including the previously outlined protection from nitrite and nitrate assault. Other tissues that depend on higher concentrations of these special polyunsaturated fats, such as the heart muscle, testicles, and retina, are also more profoundly damaged by a trans-fat-rich diet and, conversely, more positively influenced by an active omega-3-enhanced diet—the Ageless Performance strategy.

If you're battling a cholesterol problem, you're just part of the trend killing many North Americans. The only viable solution is a healthy, supplemented diet combined with an active lifestyle.

ANTIBIOTICS CAUSE CARDIOVASCULAR DISEASE

The abundant use of antibiotics that you've likely applied frequently without second thought contributes to cholesterol anomalies more than you know. If you're like most North Americans, you're an unwitting subject of large-scale experimentation for antibiotic administration. One of the factors contributing to LDL cholesterol elevation is a loss of gut-friendly bacteria, which the inadvertent use of antibiotics obliterates. These symbiotic intestinal creatures convert dietary fiber into compounds called short-chain fatty acids, producing lignan enterolactone from lignan-fiber.

Lignan enterolactone and other fiber-derived fatty acids protect against various cancers and cardiovascular diseases, including LDL elevation. Studies show that blood levels of enterolactone can be significantly lower for regular users of antibiotics compared to nonusers (41). The reason for the diminished protection is the antibiotic-induced reduction in friendly intestinal microflora. With a compromised gut, microflora, supplements, or food-nutrient sources that depend on bacterial metabolism, such as fructo-oligosaccharides and lignans, can't deliver the expected health benefits.

In addition, gut microflora act as living obstructions to pathogens such as enterococcus and yeasts like Candida albicans (42, 43, 44). The common devastation of this bacterial flora in combination with dead, processed, fiber-scant foods is the likely cause of cholesterol disease, not to mention numerous other health problems. Fiber feeds this bacterial population; the LDL-regulating short-chain fatty acids (or volatile fatty acids, as they're often called) are merely a byproduct of this feeding. In fact, some cases of hypercholesterolemia (high blood cholesterol) were once treated with the shotgun approach of antibiotic administration—namely, the extensive application of neomycin—until the risks associated with such procedures were taken more seriously (45). The objective of this treatment was to rid the body of pathogenic bacteria, making room for friendly bacteria. However, this was only a temporary solution to the problem.

Now there are new facts that bring greater sense to the multiple-disease syndrome: hypercholesterolemia has been shown to interfere with nitric-oxide synthase in the endothelial cells, and independent research has demonstrated that it's likely caused by oxidized LDL (46, 47). This means that nitric-oxide production by the cells of our blood vessels can be impaired by high blood cholesterol, subsequently inducing elevated blood pressure—one reason these two conditions, hypertension and hypercho-lesterolemia, are often experienced concurrently. Nitric oxide is central to blood-pressure regulation. Furthermore, antioxidants prevent the oxidation of LDL and assist in the regulation of normal nitric-oxide activity to better control hypertension. Arginine supplements employed to enhance nitric-oxide production and reduce blood pressure can't function at the expected capacity unless nitric-oxide synthase (the enzyme responsible for producing nitric oxide from the amino acid arginine) is free of cholesterol's inhibitive influence.

Problems such as those mentioned above can be avoided if the body's immune system functions at full capacity to result in self-sufficiency, and Ageless Performance helps make that happen. The program incorporates these co-dependent synergies to decrease the risk of drug requirement. If the immune system fails and antibiotic use is required on an ongoing basis to treat, say, recurring infection, a secondary problem develops—the destruction of gut bacteria. However, the dilemma can be avoided if orally supplemented lactobacillus and bifidus bacteria are administered immedi-ately after terminating the antibiotic cycle, if antibiotics are absolutely required—integrated complementary medicine. Such treatment inoculates the gut with friendly bacteria, keeping pathogens at bay and protecting the body from cancers, hypertension, and cholesterol elevation. The sole cause of multiple anomalies is a failure to maintain a healthy immune system, including gut bacterial flora, but few, if any, health professionals ever see this.

So what's the common expert therapy for multiple disorders as outlined above? The likely mainstream medical solution is to administer more antibiotics and/or statin drugs to lower cholesterol—a drug for each symptom. But cholesterol-lowering statin drugs have recently been recognized by medical science as cardiac muscle busters. In other words, they deplete the heart muscle of coQ10, creating an environment for cardiac arrest (48). coQ10 is critical for the oxidative phosphorylation process in the mitochondria that produces energy for cell function. However, coQ10 is involved in much more than just energy production; it's a crucial participant in gene expression and antioxidant activity. It also protects aging hearts against stress (49). Deplete coQ10 and you're in trouble. Its supplementation is essential with statin use—another example of nutraceutical and pharmaceutical synergy.

More and more post-2000 research reports recommend coQ10 supplementation with statin use. However, since statins are used in the first place to reverse cardiovascular disease, doesn't it make sense to employ Ageless Performance to alleviate the need for the heart-buster (50)? It's clear that drugs aren't the long-term answer. They should only be used short-term while a program such as Ageless Performance pumps up a self-sufficient biological system.

Has your doctor ever talked to you about intestinal flora and a diet that's supportive of this symbiotic relationship? Probably not. Healthcare practitioners are overeducated in one area of expertise, but most don't have the knowledge to appreciate alternative or complementary approaches, so it's up to you to present them or find a doctor who knows how to apply them.

Your best solution to the cholesterol problem is polyunsaturated-fat supplementation (flaxseed and salmon oil concurrently), probiotic (acidophilus and bifidus bacteria) supplementation, the right food within which these precious bacteria can flourish (the prebiotic fructo-oligosaccharides, lignans, and other natural fibers), and a comprehensive antioxidant program (51). All of this must be supported by a natural, whole diet, and Ageless Performance accounts for all of these requirements.

BUTTER CAN BE BETTER

Produced from saturated animal fat and heavy in cholesterol, butter is still a healthier choice than hydrogenated vegetable spreads. First, the saturated fat in butter isn't all that bad. It's not the culprit manufacturers of margarine make it out to be. Butter is rich in butyric acid, a short-chain fatty acid with four carbons, which doesn't aggregate or clump up in the bloodstream the way long-chain saturated fatty acids do.

Say you bundled up 100 pieces of rope, with each section about 20 inches in length. Now tie up a second bundle of 100 pieces of rope. This second bundle, however, is made up of rope lengths that are only four inches. If these two quite different bundles were stored in the trunk of your car to roll and bump around for a month or two, the bundle of long rope would eventually become quite entangled. Now try to pick out individual strands from each bundle. The bundle of long rope represents long-chain saturated fats in your blood, and it's a clumpy mess. The bundle of short rope is the aggregate of short-chain fatty acids akin to the four-carbon chain of butter's butyric acid. Release the tie of the bundle and these four-inch pieces of rope fall apart and disperse with ease. Butter is a safe fat. The only real problem with it is that it delivers dietary cholesterol.

The risk that dietary cholesterol poses is usually caused by the body's inability to cope with it and not so much the dietary supply. Endogenously manufactured cholesterol is generally a bigger contributor to levels of systemically circulating cholesterol than the typical diet is. About 40% of the cholesterol in the average North American is of dietary origin. In fact, some studies show that even high-cholesterol diets only account for about 40% of circulating cholesterol. This means that well over 50% of circulating cholesterol comes from internal bioprocessing. Interestingly, just as insulin increases arachidonic-acid production from the essential fat, linoleic acid, it also stimulates the enzyme responsible for cholesterol production (52). Controlling insulin health helps downregulate cholesterol production automatically, and one of the primary functions of Ageless Performance is to enhance insulin efficiency to lower insulin output required for normal function.

Serum cholesterol regulation isn't that difficult. It starts with insulin control and this, too, involves the consumption of the right poly and monounsaturated fats. Garlic, whether in an oil extract or whole clove (three to four cloves per day), effectively reduces serum cholesterol and inhibits platelet aggregation or clotting (53). Why use drugs? There are many alternatives. Ageless Performance is likely all you'll need and you won't have to deal with the antisocial influence of garlic overconsumption.

If bread spreads are part of your dietary intake, here's a solution that might work for you. Although I do try to avoid the need for a bread spread, when I do use one, I employ my own concoction. I call it Heart Healthy Spread, and it can be used on much more than bread. Melt it on corn on the cob, pasta, rice, steamed vegetables, popcorn, and so on.

Heart Healthy Spread consists of fresh, organic extra virgin olive oil, flaxseed oil, and premelted butter. This homemade spread has a slightly different flavor than pure butter, but it tastes great. It's soft even after removal from the refrigerator; it melts instantly on warm toast; and it supports healthy blood fats, including cholesterol, functional cell-membrane lipids, cognition, and general metabolic health. And it only takes a few minutes to make!

Heart Healthy Spread contains relatively no trans fats and no artificial preservatives. The vitamin E that's added in conjunction with the inherent array of antioxidants supplied by the fresh olive oil will help protect the delicate polyunsaturated fats naturally.

Make enough to last your family four to five days to maintain freshness and ensure fatty-acid integrity. Keep the spread refrigerated as much as possible with the lid on the container. If you wish to omit one of the vegetable oils, change the recipe to include one-third premelted butter and two-thirds olive oil or flaxseed oil, then follow the above instructions. This will change the flavor of the spread. Enjoy and share the good news with your family members and friends!

Again, an occasional meal that consists of unhealthy factors is easily tolerated once your lifestyle is such that the majority of your meals are healthy. In other words, you don't have to lug around bins full of food to a celebration to eat the way you know is healthy. You can ask to have your meals specially prepared. Restaurants today are eager to take care of your individual requests.

HEART HEALTHY SPREAD

Find an oxygen-tight, opaque container. I use a little 125 ml or a 177 ml flat, square (1.5 inches high by 3.5 inches by 3.5 inches) Rubbermaid container. Make sure it seals tightly and that light can't penetrate it.

Measure the volume by eye:

1/3 organic extra virgin olive oil
1/3 cold-pressed organic flaxseed oil
1/3 premelted butter

Stir in a pinch of salt or two if your taste buds require a saltier spread. Omitting salt is a healthier solution. Another alternative is to use one pinch of potassium chloride (half salt) and a second pinch of sodium chloride (regular table salt). This will promote a healthier mineral balance to offset some of the biological influence from sodium chloride. Now stir in one or two drops of vitamin E, preferably alpha tocopherol. Just poke a hole in one of your vitamin E gel capsules and squeeze out what you need. Don't throw away the rest of the capsule's content; consume it immediately as your supplemental dose for the day. This vitamin E will help protect the polyunsaturated fats of the spread against oxidation. Snap the lid on tightly and place the container in the refrigerator. It solidifies within an hour.

When I eat out, I ask for a variety of lightly stir-fried or steamed vegetables and eliminate the pasta, rice, or potato that often comes with an oven-baked chicken breast or fish. In effect, I double or even triple the vegetable serving. Sometimes I just eat the meal as is. Start with a large salad, with the dressing on the side. Dilute the dressing with a little olive oil, water, and vinegar—they're usually right on the restaurant table. The healthy choices are easy to make if you know what they are and if you feel you're worth it. And believe me, you're worth every bit of health and joy, and Ageless Performance is for you!

10

FATS OF LIFE

The Ageless Performance strategy is a complex array of precursor nutrients, gene modulators, and biochemical navigators for these precursors. The system focuses on the metabolic pathway, which is central to cell-membrane integrity, hormone communication, and immune response. In order for the recommendations that follow to work according to plan, *complete* antioxidant protection must be in place. This involves the laying down of the foundation detailed in previous chapters. The essential fatty-acid precursors (primary starting building blocks) and the intermediates (the secondary building blocks that result from the processing of those precursors) that are produced from these essential fats (linoleic and linolenic acids) are extremely susceptible to oxidation or destruction.

These essential fats are quite delicate, and even exposure to oxygen can cause them to go bad or rancid. A body exposed to high degrees of oxidative stress whether from poor nutrition, emotional strain, and/or environmental toxicity can't maintain the integrity of these precursors, nor can it direct their healthy integration. The polyunsaturated fats our cells produce from these essentials have been elongated and further *desaturated* or *unsaturated* by the cell's bioprocessing and are even more susceptible to oxidation. Upon oxidation these fats themselves contribute to more oxidative stress, toxicity, and disease. The antioxidant program outlined in previous chapters has many levels of activity in the corrective strategy, and these antioxidants provide far more than mere protection for fat precursors and their products of biosynthesis.

Ageless Performance is a highly specialized program that protects the genes involved in the regulation of these polyunsaturated fats. Furthermore, it guides the expression of these genes to navigate the metabolic flow that rises out of these precursors. Many factors influence this genetic expression. Just as you may be genetically coded for a certain height but nourishment will play a huge role in how that code is expressed, a shortage of essential nutrients can result in a disabled thermogenic system, leading to body-fat storage from excess calories. Our diets are calorie-rich but nutrient-poor— a perfect prescription for fat accumulation. The same thing applies to the chemistry that regulates cardiovascular performance, cognitive health, and inflammatory status. Genes initiate these processes, but food and other lifestyle factors determine how, when, and to what degree the processes ensue. And as we've seen, you can control how, when, and to what degree your genes are expressed.

One of the gene systems central to Ageless Performance is involved in the production of enzymes (cyclo oxygenase or cox) that are engaged in the metabolism of dietary polyunsaturated fats (such as those from flaxseed oil) to hormone status. Maintaining optimal function of this system is the premise for powerful prevention and therapy as well as maximum athletic performance. Optimal function simply means letting the body do what it's genetically programmed to accomplish without free-radical interference, which includes meticulous *control* of nitric-oxide systems. However, optimal function isn't operation above maximum potential, for that state only results in biological damage in the long run.

GUIDING THE FLOW

Don't confuse DHA (docosahexaenoic acid) with DHEA (dehydroepiandrosterone—commonly known as the starting biochemical for the sex hormones estrogen and testosterone). A cell-membrane building block that contributes to the cell's elasticity, DHA is one of those fatty acids produced by our cells from the elongation and unsaturation of linolenic acid, the omega-3 fat we can supplement with flaxseed-oil supplementation. When our metabolisms are impaired, our cells can't efficiently manufacture (desaturate and elongate) these complex fats from the essential fats, so supplementation with flaxseed can be futile. The fish fats common on retail shelves contain DHA and EPA premade by fish in high concentrations. Our cells take these dietary fats and fit them into our biochemical works instead of manufacturing them from essential building blocks.

One of the more unsaturated of the polyunsaturated fats, DHA is highly electric and is therefore concentrated in the brain tissue and the synapses of our peripheral nerves. This electricity, however, contributes to its reactivity. If dietary DHA and the body's ability to produce it are limited, so is neural function; in other words, cognitive and motor function can be severely impaired by DHA restrictions, which include mood and emotional experiences. Supplementation with premade DHA and EPA such as the kind found in cold-water fish oils is a solution to this problem. A study performed at Ohio State University and reported in 2001 in the *Journal of Molecular Neuroscience* demonstrated that DHA deficiency is implicated in the pathogenesis of Alzheimer's disease, depression, and attention-deficit hyperactivity disorder (ADHD).

In fact, 2002 studies indicate that DHA supplementation *prevents* the onset of Alzheimer's in rats (1). In this study, rats' brains were infused with the precursors for amyloid plaques, which are responsible for Alzheimer's-associated brain damage. The animals presupplemented with DHA were protected from Alzheimer's development. These are facts that have been speculated on in the past but are being confirmed today by new windows into molecular science. A study done in 1987 demonstrated that DHA, DGLA (dihomo gamma linolenic acid), and serum essential fatty acids were low in hyperactive children (2). Another study reported in the *American Journal of Clinical Nutrition* in 2001 confirms this 1987 finding with stronger conclusiveness (3). DHA combats bipolar disorders, as well, but supplementation with it alone isn't the answer to the problem, nor are flaxseed and salmon oil. The protective and navigational characteristics of the antioxidant component of the program are extremely important factors supporting the correct bio-incorporation of fats.

A new source of marine oil that's entered the nutraceutical marketplace has shown tremendous potential. Krill oil seems to be one of the most complete polyunsaturated fat sources available in supplemental form. Although it's new and not that popular right now, krill oil has groundbreaking research behind it that will expose its powerful benefits and make it one of the most treasured therapeutic and preventive substances available. The only problem with krill is that it's quite expensive, which means it will likely only be part of essential and conditionally essential fatty-acid supplements on retail shelves in the near future. Nevertheless, the inclusion of krill oil in fat formulation is enormously valuable.

What makes krill oil so incredible is its naturally inherent phosphatide component, its high DHA and EPA content, and its healthy natural omega-9. The omega-3 fat in krill oil in proportion to the omega-6 fat is high—about 30 to 1—which makes it a great offset for the typical North American diet. The phosphatides in krill oil are the perfect food for the nervous system— the brain, the spinal cord, and the peripheral nerves—and they include healthy levels of phosphatidylserine, choline, ehtanolamine, and inositol. Omega-9, oleic acid, is the cardiovascular protective fat found in olive oil.

But that's not all. Krill oil contains an extremely potent antioxidant component built right into its natural profile. It's one of the first natural marine flavonoid antioxidants to be found with a protective potential that's far more powerful than that of common plant-derived carotenoids employed to quash the nasty peroxynitrite radical. What's more, krill oil's antioxidant value is surprisingly as much as 80 times greater than that of vitamin E. Not only is this unique antioxidant component protective of the fats it comes with, guarding them during processing and storage, it's been shown to deliver significant antioxidant protection for the entire body. That's the kind of synergy I've mentioned throughout this book. Krill oil contains natural vitamin E, as well, but it also delivers a naturally high dose of synergistic selenium and zinc. Whole krill oil is awesome stuff!

The probable reason many marine mammals like dolphins and whales have been able to develop advanced cognitive abilities is because of such rich sources of neural building blocks. My preferred oil combination for general prevention as well as a foundation for therapy of any kind includes krill—equal parts of molecular-distilled salmon oil, krill oil, and organic, cold-pressed flaxseed oil with the addition of some extra-extra virgin olive oil. The fatty acid and antioxidant activity of this combination is exceptional. The Biologic Nutritional Research Inc. Web site (*www.biologicnr.com*) describes krill oil and other nutraceuticals in more detail with supportive research documentation.

Interesting facts now link the deficient polyunsaturated-fat levels in the dysfunctional brains of ADHD cases with the similar activities and profiles found in those addicted to cocaine. A 2002 study released by the University of Kentucky's Department of Psychology found that cocaine users have an impairment in the cognitive system related to a behavioral-response mechanism similar to that of the ADHD-diagnosed child (4). In fact, in these two groups, cocaine users and ADHD sufferers, the ability to respond to signals seems to be a bit slower and this is thought to contribute to cocaine abuse. This serves as a model for general addictive, impulsive behavior. Fat supplementation of the sort I'm detailing hasn't been proven to aid the drug-addicted individual, but I believe it can help if it's administered correctly. Ageless Performance is the right application that will enhance the body's responsiveness to biochemical feedback, especially if these systems are significantly compromised. These feedback mechanisms alert us to stop the impulsive, addictive behavior before we cross the line.

Stored emotional issues contribute to the multifactorial addiction phenomenon, as well. Address each issue and the motivating factor for the addiction is easier to relieve; deal with one of the many issues and the battle is more difficult to overcome. Treat the emotional and dietary component of the phenomenon and it can be beaten. Do what most do and deal only with the behavioral symptom—the desire—that's a consequence of the deeper emotional and/or nutritional deficit and the addiction becomes a persistent battle and the desire never goes away completely.

Polyunsaturated fats, remember, are more susceptible to oxidative stress, which makes them more delicate than saturated fats. Because it's highly saturated, butter can be left on a counter without going rancid. The fat in it isn't vulnerable to the elements and free radicals. However, if flaxseed oil is exposed to air, light, heat, and free radicals, it will go off or become deactivated. The same applies to DHA- and EPA-rich fish oils. As described above, these fish-derived, extremely unsaturated polyunsaturated fats have even greater numbers of double bonds than essential fats. Again, double bonds are the points of "unsaturation," so to speak, and they're the factors that lend this kind of fat its greater electrical potential.

DHA is found in high concentrations in nerve tissue, cardiac muscle, and the retina of the eye. The greater quantity of these reactive fats in these tissues explains why the human nervous and cardiovascular systems are extremely vulnerable to disease as we get older. Our production of protective antioxidants declines with age, making these fats and the tissues they infuse abundantly most vulnerable. Brain tumors have much lower levels of tissue DHA (omega-3) and higher linoleic acid (omega-6) than the surrounding healthy tissue (5). Research in the past few years such as that evident in a 2002 U.K. study has unveiled powerful anti-cancer activity for omega-3 polyunsaturated-fat supplementation, including inhibition of breast cancer (6).

A deficiency of these special fats most readily causes disease in the tissues that are dependent on higher polyunsaturated-fat concentrations—the heart, neurons, retina, and testes. DHA and other polyunsaturated fats like it also constitute the membrane building blocks of every cell in the body, imparting electrical potential, flexibility, and hormone communication throughout. From these essential fats our cells eventually manufacture autocrine hormones. These are the eicosanoid-hormone messengers mentioned earlier—prostaglandins, prostacyclins, thromboxanes, and leukotrienes.

To reiterate, these specialized hormone molecules have a wide range of activity, including immune, inflammatory, cardiovascular, cognitive, and general metabolic influences. An imbalance of the essential fat precursors can result in off-kilter hormone response and subsequent disease. This disjointed cellular fat chemistry, as we've seen, can be a direct reflection of an imbalanced diet. Balancing the diet is the first step toward rectifying this problem; blocking the environmental toxicity that interferes with this chemistry is the second part of the solution.

Unlike the endocrine-hormone system, the autocrine influence is localized and short-lived. However, autocrine hormones are very powerful and usually more potent than their endocrine cousins such as insulin and thyroxine. The inflammation you might experience is a result of the combined activity of different autocrine hormones—in effect, a mix of the essential fat-derived hormones. A cell can release multiple autocrine hormones on an ongoing basis in response to persistent triggers. The chronic inflammation you might not be able to control is likely a result of the *wrong* combination and the *wrong* proportions of these hormones—proportions that stem from poor diet and/or environmental interference in the chemistry.

Whether it's pain, inflammation, blood clot, or asthma attack, the biological response is caused by multiples of specialized autocrine hormones. Cells are designed to produce in excess of 100 of these hormones in carefully planned, precisely balanced proportions. Some of these hormones oppose the activity of others, while some boost one another. These finely tuned chemicals produce a symphony of activity or self-regulation of the bodily systems in response to various stimuli. Self-regulation is impossible when the starting materials aren't available or when the chemistry is blocked. Essential-fat and other omega-3-fat supplements, such as the previously mentioned fish fats, deliver the precursors, and the complex antioxidant system of Ageless Performance stops the interference and navigates the precursors down their destined paths. Self-regulation, however, is only possible when all the vitamins and mineral co-factors for enzyme function are also provided abundantly in the diet.

Treating this imbalance is the corrective therapy. Treating the symptom of disease—the symptom of the imbalance—with our common drugs only masks the underlying problem. A disproportionate hormone release is often characterized by inflammation that spirals out of control. ASA and other NSAID administration is a good example of compensation for this eicosanoid-hormone imbalance.

Ongoing ASA administration to combat cardiovascular risks such as blood-clotting is also a need created by this imbalance. ASA blocks the excessive production of thromboxane, an eicosanoid hormone whose production can be limited naturally if we choose to do so. This natural correction isn't compensation for dysfunction the way ASA might be. The correction I'm referring to is the balance we're supposed to have in the first place, balance that can only be attained with a proper diet and a healthy lifestyle.

The need for ASA in our typical thermogenic, weight-management drug strategies is a requirement created by this same imbalance. The prostaglandin hormones that interfere with our natural ability to burn fat are a result of fatty-acid processing in cells gone awry. The same corrective balance that alleviates cardiovascular risks and chronic inflammation can help fix weight problems, too.

However, singular supplements are no more a corrective strategy than pharmaceutical symptomatic relief is. Gamma linolenic acid (GLA) supplementation with primrose or borage oils is a good example of how singular supplements just don't cut it. In fact, they can advance disease.

GLA FROM PRIMROSE OR BORAGE OIL

GLA is the special fatty acid we often supplement through primrose or borage oil. This fat fits right into the subject at hand. Insufficient cellular GLA levels are common among those suffering from biochemical imbalances that can lead to and are characteristic of diseases such as chronic inflammation, diseases of cognition like ADHD, and cardiovascular conditions such as hypertension (7, 8). GLA supplementation has even been shown to induce abrupt occlusion or blockage of the vessels that feed tumors (9, 10). In fact, a study as recent as 2002 performed in the Oncology Division at the University of Octubre in Madrid, Spain, revealed powerful synergistic value contributed by GLA when combined with the chemotherapeutic agent vinorelbine on the treatment of breast carcinoma. The cell-kill ability of the drug was greatly modulated by GLA, promoting tumor-cell chemosensitivity. The potential is tremendous, lowering the required toxic chemotherapeutic dose and term and, obviously, the associated side effects (11). An example, again, of powerful nutraceutical and pharmaceutical synergy that's irrefutable.

However, for general prevention I'm not certain that GLA supplementation is safe unless the fatty acid is taken with a complete strategy. It definitely shouldn't be used on its own. GLA deficiency in the cell is likely a result of the environmental and dietary interference with the natural processing of essential fats in our bodies. Although orthomolecular supplementation of GLA is effective against some diseases, day-to-day use can be hazardous.

In most cases GLA supplementation (borage or primrose oils) can fuel more disease if unhealthy dietary habits aren't changed at the same time the oil is administered. GLA is an omega-6 fat produced in our cells from linoleic acid, the essential fat that flaxseed oil can supply. We usually get more than the required share of linoleic acid from our North American diet. GLA can be converted into arachidonic acid in the cells, and an overconcentration of this latter substance has been implicated in the development of multiple diseases, including hyperinsulinemia, an oversecretion of insulin (12, 13, 14). In fact, the oxidation of arachidonic acid in the body is a culprit in the development of diabetes, based on the fact that it provokes unnecessary insulin secretion. Red meat and whole-fat dairy products are loaded with arachidonic acid. If you consume them abundantly and expose yourself to free-radical stress, you could be setting yourself up for a Type II diabetic state as well as pancreatic burnout, especially if the rest of your lifestyle is poor.

Primrose and borage oil supplements are commonly recommended to women suffering from pre-menstrual syndrome and symptoms of menopause. Again, this crude strategy fails to address the deeper problem that contributes to GLA deficiency in the cells, and it can add to a dangerous end result unless a complete program is applied. In order to prevent GLA's promotion of disease, precautionary measures must accompany primrose and borage supplementation, and very few formulations or advocates of GLA incorporate these critical protocols. If cellular processing of fatty acids functions according to evolutionary design, GLA supplementation isn't necessary at all. GLA isn't an essential fat, though many people refer to it as such.

A high-glycemic-index diet, one that rapidly pumps sugar into the blood and drives insulin way up, can interfere with GLA production from linoleic acid. The high-glycemic-index diet promotes hypertriglyceridemia, which is now known to obstruct the enzymes involved in the processing of essential fats, thus abetting the depletion of natural GLA levels in cells (15). Insulin resistance has been demonstrated conclusively in recent studies to impede severely the insulin-dependent activity of the desaturase enzymes involved in the bioprocessing of essential fats in cells (16). The typical North American diet is rich in arachidonic acid, is loaded with saturated fat, and is high in glycemic index, and it promotes insulin resistance. It's easy to see how the North American diet inflicts a multifaceted pounding on our bodies, desecrating the fatty-acid pathway and the hormone-communication system it's responsible for, advancing disease and biological age.

Supplemental GLA itself isn't a dangerous element, though; in fact, if it's processed in the body the way it's supposed to be, it can deliver impressive anti-inflammatory potential and cognitive support. A building block with powerful anti-inflammatory hormone activity, GLA is vital to neuron function via its induction of PGE$_1$ or Type 1 prostaglandins (17, 18, 19). In fact, studies demonstrate that there's a direct impairment of the metabolism of PGE$_1$ in the brain of schizophrenics along with reduced levels of both omega-3 and omega-6 fats. Supplementation of these deficient fats shows promising results for victims of schizophrenia but, again, GLA augmentation alone doesn't work and it's potentially harmful (20).

If GLA is converted by the dysfunctional metabolism to arachidonic acid, the imbalanced eicosanoid-hormone system is further exacerbated to increase the risk of production of hormones that clot blood, induce inflammation and pain, and block the ability to burn away body fat via thermogenesis. As GLA is shuttled away from the production of an anti-inflammatory hormone, it heads down the wrong path and creates more disease-instigating hormones. Cognitive disorder can also be further compromised in this way, and that's why the results from the administration of these GLA therapies are so hit-and-miss—some get nominal results but most get nothing positive out of the strategy and many provoke underlying danger. The upcoming schematic of this pathway clarifies these details.

If we all addressed the common biochemical imbalance that precedes eicosanoid-hormone output by our cells, the symptoms of disease that are so common today wouldn't require masking, and pharmaceutical sales would suffer significantly. That's a bitter pill these drug companies don't want to swallow. However, most of us do nothing to change this trend and seem to do everything just right to support the need for pharmaceutical symptomatic relief.

The association between a shortfall of cellular GLA and the prevalence of disease isn't groundbreaking news. GLA supplementation with primrose and borage oils has been widely advocated for years, but the limited success experienced with its administration is also quite typical.

Mineral deficiencies and imbalances that are quite common in the processed diet also result in impaired enzyme function and weakened polyunsaturated-fat metabolism. A proper diet and a complete nutrient supplement program are critical to a positive outcome from such therapeutic and preventive programs. The bottom line is that it doesn't matter how hard we try to correct these cellular imbalances with supplementation—

an unhealthy diet will force an unhealthy outcome from supplementation. Most of the time, luckily, supplementation amid a poor lifestyle only results in futility. However, GLA supplementation can promote disease.

There are certain precautionary measures we can take with GLA supplementation. Supplemental salmon oil slows down cellular production of arachidonic acid from GLA, thus protecting the body (21). Krill oil, with its high EPA content, does the same. Curcumin blocks gene/enzyme activity that produces inflammatory hormones, and this, too, prevents GLA from instigating a dire outcome. Grapeseed extract protects fats and obstructs inflammatory and other disease instigators. Supplemental alpha lipoic acid, like curcumin, guards the cells against incorrect GLA metabolism by impeding gene/enzyme activity (COX-specialized enzymes) that leads to inflammatory hormones. And supplemental protein stops GLA conversion to arachidonic acid by way of glucagon secretion. Dietary protein induces secretions of glucagon, a hormone that inhibits insulin secretion and desaturase activity (enzymes processing fats) that's insulin-dependent (22). Overall, a low-glycemic-index, high-protein diet blocks GLA conversion to the detrimental arachidonic acid via insulin down-regulation. These precautionary measures are critical preventive and therapeutic activity, and they're absolutely imperative if GLA is supplemented. They're the crux of Ageless Performance.

EXCESS INSULIN SECRETIONS— INFLAMMATION AND CARDIOVASCULAR DISEASE

Arachidonic acid is the precursor omega-6 fat for prostaglandins, prostacyclin, thromboxane, and leukotriene, the autocrine hormones that, when mismanaged, contribute to the development of our epidemic diseases. An imbalance of these hormones induces tissue responses such as clotting, inflammation, constriction of vessels and bronchial tubes, and the development of atherosclerosis and vessel blockages.

Independent studies have presented conflicting data about how insulin affects the balance of polyunsaturated fats and the related hormones in cells. Some research such as a study done at Cambridge University in England suggests that insulin doesn't have a direct effect on the enzymes that influence arachidonic-acid levels (23). This study indicates that fat uptake is altered to create a cellular imbalance that leads to a higher arachidonic-acid level in the cell from absorption of arachidonic acid that pools from dietary sources. The high arachidonic-acid levels can prompt a predisposition for disease. However, other studies such as one done in Sweden in 2000 point out that the metabolism of linoleic acid is disturbed when insulin resistance advances, impeding natural GLA production while speeding up other conversions that induce arachidonic-acid production in the cell (24). An Ohio State University study shows via in vivo human research that desaturase activity is insulin-dependent and that when too much insulin circulates the enzymes are overactive, again overproducing arachidonic acid in cells (25).

Other human studies confirm the activity found by Ohio State: that the conversion of DGLA to arachidonic acid is dose-dependent on insulin—the more insulin, the greater the rate of conversion (26, 27). What this means is that increased insulin causes more unnecessary inflammatory and blood-clotting hormones. This process occurs in Type II diabetic or insulin-resistant individuals—more insulin, more enzyme activity, more arachidonic acid from GLA and a greater predisposition for the associated diseases. It's easy to see how diabetes, or insulin resistance for that matter, contributes to the associated secondary diseases characterized by Syndrome X. It's easy to see how hazardous uncontrolled GLA supplementation can be.

Now let's have a look at the pathway we've been discussing.

Just as hormones are manufactured from the omega-6 fat, arachidonic acid, they're also produced from omega-3 fats like EPA (fish oils). Krill oil is abundant in EPA, as is salmon. Generally the hormones our cells make from omega-3 fats oppose the physiological effects of the omega-6-fat-derived hormones—the hormone influences from arachidonic acid. However, if everything works according to design in the cells, the omega-6 fats can be used to generate hormones that combat the inflammatory ones, as Figure 12 reveals.

Insulin resistance pushes the omega-6 essential fats to arachidonic-acid formation. As we age, insulin resistance can advance, which is another way we become more vulnerable to inflammation, cardiovascular disease, and accelerated biological aging. The Aspirin a day that might be needed to prevent heart disease blocks the production of harmful hormones such as PGE_2, derived from arachidonic acid, giving opposing hormones such as PGE_1 and even PGE_3 a chance to deliver balancing or counterregulatory influences.

As I've already mentioned, studies conclude that the refined, sugar-rich, high-glycemic-index North American diet advances frequent and excessive insulin secretion and, in due course, leads to insulin resistance and even diabetes. Insulin resistance is a common fact of life and a condition that contributes to overproduction of the PGE_2 hormones and to many diseases, but we don't have to submit to this biological vulnerability. We can do something to limit its advancement and the development of Type II diabetes. In fact, we can even reverse the damage that may have already occurred. By doing so we slow and even reverse biological aging.

Type II diabetes is essentially a progressed state of insulin resistance.

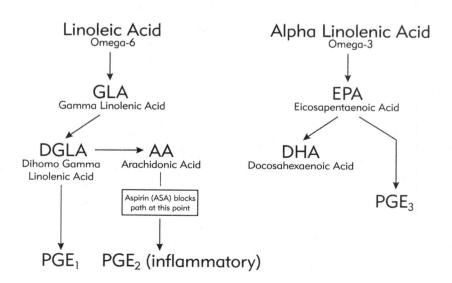

FIGURE 12:

Bioprocessing of Essential Fatty Acids in the Body

Linoleic Acid
Omega-6

GLA
Gamma Linolenic Acid

DGLA ⟶ AA
Dihomo Gamma   Arachidonic Acid
Linolenic Acid

Aspirin (ASA) blocks
path at this point

PGE_1 PGE_2 (inflammatory)

Alpha Linolenic Acid
Omega-3

EPA
Eicosapentaenoic Acid

DHA
Docosahexaenoic Acid

PGE_3

The higher insulin output that results from these conditions misdirects the essential fats to load cells in preparation for an outburst of inflammatory hormones. Now all that's needed is a trigger, and diet and environment can provide that, as well. Again, daily ASA in preventive protocols might be required because insulin accelerates the production of arachidonic acid from DGLA. Figure 12 clarifies this activity. At the same time the oxidative stress that this poor glucose regulation imparts also speeds up the enzyme activity that converts arachidonic acid to the *irritating* PGE$_2$, the Type 2 prostaglandin. This involves the free-radical activation of NF-kappa-B, the gene accelerator. All of this activity promotes uncontrollable inflammation. Aging is a function of inflammatory activity.

Many of the common nutraceutical supplements used as preventive or therapeutic agents in the health industry have a tremendous positive influence on the metabolic pathway essential fatty acids conduct themselves down. In other words, many of the common supplements support the balanced processing of eicosanoid hormones from essential fats, the fats we might get from supplemental flaxseed oil.

As much as one factor like alpha lipoic acid might have a positive influence, it can't provide all of its powerful therapeutic potential on insulin function and gene activity if the diet is full of interference. We must also supply abundant essential fats in the diet to get the metabolism rolling in the right direction, but even these two strategies alone can be pointless in a metabolism festering with inefficiency and disease. Curcumin, as we've seen, is a powerful protector of the genes involved in the regulation of these fats. Grapeseed extract plays a role in enzyme operation in this same fatty-acid pathway. Fish oils, bromelain, and the array of antioxidants described all converge on this pathway to improve the conditions for essential-fat metabolism or the processing of linoleic and linolenic acids in cells. Vanadyl sulfate may be a power-punch, insulin-improvement strategy required in the case of severe insulin resistance.

Apply all this together and systems will be set straight. Apply these supplements in part and the momentum of a dysfunctional system will be difficult to shift in the correct direction. Ageless Performance is designed as a potent therapy and an impermeable defense system. The program simply empowers your own intrinsic systems to do what they're supposed to do when they're free of self-imposed restrictions. The program is a comprehensive system that depends on its multifaceted design for potency. A missing factor results in a reduced preventive and therapeutic potency.

Studies show that excessive insulin secretions stimulate the enzyme nitric-oxide synthase, promoting excessive nitric-oxide production, as well. In fact, nitric-oxide-synthase activity is dependent on insulin; without insulin it doesn't produce nitric oxide (28). As much as oral arginine loading in an effort to pump up nitric-oxide levels in the cells lining the blood vessels is known to support blood-vessel health, including anti-clotting activity, if nitric oxide is left uncontrolled to react with free radicals, it gives rise to peroxynitrite radicals and disease. An example is the inflammatory effect of peroxynitrite in the gut (29). Earlier I mentioned that without antioxidant supplementation, arginine augmentation can be perilous. The potential for peroxynitrite production is the reason.

A 2002 study performed at the Cook County Hospital, Department of Medicine, in Chicago, Illinois, demonstrates how delicate this system is (30). This study clearly indicates the activity of resveratrol on carcinogenesis of the gut. Resveratrol, a powerful antioxidant phytochemical, is shown in this study to stimulate nitric-oxide synthase in the gastrointestinal tract to induce the production of *low levels* of nitric oxide. Low levels of nitric oxide are antioxidant in nature. The study confirms that this is the activity responsible for the protective and restorative effect on the gut mucosal cells by resveratrol, but it also illustrates that the phytochemical inhibits the development of reactive oxygen species or ROS, which causes the conversion of nitric oxide into the dangerous peroxynitrite radical. Resveratrol promotes nitric-oxide activity but also regulates it.

Peroxynitrite radicals motivate the activity of the COX enzyme, precipitating the conversion of arachidonic acid into inflammatory prostaglandins—the same prostaglandins and other eicosanoid hormones that may require daily doses of ASA as a blocker (31). Alpha lipoic acid and its newly produced analogues such as selenolipoic acid down-regulate nitric oxide, helping to control the potential ill effects of arginine overload (32). Glucagon, the hormone that dietary protein induces, was also shown in a recent study to down-regulate nitric oxide, aiding in the management of peroxynitrite activity in the cells of the pancreas (which secrete insulin) and protecting their longevity (33). Melatonin is an enhancer of insulin function and assists in the normalization of the activity of desaturase enzymes (34). Conjugated linoleic acid (CLA) is another common nutraceutical compound that, according to a 2002 study, down-regulates the production of PGE_2 and nitric oxide, reducing the risk of disease (35). All of these nutraceuticals applied together provide a powerful therapy strategy against disease and a complete biological preservation system. Combined they're potent; singularly they're weak. Partial use of the group will result in proportionally weakened therapy and prevention. The point is clear: therapy and prevention with nutraceuticals requires strategic programs.

SUMMARIZING THE FACTS: EPA AND DHA FROM FISH OILS

We've touched on the value of marine oils many times throughout this book, so let's look at this category with a little more focus. Fish is recognized today as a preferred protein source for more reasons than just the protein quality. Fish fat delivers a variety of the polyunsaturated fats that fit right into the chemistry discussed in previous pages.

Marine fats are different from flaxseed fats, but they, too, have a positive influence on the hormonal balance the body produces from linoleic and linolenic acids, the essential fats from flaxseed oil. The fish fats of value in most fish oils are eicosapentaenoic acid (EPA) and docosahexaenoic acid (DHA). These marine-source fats contribute to therapy and prevention in multiple ways.

A limited supply of EPA and DHA in the cell results in compromised membrane integrity and dysfunctional hormone communication. As we've seen, the EPA and DHA from marine oils are premade membrane components that, when supplemented, don't have to be manufactured from essential fats in our cells. They give our cells a bit of a head start with regard to maintenance and recovery of tissues when the diet supplies them abundantly. The fats from fish oils function with other polyunsaturated fats such as arachidonic acid as crucial structural components of cell membranes. In other words, they're building blocks for cells, just as individual bricks go together to make a wall. Previously we saw arachidonic acid described as a kind of bad guy supporting the production of hormones that can promote the symptoms of disease that are inflammatory in nature. However, just like DHA, arachidonic acid is an important building block for the construction of cell membranes, keeping them free-flowing and healthy. The problem arises when arachidonic acid (omega-6 fat) in these cells predominates over omega-3 fats such as DHA. Imbalance is the real problem, and not so much arachidonic acid's presence.

Since our diets are typically loaded with arachidonic acid and the components used to make it such as linoleic acid (omega-6 fat), a predisposition for the symptoms of disease is set in our cells. The typical North American diets tend to deliver an omega-6 to omega-3 fat ratio of more than 20 to 1. Furthermore, as I've already detailed, the processed diet fuels arachidonic-acid conversion into inflammatory and clot-producing hormones. This includes gene acceleration by free radicals.

However, these disease-promoting fat proportions can easily be changed with a diet that limits omega-6 fat sources and is supplemented with omega-3 fats. That's what Ageless Performance is about. This first corrective step is easy to apply by reducing consumption of red meats and high-fat dairy products, which in turn decreases the levels of incoming arachidonic acid and other omega-6 fats. Marine oils such as those from krill, salmon, and tuna supply an abundance of EPA and DHA. So the next step is to eat more wild seafood and supplement with these special marine-source fats (molecular-distilled versions only). These simple strategies will provide the desired adjustment in cellular balance.

Marine oils play an important role in this process as more than just building blocks for cell-membrane construction and hormone precursors. EPA and DHA from fish oil are farther along the desaturating pathway, which means they're more unsaturated than linolenic acid and therefore a lot more vulnerable to oxidation or destruction by free radicals, air exposure, heat, and light than linolenic acid from flaxseed is.

The consequence of this vulnerability is a greater need for antioxidants to protect these fats when we supplement marine oils. Since our membranes are fabricated from these very delicate fatty acids, they, too, are highly susceptible to degradation by free radicals and environmental toxicity.

Antioxidants, antioxidants, and more antioxidants are necessary to shield us from this scourge. I can't overstress enough the importance of antioxidants in Ageless Performance, and not just one element but the entire strategy. That's especially so after age 30.

If you're leading an active lifestyle, the accompanying oxidative damage in your body results in more frequent inflammation; you experience it as soreness, stiffness, and fatigue. The muscle tenderness that may develop over a few days after intense training or a full weekend of yard work is a result of this oxidative stress on the membranes of the muscle cells. Left uncontrolled, this cell damage accumulates and eventually causes irreparable harm.

We generally rely on anti-inflammatory drugs like Aspirin or Ibuprofen to pull us out of this misery when, in most cases, poor hormone balance was the cause and drug use simply blocks the overproduction of hormones. The healthier solution is better hormone balance and antioxidant protection. When you embark on that strenuous workload with balanced cell-membrane fats and a full antioxidant status, the pain and stiffness aren't likely to be as severe if at all noticeable. This indicates less oxidative stress on the body.

Let me remind you that inflammation occurs in our bodies at different levels. Subclinical levels of inflammation actually increase aging, which means if we maintain a state of fatty-acid and hormone imbalance in our cells, we might be supporting inflammatory activity we don't even feel. Depleted antioxidant status contributes to the same. Slowly but surely this activity prevents the body from functioning normally. The subclinical inflammation goes unnoticed until it shows up as premature wearing of cartilage and other connective tissues.

As I've already mentioned, DHA is especially concentrated in higher levels in the retina, the terminal ends of neurons at the presynaptic junctions, the heart, the testicles, and brain tissue. These tissues are involved in a profusion of activity. Here cell membranes must be highly malleable, supple, and electrically active. These tissues are also more vulnerable to oxidation because of the high polyunsaturated-fat content. They must be maintained in balance and protected from free radicals in order to maintain their normal activity and youthful biological age. It's clear why cognitive faculties, eyesight, heart, and sexual health decline rapidly with age. But they don't have to.

Scientists search high and low for drugs that can cure diseases that arise out of dysfunctional chemistry, and often all they come up with are "remedies" that merely provide symptomatic relief. I'm often told that consumers typically look for quick fixes, and the common pharmaceutical drugs do just that. We've accepted these quick fixes because they're readily available and they're acceptable. Fix the disease with one pill per day for one week, we're told. A simple solution, right? Wrong. Most often the short-term "remedy" becomes a long-term prescription. As we've seen, the simple solution doesn't derive from treating symptoms with prescription pills; it's achieved by changing our ways. Ageless Performance is that simple change—a dietary correction that promotes cellular balance and self-sufficiency.

Supplementation with omega-3 fats is critical to optimal health. The essential linolenic acid is required for obvious reasons, but the need for omega-3 fish fats like EPA and DHA isn't so obvious. In a sense, EPA and DHA from marine oils also help prime the fatty-acid system that manufactures eicosanoid hormones. In cases where the system isn't able to generate its required EPA and DHA, marine-oil supplementation, as we've seen, helps to meet the need so that hormones that oppose the arachidonic-acid-derived hormones can be produced from readily available EPA.

EPA delivers another powerful influence to this system. Interestingly the omega-6 and omega-3 fats of the pathway seen in Figure 12 use some of the same desaturase enzymes for intracellular processing. These enzymes, as their name indicates, desaturate the essential polyunsaturated fats linoleic and linolenic acids, making them more unsaturated and producing the subsequent fats. Since omega-6 fats compete against omega-3 fats for the same enzymes, an abundance of omega-6 fats can take opportunities away from omega-3 fats for conversion into their balancing hormones. This compounds the state of hormone imbalance. And, as we know, the common North American diet has an abundance of omega-6 fats.

However, if we supply more omega-3 linolenic acid and more EPA from fish oils, they'll use up desaturase enzyme activity so that it's less available for omega-6-fat processing and arachidonic-acid production (36, 37). This strategy not only limits arachidonic-acid production but leaves more GLA available for the manufacturing of PGE_1 anti-inflammatory hormones that also oppose some of the arachidonic-derived hormone activity. Marine-oil supplementation is a lot like the strategy used to fight forest fires in which a purposely set brushfire burns up the fuel that an approaching wildfire would have used to advance with. Once the wildfire reaches this deficient spot, it can't move forward. That's how EPA-rich salmon and krill oils work in synergy with GLA supplementation to make the latter safe and more effective.

Once more, the right marine fats are abundantly available from krill, salmon, tuna, and mackerel but, remember, consuming these fish after they've been cooked to death won't supply abundant levels of active DHA and EPA.

CLOSING FAT FACTS

Polyunsaturated fats, such as those found in supplements of flaxseed and fish oil, reduce blood viscosity; that is, they thin the blood by dispersing cells and reducing the risk of clotting (38, 39, 40). This dispersion effect is attributed in part to the fact that these unsaturated molecules tend to repel one another in the blood due to their electromagnetic energy patterns. However, studies confirm a powerful pharmacological activity in the chemistry of the platelets, the cells involved in the clotting mechanism.

Saturated fats, such as those abundant in beef, pork, and whole dairy products, tend to aggregate or clump together in the blood, producing thicker, more viscous blood when they're consumed frequently. The previously discussed polyunsaturated omega-6 fat, arachidonic acid, contributes to this bloody sludge in a different way. Arachidonic-acid accumulation, as I've clearly outlined, clots blood by supporting the biosynthesis of hormones—thromboxanes—that induce platelet aggregation and blood coagulation. Earlier we saw that magnesium deficiency can also result in platelet aggregation. Poor diet causes diseases in many ways, and magnesium deficiency, essential-fat shortages, insulin resistance, and excessive dietary saturated fat can all contribute to a cardiovascular problem cumulatively. The typical North American diet is a perfect prescription for this cumulative activity—a design for disease.

Omega-3 polyunsaturated fats, DHA, EPA, and alpha linolenic acid combat the diet-induced problem by first dispersing blood when they enter the bloodstream. This imposes an immediate effect. Second, these corrective fats help instill cellular fatty-acid balance to bolster the production of hormone balance, down-regulating thromboxane production from arachidonic acid.

I've used small amounts of Aspirin or ASA (20 to 25 mg two times daily) in a cyclic pattern in conjunction with high doses of blood-thinning marine oils. The objective for the ASA use in my case was to support a thermogenic program, and as we've seen, the 20 to 25 mg dose can act as a powerful antioxidant. Higher doses increase the common risks that ASA can deliver. However, I must caution you to be careful when combining these two strategies, especially when ASA is employed in high doses. Typical adult-dose ASA tablets contain more than 300 mg, with smaller baby-dose tablets delivering 80 mg.

Wound healing can be delayed if blood becomes too thin, and utilizing both an abundant dose of polyunsaturated-fat supplementation and a lot of ASA can excessively thin the blood. Bleeding time can be extended with the use of ASA, just as it can with the application of marine oils. One isn't more dangerous than the other. Combining the two strategies has a cumulative effect that can be unsafe. In my opinion the 20 mg daily ASA dose is more than enough for fat loss and prevention of inflammation and cardiovascular disease as long as the Ageless Performance strategy is applied concurrently to alleviate the side effects associated with excessive ASA.

The same precautions must be taken by people using other "blood thinners" such as Coumadin. Extreme polyunsaturated-fat supplementation can present a problem when used concurrently with the aforementioned prescription drug, which is no different than the fact that ASA therapy mustn't be employed inadvertently while on Coumadin. Furthermore, vitamin E supplementation *must* accompany polyunsaturated-fat augmentation as an antioxidant, but vitamin E can lower blood viscosity, as well.

If you're taking pharmaceutical anti-coagulants or anti-clotting drugs, make doubly sure your prescribing physician is aware of any adjunctive nutraceutical strategies you're applying. Most medical professionals will immediately insist you don't combine any nutraceutical supplement with a drug program. Their rationale is usually based on the fact that they don't know enough about nutraceuticals. Some health professionals might even advise against using a basic multi-vitamin/mineral formula. If your doctor suggests that a basic multi-vitamin/mineral isn't important and even advises against it, find an MD who has some knowledge of nutraceuticals, preferably one who has experience with alternative and complementary therapies.

These nutraceutical strategies help rectify the cause of our most common diseases. If you decide to stay on pharmaceutical drugs exclusively, you'll inevitably develop other diseases that you'll need more drugs for. ASA or any other pharmaceutical you might be using to combat these imbalances aren't acceptable alternatives to a self-sufficient metabolism. If you employ the right corrective nutraceutical program, you might never have to go back to using compensatory drugs. In addition, you'll prevent the development of other diseases that will arise from the same biochemical dysfunction that caused the first problem. The choice is easy to make.

Believe it or not, there are thousands of reported poisonings and even deaths in North America attributed to ASA and acetaminophen use each year, but no such occurrences have yet to be recorded resulting from marine-source or flaxseed oils (41, 42, 43, 44). We've already seen that N-acetyl cysteine, an amino acid nutraceutical, displays powerful protective and therapeutic activity against acetaminophen toxicity. In fact, it's one of the most effective antidotes known to medicine for the prevention of liver damage and death from acetaminophen overdose. Pre-exposure to grapeseed extract is also known to shield against this sort of toxicity (45). Prevention is the best cure.

On the other hand, in *small* doses ASA does reduce the risk of colon cancer, making it a preventive pharmaceutical (46). Studies indicate that a body depleted of intracellular glutathione is at a much higher risk of hepato-toxicity or liver poisoning from even suggested doses of acetaminophen (47). Ageless Performance is geared toward providing saturated levels of intracellular glutathione; it's structured to raise all antioxidant fronts to levels that protect cells from toxins that have been identified as silent killers; it's the only real hope for optimal health and fitness; and it's the most powerful and cost-effective health insurance you can employ.

About 70,000 deaths annually in Britain are attributed to paracetamol (British acetaminophen) toxicity. s-adenosyl-methionine, or SAMe, is also recognized as a safe and powerful detoxifier of acetaminophen toxicity and, as previously disclosed, it's also a valuable analgesic agent—as potent as Ibuprofen or piroxicam (48). So why use acetaminophen?

Wild-yam extract also appears to have tremendous protective influences on the liver and kidneys against such toxicity (49, 50). In fact, diosgenin, an active component of wild yam, has recently been shown to be a powerful cyclo oxygenase (cox) *promoter* in cancer cells. A 2001 study demonstrates that accelerated cox activity in carcinomas is responsible for an overproduction of PGE_2, thus poisoning the cancer cells to death. This cancer-specific activity is a lot like the previously described excessive PGE_2 production in healthy cells that poisons and impairs the body (51). But these strategies are most powerful when applied during early stages of disease, and this makes them most effective as preventive strategies because diagnosis that's early enough isn't common. If you're at risk, prevent the onset and apply the program at the end of this book. Are you willing to take the chance that you're not at risk? The odds are dead against you.

How is it possible that household pharmaceutical drugs like acetaminophen, ASA, and even statins (administered to lower cholesterol) make it into our health-care programs as *primary* strategies while nutraceuticals aren't recognized as therapeutic choices when they don't present the same dangers? The answer is easy. Pharmaceutical companies aren't going to make a case for nutraceuticals. So nutraceutical scientists must do what the pharmaceutical industry does: provide medical schools with the proper knowledge. And we must also collaborate with conventional medicine to make sure the two synergistic sciences don't remain separate.

Human health care encompasses the physical, mental, emotional, and spiritual, and the science that's most effective is the one that's preventive, not reactive. Ageless Performance is the preventive foundation of this science.

We must strive for a convergence of nutraceuticals and pharmaceuticals—one science, one focus, one system, a single human health care.

11

CLEARING THE PATH

Clearing the way through an overgrown forest can be an arduous task. Fallen trees, out-of-control bushes, ivy, and weeds can shut down a path in no time at all. Although the task can be laborious, once the path is cleaned up, maintaining it is quite easy with an occasional cutting back. The clearing of the biochemical pathway responsible for essential-fat metabolism is no different. Years of abuse and neglect result in path blockages, giving rise to unfamiliar detours that lead to mistaken destinations, the wrong hormones, and inevitable pathological conditions.

The tumultuous environment and limited nourishment that most of us are exposed to today require the application of an aggressive compensatory strategy even as a health-maintenance program. The degree of program intensity needed to regulate or heal disease depends entirely on the individual metabolic state and lifestyle you decide to lead, which includes the mental and emotional anguish *you decide* you'll impose on yourself.

Ageless Performance is much more than a preservation system. It takes its place in your cells during the course of natural tissue turnover, replacing old tissues with new, nutrient-rich, nutrient-balanced ones. Like a splint or a cast that holds a limb in place to ensure correct alignment during bone repair, Ageless Performance guides the correction of the biochemical paths that make up the body's metabolism, conducting the metabolic system toward the right alignment. This can't take place overnight; persistence and perseverance are important.

Regular or competitive training results in increased tissue turnover, incremental subclinical inflammation, and more oxidative stress than the kind a sedentary individual experiences. This requires that a more densely packed nourishment be made available for tissue reconstruction and metabolic-pathway maintenance. Ageless Performance fits the active individual's requirements, as well.

Don't think for a minute that anti-aging isn't your gig. Anti-aging isn't about living forever; it's about living life to the fullest for as long as possible, and that requires the ongoing maintenance of both mental and physical health. Getting older is a natural occurrence we all face, but there's no reason why you should allow your body to age unnaturally due to self-imposed metabolic restrictions. Ageless Performance removes these restrictions and replaces them with positive nutraceutical guidance.

Our bodies are on missions of perpetual turnover, and with each step they try to maintain their genetic codes' instructions. For the majority of us the programmed directive is optimal biological health. The physical outcome from our genes, however, is a function of the codes, the influences on these instructions, the nutrient building blocks available for transcription of the codes, and the environmental and dietary chemicals that form the downstream chemistry from them. If building-block nutrients are limited, genes can't produce their metabolic instructions. And according to the newest research, if the right nutrient keys aren't available to activate these codes, the genes become dormant. In addition, as we now know, the free-radical scalding delivered by our environment and food supply can also significantly manipulate gene instruction. Downstream chemistry can be impaired or rerouted by toxins and free radicals, as well. If the food supply doesn't provide the antidote antioxidants in requisite quantities to protect genes from the multiple influences, their codes can be altered at any point along the vast and complex stream of chemistry.

Traditions, customs, and other habits learned within the family can be maintained lifelong to mold biological chemistry and convey the same outcome day in and day out, generation after generation. For this reason similar characteristics are molded within you just as they are in your brothers, sisters, mother, father, grandparents, uncles, aunts, cousins, and so on. Not only do many in this familial group have comparable genetic characteristics, but they've all probably adopted common lifestyle habits that shape these analogous codes with shared chemical influences.

All you have to do to change the mutual outcome is remove the negative chemical consequences that might be factors in your life—your body will do the rest. Ageless Performance is designed to free the body from these bindings and release the genetic potential we were intended to experience. This built-in potential includes impressive physical healing, impermeable prevention, incredible mental health, potent immune-system activity, optimal metabolic efficiency, and outstanding athletic performance.

Keep in mind that an athlete resides somewhere inside you. Athletic ability was essential to our survival during the hunter-gatherer stage of our evolution, and within you today it pulsates with the need to perform. Physical activity/exercise is natural, but most of us have abandoned it while inducing unnatural events within our bodies that aid and abet disease. Although very little space is spent on exercise in this book, understand that it's an important part of any health-restoration and maintenance program and expect that your body and mind are begging for some sort of regular physical exercise. Only after you've become engaged and persisted for some time on a proper program will you realize just how valuable exercise really is.

If your state of imbalance today is severe, correction might require a full year of aggressive Ageless Performance administration. Clearance of the overgrown path will take a lot of time and many synergistic nutraceuticals, but once the way is cleared, maintenance will be easier and will take much less supplementation. Chronic disease is indicative of severe imbalance; Type II diabetes, arthritis, colitis, uncontrollable asthma, and cardiovascular disease are conditions of metabolic disarray. Very few cases of today's epidemics are caused by true genetic anomalies that can't be reversed. The likely case is that your condition can be undone but not overnight, and in chronic cases definitely not in one month. Be patient and persevere; results will eventually become apparent.

ANTI-AGING MEANS AGGRESSIVE PREVENTION

Anti-aging and preventive programs are in essence the same thing. The anti-aging strategy is essentially a more aggressive version of the basic preventive program. The aggressive nutraceutical supplement portion of Ageless Performance might be required indefinitely to prevent disease if your dietary habits include the regular consumption of processed and refined foods. The more mental and emotional strain and environmental and dietary chemical toxicity you impose, the more assertive the combative strategy has to be. Obviously the best strategy lies in limiting the negative influences while applying the positive nutraceutical guidance and protection—healthier dietary and other lifestyle habits in addition to the nutraceutical supplement program.

Mentally and emotionally stressful lifestyles aren't much different in terms of their taxation on the body than physically demanding lifestyles. Mental stress increases nutrient demands, but keep in mind that this *stress* factor is as much a function of the event itself as it is a part of how we deal with or internally process the *stressful* incidents in our lives. As I've outlined in previous chapters, we really do have control over how these episodes manifest themselves in our biochemistries.

A higher degree of contact with environmental toxicity—exposure to radiation, adhesives, plastic residues, fuel emissions, cigarette smoke, et cetera—will boost nutrient requirements and create a need for the entire aggressive corrective program on an ongoing basis. As much as these environmental poisons alter metabolic pathways to cause illness, they impair our inherent abilities to prevent and recover from disease.

Physically demanding lifestyles require the full, continual application of Ageless Performance. For those people who live relatively less-demanding lifestyles, the corrective period (six months or so) of the program may be followed by a reduced version of Ageless Performance to battle pathway disintegration. The aggressive corrective period can be repeated every six to eight months for a period of a month or so to top off nutrient stores and support insulin efficiency in case it has decreased. With the passing of years, remember, insulin efficiency declines, setting in motion imbalances that include damaging eicosanoid/autocrine hormone cascades. These hormonal problems also result in inferior nutrient absorption and metabolism, promoting nutrient depletion. I reset my insulin function approximately once or twice a year by administering a six- to 10-week cycle of vanadyl sulfate. I also take higher doses of many of the vitamins, minerals, and protein supplements during this period to help restore any partially depleted nutrient stores in my body. This total-body reset is part of my preventive protocol. People hitting their late thirties might require the same on a regular basis.

The dose-specific prioritized summaries in Chapters 6 and 15 contain fairly aggressive corrective strategies, though some diseases require a few additional specialized tactics, which are outlined in Chapter 16, "Condition-Specific Therapies." Apply the program at the level you're comfortable with. Use the prioritized tables to progress through the different levels of the program appropriately so as not to cause missing links in your strategy. Don't start the program by using supplements detailed in the tables without employing the entire array of supplements and protocols that precede the choice.

For example, don't use megadoses of curcumin without first addressing the issues that come before it such as the inclusion of a multi-vitamin/mineral and the elimination of the processed, high-glycemic-index diet. In this case there's no danger in skipping the protocols; curcumin's corrective activity will simply be impaired by the high-glycemic-index diet. If you begin to use a supplemental whey protein isolate daily without changing the diet from processed to whole, the corrective results and athletic performance won't be optimal. I suggest you use a multi-vitamin/mineral regardless of the type of diet you have. Understand, however, that this multi-vitamin/mineral formulation will do little for your body while it battles the turmoil caused by a processed diet.

The danger is in applying aggressive essential (flaxseed) and salmon (omega-3 DHA and EPA) or other marine oils without first laying down the foundation. This foundation includes the co-factor system supplied by the multi-vitamin/mineral; the removal of the high-glycemic-index diet's influence; and the application of appropriate navigational factors such as alpha lipoic acid, curcumin, supplemental protein, and other insulin augmentation such as chromium supplementation. Without these navigational factors, people who use these fats will experience little or no positive results, but some will manifest toxicity. This is the chemistry involved when researchers point to the dangers of polyunsaturated-fat supplementation. These fats aren't dangerous; they're as vital as oxygen to our cells. It's only that their deficiency doesn't result in death as quickly as oxygen depletion can. However, just as inadvertent doses of these electrically active fats can cause cell damage and even cell death, oxygen overload in a free-radical-saturated cell will also kill. With higher doses of the fats, extra vitamin E supplementation to enhance the multi-vitamin's payload of vitamin E will also be required as protection. Again, all of this information is clearly displayed in the prioritized summaries in Chapter 15.

If you can afford to do so, my recommendation is that you practice these corrective strategies indefinitely as an aggressive preventive or anti-aging program. Since we're not always aware of each and every environmental factor we're assailed by, it's wise to be prepared. We've read about the science that confirms that presaturation of the body with these protective strategies reduces and even prevents the damage, disease, and death associated with exposure to common poisons, even those toxins that might be required in the form of pharmaceutical drugs. Pharmaceuticals are typically composed of chemistry that's foreign to our universe. The application of the drug might be essential to immediate health one day if it hasn't already, but the pharmaceutical "medicine" usually imposes secondary strain on the body.

We don't know when we'll need this assistance and we don't know precisely how these side effects will influence us when trauma or surgery occurs. In fact, many of the new drugs, those introduced in the past few years, won't be properly assessed until they've been in the global market for as much as five or six years. Only then will the long-term effects be accurately determined; only then will we know the true implications of their use. So get on Ageless Performance and be prepared.

THE COMMON PATH TO RECOVERY

We've already discussed in detail the pathway that links our epidemics to a common root of biochemical origin. The evidence clearly reveals the reason why many of us can suffer from multiple disorders without resolution of any single one. These disorders are merely symptoms of underlying biochemical imbalance that we fail to identify and treat because we've been brainwashed to believe that the only possible action we can take is that of symptomatic relief.

When we choose to mask one symptom of this imbalance with drugs as in the case of chronic inflammation with corticosteroids, other conditions such as serum lipid anomalies like cholesterol elevation can develop. Soon after, blood pressure might rise, as well. Not too long after that, mental function could decline significantly and signs of diabetes might appear. These are symptoms that manifest themselves out of a common biochemical dysfunction, and insulin resistance and impaired essential fatty-acid metabolism is that shared root. Instead of addressing each sign of disease with multiple drugs, the common root can be fixed to eliminate all of these disorders in one clean sweep with Ageless Performance.

MALNUTRITION IN NORTH AMERICA

Emaciated to skeletal definition, the malnourished live a slow and unforgiving death. In North America, just as in Third World countries, people are dying from malnutrition, but the clinical symptoms are so different from those of developing-world cases that we fail to identify the underlying similarity.

Our food delivers more than sufficient macronutrients (protein, carbohydrate, and fat) and calories to overfill our adipocytes, or fat storage cells, and maintain minimum muscle mass. However, the typical North American diet severely lacks vital micronutrient essentials and is rife with damaged nutrients that result in metabolic impairment, disease, and death. Sounds like malnutrition, doesn't it?

Since every cell in the body relies on the common chemistry we've seen so far, they're influenced positively by Ageless Performance's multifaceted corrective strategy. However, the effect penetrates deeper than just the fatty-acid/hormone process. Although this system is crucially delicate and is most commonly afflicted by nutrient limitations and environmental toxicity, all of the other biochemical pathways that support life rely on the same indispensable nutrients. Even minute shortages, as we've seen, can result in profound metabolic havoc.

Just as your car can be equipped with the most expensive, highest performance engine and drive-train components, without a steering wheel you're in trouble. Stripped of rubber tires, you can't grip the full potential of the performance. The smallest, least complex factors play critical roles in this matrix of dependent systems. These smallest factors are missing in multiples in our modernized lives. Our First World malnourishment, the deficiencies in our North American countries, has a much different character than that found in the nations of our calorie-deprived Third World brothers and sisters. But the end result—death and disease—is remarkably similar, though the process toward the final outcome is more prolonged for us.

DEEPER INTO EICOSANOID HORMONES

Let's take a look at an extension of the metabolic pathway we've been examining to get a better understanding of the dynamics that ensue after the fats gain hormone status. Prostaglandins, as we've seen, are a category of eicosanoid hormones that are produced from these different fats. As previously discussed, there are various types of prostaglandins with varying degrees of the same activity, and there are completely different categories that exhibit quite dissimilar functions.

These assorted prostaglandins are categorized and identified as follows: PGA, PGB, PGE, PGF, PGG, PGH, and PGI. Subclasses of these categories further distinguish highly specialized activity (i.e., PGE_1, PGE_2, and PGE_3). Interestingly many of these prostaglandins are variations of previous ones in the same pathway. In other words, the production of one prostaglandin can depend entirely on the availability of its predecessor. Minute biochemical changes to this predecessor material can lend the new chemical a wholly distinct property.

The chemistry of emotional strain intensifies oxidative stress, which in turn accelerates the cyclo-oxygenase or COX enzyme, inducing the manufacturing of more inflammatory PGE_2 and clot-promoting thromboxane or TXA (1). This one-way stress can induce disease. If you study the prostaglandin processing in Figure 13, which follows, you'll see that PGF and PGI are actually made from PGE_2. If we were to block production of PGE_2, say, with aggressive ASA administration, we'd also arrest the creation of PGI and PGF.

In fact, megadoses of ASA inhibit COX (the enzyme that facilitates arachidonic-acid conversion to hormones), which itself hinders the production of all hormones in the path stemming from arachidonic acid. That's how anti-clotting activity from ASA administration occurs. However, this is also how drugs can cause damage in the body when used in high doses and for prolonged periods. For example, blocking these prostaglandins, say, with megadoses of ASA or other nonsteroidal anti-inflammatory drugs (NSAIDS) over time imbalances the entire system and harms the intestinal lining. These drugs can also injure the kidneys and liver. The kidneys depend on PGE_2 for normal function; impede it and these vital organs fail (2, 3).

That's why there's a variety of cox1 and cox2 inhibitors in the pharmaceutical industry today. cox2 drugs like Celecoxib are said to stop the production of prostaglandins and other eicosanoids in all tissues except for the gut and kidneys, sparing them from the blanket COX-inhibiting activity ASA might evoke. So, you say, selective COX inhibitors are safer drugs, right? Think again.

Research in 2001 demonstrated that these so-called newer and protective cox2 inhibitors still affect the kidneys negatively; now it's suggested they should be "prescribed with caution" until further investigation. By damaging the function of the kidneys, these drugs can actually induce hypertensive states, which abolishes the rationale that deemed the drugs innovatively superior. Yet the cox2 drug is still sold at a premium that far exceeds other anti-inflammatories such as Ibuprofen and Aspirin without the original scientific foundation the drug companies said they had.

The fact that the new cox2 drugs spared the gastrointestinal tract and kidneys was an amazing revelation that skyrocketed sales and made other anti-inflammatories such as ASA obsolete, since it and other older, more traditional drugs block COX activity throughout the body without specificity. Still, cox2 selective drugs might not be as effective as ASA in protecting against cardiovascular disease (4). After the new, more selective COX drugs were approved, and you and I were used as study subjects, it was discovered that the research relied on to approve or designate the drugs as newer and safer anti-inflammatories wasn't correct. Nevertheless, these drugs made it into the marketplace with claims of greater safety and are still perceived today as such.

So perhaps you think there's still a benefit in using a cox2 anti-inflammatory over a traditional anti-inflammatory like ASA because cox2 drugs don't negatively influence the gastrointestinal tract. Well, the research demonstrating the sparing of the gastrointestinal tract by cox2 is now being questioned, as well, because even more recent studies show that this *might* not be an accurate conclusion. A clutch of studies demonstrates that cox2 selective drugs do, in fact, interfere with ulcer healing (5, 6, 7). Keep in mind that impaired ulcer healing is different than ulcer induction. These studies and many more indicate that cox2 inhibitors *might be less likely* to cause gastrointestinal toxicity. However, the new research also shows that once gastrointestinal damage has been experienced, cox2 not only impairs recovery, it actually aggravates the condition. This implies there's a method of activity for cox2 that negatively influences the gut and that perhaps longer-term use will reveal the true nature of the drug. And guess who will be used in the long-term study? You and I, of course.

The immediately apparent problem is that most users of anti-inflammatories who employ cox2 because of previously experienced gastrotoxicity caused by traditional drugs expect the newer, more advanced selective cox2 to be safer. To their surprise, though, the damage is only made worse by cox2. My point should be very clear. Again, the preventive Ageless Performance program prepares the body with a self-sufficient chemistry that eliminates the need for these drugs and frees us from their consequences. This efficient chemistry also allows the body to recover from acute anti-inflammatory conditions with lower doses of drugs, if they're needed at all, and shorter terms of use, providing reduced incidence and intensity of side effects. Ageless Performance decreases the risk of becoming a test subject for the global pharmaceutical research network. The statistics collected by our medical practitioners are employed to assess the viability of new drugs in the real world. An unexpected reaction that we might have to a new drug can become a reason for banning the drug or using alternatives with lower risks. Ageless Performance makes sense: by balancing this complex system, life can become a completely new experience, and our chances of being turned into lab rats are lessened.

The following flow chart in Figure 13 discloses how other hormones are related in the pathway and how this "all or nothing," hormone-blocking

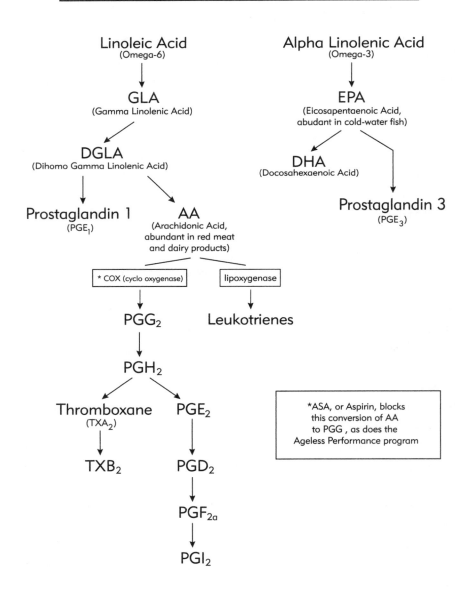

FIGURE 13:

Essential Fatty-Acid Conversion to Eicosanoid-Hormone Status

Linoleic Acid
(Omega-6)

Alpha Linolenic Acid
(Omega-3)

GLA
(Gamma Linolenic Acid)

EPA
(Eicosapentaenoic Acid,
abudant in cold-water fish)

DGLA
(Dihomo Gamma Linolenic Acid)

DHA
(Docosahexaenoic Acid)

Prostaglandin 1
(PGE_1)

AA
(Arachidonic Acid,
abundant in red meat
and dairy products)

Prostaglandin 3
(PGE_3)

* COX (cyclo oxygenase)   lipoxygenase

PGG_2 Leukotrienes

PGH_2

Thromboxane PGE_2
(TXA_2)

TXB_2 PGD_2

PGF_{2a}

PGI_2

*ASA, or Aspirin, blocks
this conversion of AA
to PGG , as does the
Ageless Performance program

effect can have profound consequences. The origins of thromboxane and leukotriene are made more apparent in the extension of this biochemical pathway, as well. Thromboxane, produced from the same precursor inflammatory PGE_2 is manufactured from, is the hormone compound that promotes platelet aggregation or blood coagulation. Leukotrienes are also created from arachidonic acid and are involved in asthmatic response. Notice how profound the overall effect of excessive ASA administration can be.

Earlier we saw that prostaglandin from the Type 2 series of autocrine hormones (PGE_2 from arachidonic acid) inhibits the activation of thermogenic brown fat cells, the cells that help us burn away excess dietary and body fat (8, 9). When our natural hormone chemistry tries to activate thermogenesis in response to a fat load in the blood from a meal, PGE_2 gets in the way and blocks activation. This, in fact, is where ASA in the common ECA stack (*E*phedrine, *C*affeine, *A*spirin formula) works its thermogenic potential.

Ephedrine has a noradrenergic effect on the neuron that controls or communicates with the fat-burning brown fat cell. This noradrenergic activity is the ability to induce secretions of noradrenalin, or norepinephrine, from the neuron. In essence, noradrenalin/norepinephrine contact on the brown fat cell membrane receptor is the signal that actually turns the brown fat cell on, stimulating thermogenic activity and triggering the natural fat furnaces. When fat accumulates in the blood, this very system is set off naturally—noradrenalin is secreted, activating the brown fat cell that chomps on fat and rids the body of excess calories from the meal as heat. PGE_2, the hormone most of us overproduce due to our North American lifestyles, blocks the neurotransmitter, noradrenalin, from contacting the brown fat cell. It competes with noradrenalin, and the brown fat cell never gets the signal to turn on the furnace. ASA simply impedes PGE_2 production to allow ephedrine (an active factor in the herb ephedra) to stimulate the brown fat cell on the surface through that norepinephrine secretion (9). Today ephedrine has been replaced in this common combination with a safer noradrenergic herb, citrus aurantium (CA). Caffeine supports the stimulation by blocking other inhibitive enzymes (phosphodiesterase) and promoting noradrenalin/norepinephrine activity inside the cell (10, 11, 12).

The multiple blocks in this system are why ephedrine doesn't work well on its own as a weight-loss agent. Caffeine must be made available to obstruct the phosphodiesterase enzyme. Then again the system is further enhanced by the addition of ASA, which blocks more than just PGE_2. Looking at the pathway in Figure 13 again, you'll notice the prostacyclin PGI_2. It, too, is a key component of fat-building activity (13). ASA prevents this prostacyclin from doing its accumulative work, as well. The over-production of these hormones makes fat loss difficult, causing us to work harder and calorie-deprive ourselves more than we have to. If weight management is your problem, this could very well be the chemistry you're battling. Ageless Performance makes that chemistry work in your favor. As a result, weight management is easy and almost effortless.

Studies have also demonstrated that nitric oxide is involved in the thermoregulation of brown adipose cells, which means this highly reactive nitrogen compound takes part in weight-management chemistry (14). Overactive nitric-oxide synthase, the enzyme that manufactures nitric

FIGURE 14:

Biochemical Activation of Thermogenesis

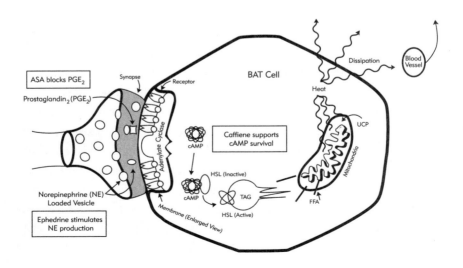

oxide from the amino acid arginine, interferes with the activation of brown fat and, as we get older, our bodies become less efficient in the control of nitric oxide. Maintaining nitric-oxide regulation helps our bodies manage fat, and the antioxidants used in Ageless Performance are crucial to this process. As we've seen, though, pumping up the body with the nitric-oxide precursor arginine isn't the key to a healthier metabolism. Arginine overload might be effective in handling blood pressure, but as we've already seen, other body tissues and processes are inversely affected by the incremental nitric oxide, including thermogenesis.

Nitric-oxide regulation is one of the keys to youthful biological function, and many of the nutraceuticals that are part of Ageless Performance help control nitric oxide. Pycnogenol (a pine-bark extract with similar activity to grapeseed extract) induces nitric-oxide production in nitric-oxide-deprived endothelial cells of blood vessels (15). This is the sort of nitric-oxide induction and site-specific elevation required for the healthy regulation of blood pressure. This strategy doesn't increase the nitric-oxide load throughout the body. Proanthocyanidins have also been shown to help down-regulate the conversion of arachidonic acid into the subsequent inflammatory, fat-promoting, blood-clotting hormones. Pycnogenol and/or grapeseed extract should be part of a daily supplement program for general protection. Ageless Performance includes this valuable preventive activity.

These potent natural extracts also assist in the down-regulation of lipoxygenase, the enzyme displayed in Figure 13 alongside cyclo oxygenase or cox. This additional activity apparently enhances asthmatic conditions (16). The aforementioned study, incidentally, further reveals that pycnogenol inhibits an enzyme called xanthine oxidase, which demonstrates its ability to down-regulate uric-acid accumulation and crystallization in joints, a problem characterizing gout. Folic acid is also a powerful xanthine-oxidase inhibitor. The anti-inflammatory and anti-xanthine-oxidase characteristics of pycnogenol, grapeseed extract, and folic acid make them vital in the battle against gout—500 to 800 mg of a standardized flavanol extract (pycnogenol and grapeseed) combined daily with 2 to 5 g of folic acid each day will do the trick. Ageless Performance has so many health benefits simply because it helps normalize biological operation.

PHARMACEUTICAL COMPENSATION WITH ASA: ANTI-AGING PROTOCOL?

Aspirin or ASA, as I've outlined previously, works its cardiovascular preventive wonders by blocking COX activity, therefore thwarting production of the pro-inflammatory PGE_2 and the clot-inducing thromboxane TXA_2 (17, 18). Acetaminophen, the active ingredient in Tylenol and other such pharmaceuticals, inhibits inflammation by retarding PGH (see Figure 13) activity (19). It's through this chemistry that these pharmaceutical substances have powerful analgesic, anti-inflammatory, fever-reducing, and cough-suppressing activity, as well. In pharmaceutical reference guides such as *The Compendium of Pharmaceuticals and Specialties*, ASA is said to "interfere with the production of prostaglandins in various organs and tissues through the acetylation of the enzyme cyclo oxygenase."

In other words, when COX is acetylated, it's inhibited and can't catalyze the conversion of arachidonic acid into eicosanoid hormones that we tend to overmanufacture when our diets are unhealthy and our metabolisms malfunction. However, chronic overproduction and imbalance of these hormones can be alleviated in most of us with a little lifestyle change, the essence of the Ageless Performance program. The twisted nature of this chemistry impairs the free flow of our preprogrammed genetic health. As a result, we require the chemistry-bending assistance of the pharmaceutical blockers described above.

The activity of ASA isn't the same as the natural salicylates found in herbs such as white willow bark and other herbal and food sources. In order for these natural salicylates to work the way ASA does, they must be acetylated, hence the name *acetyl*salicylic acid. Those thermogenesis-promoting, fat-busting stacks that include white willow bark instead of ASA with the common caffeine and ephedrine sources don't have the same effect as those that include ASA.

White willow bark salicylates can't acetylate COX the same way ASA can and therefore aren't able to arrest the activity similarly (20, 21). Interestingly studies have shown that ASA is metabolized eventually into salicylic acid in the body. The acetylsalicylate will acetylate COX, as we've seen, but the biochemical influence doesn't end there. Salicylates do induce COX inhibition, as well, but not nearly with the potency of ASA. So how does the salicylate work?

In post-2000 studies salicylates were shown to down-regulate NF-kappa-B activity (22). As noted earlier in this book, NF-kappa-B activity stimulates the genes that produce COX to promote the production of disease-instigating prostaglandins and thromboxanes. By inhibiting NF-kappa-B activity, COX-related gene activity is slowed down and COX activity is reduced, but through a different method than acetylation.

ASA displays two rounds of activity in this system at two different levels—COX inactivation (by acetylation of the enzyme) and reduced COX production (by decreasing gene activity). It's this NF-kappa-B down-regulation by white willow bark and other food sources of salicylates that provides milder anti-inflammatory activity but takes more time to induce than the more immediate inhibition by ASA acetylation. And it's this NF-kappa-B suppression that prompts me to advocate long-term use of low doses of ASA—20 to 25 mg daily. The NF-kappa-B inhibition by low-dose ASA administration, in particular the salicylate, is likely due to antioxidant activity on the NF-kappa-B complex that I mentioned earlier. In fact, studies have indicated that low-dose ASA can neutralize the hydroxyl radical in the biological system with much greater potency than ascorbic acid, glutathione, or cysteine (23). Antioxidants, as we know from the many studies previously cited, down-regulate NF-kappa-B, which is one way to maintain cellular health and biological age in a youthful state.

The prostaglandins we have to block in order to promote natural fat incineration are produced in extraordinary levels due to a metabolic imbalance that can exist at various levels in our bodies. This same imbalance causes chronic inflammation we can measure or feel, cardiovascular risks such as clotting that might or might not be apparent, but it also creates subclinical inflammation that we're not aware of that can promote acceler-ated aging if it's allowed to fester. Fix this common metabolic pathway and many health issues will miraculously rectify themselves and we can look and feel much younger. However, the reestablishment of balance might take a few months to instill and involves a lot more than low doses of ASA.

ASA's activity is very much like that of alpha lipoic acid except that the effect of the latter isn't as immediate as that of the former. As we've seen, alpha lipoic acid inhibits gene biosynthesis of cox by protecting the NF-kappa-b complex, as well. This is a similar activity to the above description of salicylates—the metabolized version of ASA.

Since the relative activity of alpha lipoic acid as well as natural salicylates is slower than ASA's inhibitive action on cox, healthy doses of alpha lipoic acid and other herbs with similar activity are required daily to *prevent* the momentum from reaching a state of overactivity for the cox enzyme. Once the momentum is in fast-forward, having gathered speed over decades, it's more difficult to pull back. This is the nature of the preventive system as opposed to the reactive one. The need to use pharmaceutical drugs is often essential because of the fast pace in which the unnatural biochemical momentum advances. Pharmaceuticals are designed to promote genetic correction and balanced hormone production, which take time to instill and persistence to maintain. On the other hand, the reactive symptomatic relief promulgated by megadoses of ASA and other NSAIDS can act quickly but doesn't inspire self-sufficiency.

Self-sufficiency certainly beats the many side effects we expose ourselves to with ongoing drug use. There are a host of adverse effects listed in *The Compendium of Pharmaceutical Specialties* even for Aspirin, including gastrointestinal bleeding, ulceration, nausea, vomiting, heartburn, hearing loss, liver damage, kidney impairment, and vertigo. The *Compendium* is a reference guide used by pharmacists and medical doctors. So would we find the nutraceutical recommendations mentioned in this book in the guide? Unfortunately, no.

The *Compendium* refers to metabolic pathways and the metabolites we've been exploring and describes prostaglandins as follows: "[they] are themselves powerful irritants and produce headaches and pain." This statement is incorrect, and it's disturbing that a health professional's guide would contain such a crude description of prostaglandins. These hormones aren't the irritating bad guys of the body. They're powerful regulatory eicosanoids that function within a delicate balance. Imbalance is the irritant.

As I've described, prostaglandins work in synergy with other hormones that enhance or oppose their cellular influence. When this system functions according to normal biological design, the total hormonal influence (in this case the autocrine effect) is a balanced response to a physical or chemical trigger. A mild inflammatory response, as opposed to a chronic, uncontrollable condition, for example, might be experienced for a short period when balance is in place.

Self-sufficiency of this system is paramount to longstanding health and maximum athletic performance. ASA megadoses of 350 mg or more per day must be used only when extreme measures are required and as a temporary Band-Aid to make life tolerable while the natural balance required for normal function is reinstituted by a comprehensive program such as Ageless Performance.

LEUKOTRIENE AND ASTHMA

If you look just right of the COX enzyme displayed in Figure 13, you'll notice the enzyme lipoxygenase, which is responsible for the synthesis of leukotriene hormones. Derived from the omega-6 fat arachidonic acid, leukotrienes have a potent influence on the cardiovascular system and are produced in varying types with different activities. This hormone generally constricts the smooth muscles of the skin and the respiratory, vascular, and intestinal systems (24, 25, 26). Leukotrienes are the chemicals responsible for clamping down on the respiratory tract during an asthma attack. The fatty-acid metabolism we've been so immersed in is highly involved in this system, as well. Regulation of this fatty-acid chemistry helps control the response to asthma triggers.

We've discussed eicosanoids such as prostaglandins and thromboxanes extensively, but we haven't looked at leukotrienes in detail yet. The same system that can result in thermogenic breakdown, chronic inflammation, and the choking of blood vessels takes part in the restriction of the body's air supply. The distinction between leukotrienes and prostaglandins, as Figure 13 indicates, is that a different enzyme produces the former, though they all come from the same cell-membrane precursor, arachidonic acid. Not only do leukotrienes have a constrictive influence on the bronchi, but they participate in the inflammatory response with prostaglandins and can also increase the clotting potential thromboxane induces by narrowing vessels (27, 28). Once again, we see another resolvable disease, in this case asthma, that's reached epidemic proportions for multiple compounding reasons, many of which are avoidable.

The omega-6-rich, omega-3-poor diet is one factor that contributes to the problem for causes already outlined. The increased level of air pollution is another of the more obvious factors involved in the higher frequency with which asthma presents itself. Our finite ecosystem can't cope with the incompatible compounds born from our technology, and today more than ever we're exposed to intolerable irritants through food, water, and air.

The trigger to an asthmatic response might be polluted air, mold, pollen, chemicals, dust mites, or dander, but the inability of the body to cope with the irritation can be caused by the biochemical predisposition infused in the cell by fatty-acid imbalance. As we've seen, Ageless Performance can help reestablish balance to this fatty-acid metabolism and reduce the severity of chronic asthma and even eliminate it in some cases. Relating asthma to a dietary influence is hard to accept, since it's more logically connected to air intake and the irritants found in the atmosphere. However, leukotriene production is associated with cellular levels and metabolism of arachidonic acid, firmly linking the response to diet.

Diet can lay down the foundation for asthma by hypersensitizing cells to the triggers. The problem might be that the body isn't prepared to deal with irritation with a response that's regulated. In the case of asthma, dietary-based corrective strategies don't normally provide immediate relief the way powerful drugs can. This also makes the concept of dietary correction difficult to accept as a solution. However, even with pharmaceutical regulation of asthma a two-part program constitutes the method of treatment: (1) a fast-acting broncho-dilating medication to provide immediate or acute relief from asthma attack, and (2) a long-term, slower-acting "control" medication. A corrective nutraceutical program *must* be part of this second, long-term control program. Ageless Performance helps reestablish the balance of membrane and cellular fats to aid in down-regulating the response to asthma triggers—both frequency and severity.

The key to long-term recovery from disease is to allow the body the opportunity to self-regulate these responses so that outside intervention isn't required. It's not possible, no matter how hard one tries, to emulate precisely the feedback systems of the human body. Timed insulin injections, broncho-dilators, and the administration of other hormones will never replace the biochemically regulated timing and feedback mechanisms the body is naturally equipped with. Regulation of these systems should be left as much as possible to nature, and the only way that's achievable is through an adequate supply of quality fuels, building blocks, and natural navigation systems. High-glycemic-index diets, which boost arachidonic-acid production, contribute to asthma attacks, as well. Stick to the low-glycemic-index strategies of Ageless Performance to decrease the intensity of this influence. Grapeseed extract also inhibits lipoxygenase, the enzyme responsible for leukotriene production. This activity reduces the intensity of the asthmatic response (29). As you can see, Ageless Performance covers a lot of ground.

As many as 10% of Canadians suffer from asthma—close to 3 million—and the numbers are rising fast. Unregulated asthma can lead to multiple additional health consequences, including death. But Ageless Performance allows us to manage this condition, letting us catch our breath.

Athletic performance relies considerably on these same systems in many ways. Regulation of inflammation can promote recovery from training and enhance the potential of competition intensity. The direction of broncho-activity is critical to performance potential. Maintaining a functional eicosanoid system helps optimize broncho-activity, increasing the possibilities for sport performance. In fact, hydration plays a huge role in broncho-regulation during intense exercise. Recent studies demonstrate that exercise-induced asthma or broncho-spasm is exacerbated by the drying out of the tracheal lining, which in turn advances the production of inflammatory histamines, leukotrienes, and prostanoids. By maintaining hydration throughout an event, especially one in which exposure to environmental pollution might be high, exercise-induced broncho-constriction is less severe and performance potential greater (30, 31).

Studies show that excess sodium-chloride (table-salt) consumption exacerbates exercise-induced asthma, diminishing performance potential in sport. However, dietary-salt restriction improves asthmatic conditions, shedding light on the *likely possibility* that excess sodium chloride also aggravates the asthmatic condition of the sedentary individual (32, 33).

Efficient broncho-regulation is an important factor in athletic performance whether asthma is a contending disease or not. Ageless Performance optimizes the oxygen flow for exceptional performance in this way, as well.

YOUR HEALTH IS IN YOUR HANDS

If you're on ongoing megadoses of ASA administration or other drugs such as corticosteroids for asthma regulation, you have to ask why it is that your body can't function normally without a crutch. What are you doing to maintain this crippled state? It's time to take charge of your health and make the changes required that will allow you to throw away the crutch that's disabling your entire biochemical framework.

As technology advances and time reveals the truth, many pharmaceutical drugs are shown to have serious side effects that necessitate the use of other drugs to relieve these secondary problems. Do side effects like lost libido, depression, and internal bleeding alarm you? They should. Synthetic chemicals aren't designed to fit into the bioenergetic scheme of life. You should avoid medical intervention as much as possible and allow your body to employ its miraculous systems—the genetically programmed potential within. More than 10,000 deaths each year in North America are attributed to medical errors.

I'm not saying that medical intervention is always a horrific experience. Many of us will require it to save our lives at one point or another. However, avoiding this trauma definitely results in a lower risk to overall health and involves leaving the healing of body and mind to a self-sufficient biological system. But if the biological system has gone awry, intervention becomes an alternative essentiality. That's right. Medical intervention is the alternative medicine; naturally induced self-sufficiency isn't alternative—it's primary care.

Colitis, Crohn's disease, arthritis, back pain, or other chronic inflammatory conditions might require prednisone for relief or survival. Advanced atherosclerosis, arteriosclerosis, and the risk of arterial occlusion require daily administration of megadoses of ASA to diminish the danger of death. These facts might be true, but lifestyle habits/choices can contribute to the problem in the first place, and in many cases they've exclusively led to the necessity of these drastic measures. You can also make the right choices with the information at hand.

In cases where disease has progressed to a debilitating stage, more of Ageless Performance should be administered, preferably the entire program, which is expanded on in upcoming pages. Whatever your choice, the solid foundation of a whole, fresh, balanced, low-glycemic-index diet must always be in place. The general diet will be detailed in the pages to come. The various condition- and goal-specific diets will be described in the last section of this book. I urge you to get yourself and your family on Ageless Performance. It will be a life-changing experience I hope you share with everyone you know.

12

THE GLYCEMIC FACTOR

You've seen how our food is much more than a source of building blocks and fuels. Each meal initiates a cascade of hormones that permeates every molecule of our bodies. You've seen how a meal can stimulate glucagon and insulin secretions and how they in turn influence other metabolic pathways.

The chemical cascade that involves the metabolism of essential fats is a small sample of the sort of activity that ensues when we eat something. Food is a powerful drug that affects the state of being, both physical and mental, with every mouthful. In fact, this druglike process forms addictions that often give rise to the need for common synthetic pharmaceutical drugs to counteract the ill effects.

If you're riddled with disease or simply can't get your health on the path you expect it to take, learn from the ordeal. Don't just continue doing what doesn't work. Set out in a new direction. This requires that you adopt a powerful role that involves far more than willpower, and if you're prepared to assume this life-changing step, a lot more positive shifts than better appetite control and efficient weight management will happen.

As we've read, emotional duress often triggers profound biochemical cascades in the body as well as in the brain. This chemistry results in bioenergetic anomalies that can seed many of our common diseases. These triggers have been shown to initiate neurological activity that results in behaviors we seldom realize stem from emotional roots. Binge eating is one such common conduct, but it's not much different than workaholism, alcohol and drug abuse, and many other obsessive behaviors. These compulsions are eventually accompanied by the influence of biochemical addictions that the chosen behavior delivers. The addiction is essentially relief from the underlying pain delivered by the powerful drug chemistry whether from food, nutraceuticals, or pharmaceuticals. The typical, uncontrolled binging with the convenience of processed foods promotes more biochemical disarray to propagate the dysfunction further. High-glycemic-index foods are powerful drugs.

We can make positive impacts in our lives by uncovering the deeply buried emotions that propel us to eat high-glycemic-index foods, to work fanatically, to numb pain with opiates, to have a drink, or to smoke a joint. That's right—we have to feel the emotional turmoil that lies deeper than the impulse that drives us to compulsive behaviors. Our cravings may simply be attempts to fill voids that are the result of a lack of self-love or other emotional issues. High-glycemic-index, processed foods are accepted drugs that can have as tight a hold on our minds and bodies and do as much damage as more conventional recreational drugs.

Fighting a carbohydrate or other drug addiction with willpower alone is frequently a losing battle because the underlying festering and nutritional depletion progress to unforgiving levels. Dealing with the cause of such emotional triggers is much like the biochemical correction of disease induced by the dietary and supplemental components of Ageless Performance. As we'll see in Chapter 14, "State of Mind Matters," this mindfulness of emotion can affect many aspects of our lives and play a huge role in the prevention of disease as well as foster relationship and confidence building.

Emotional duress might instigate our eating habits, but passively giving in to high-glycemic-index foods only further promotes biochemical confusion, which can exacerbate emotional duress, leading to a classic vicious circle. We can decide to apply a different method of nourishment to help break the cycle or address the emotional turmoil that fuels the need to feed uncontrollably from deep within. Either strategy will help us achieve our goals, but if we tackle both the emotional and the nutritive, the comprehensive strategy will be more positive in all aspects of our lives. For the rest of this chapter we'll focus on the nutritive strategy, while in Chapter 14 we'll concentrate on the emotional aspect in more detail.

Ageless Performance is designed to encourage the right nutrient navigation. It delivers the correct building blocks and fuels. Just as important, it prompts the necessary hormonal cascade, one that promotes a healthy direction for the nourishment of food. The glycemic factor plays a big part in the direction of nutrients to either support or derail maximum biological health and optimal athletic potential.

We've already touched on the nature of the glycemic index of foods and its influence on metabolic health. As I've already pointed out, the glycemic index is a value assigned to food based on its ability to raise blood-sugar levels. A high value indicates that upon consumption food can cause blood sugar to increase quickly and drastically, whereas low-glycemic-index nourishment unloads sugar into the bloodstream more slowly and in smaller quantities.

High-glycemic-index food elevates insulin—the sort of extraordinary secretions we have to avoid if we want to prevent disease. As we've seen, this insulin bombardment advances the development of premature insulin resistance, diabetes, and the related secondary diseases that characterize Syndrome X—in other words, cardiovascular disorders, dementia, chronic inflammation, obesity, and asthma.

Sports-nutrition companies rave about the insulinogenic, or insulin-secreting, potential of their formulations. An insulinogenic response is said to enhance the absorption rate of creatine and other nutrients by our cells. High-glycemic-index sugars such as dextrose and maltodextrin, and high-glycemic starches from processed potatoes and rice, are often added to creatine formulations to force the body to produce more insulin. But, of course, this can also promote more disease!

For years I've battled this trend. If you're into sports, this type of nourishment will only slow you down, despite hyped claims to the contrary. Certainly sugar-spiked creatine might be absorbed more rapidly, but insulin resistance is bound to set in if cells are frequently pounded with this load. Furthermore, with the advancement of this inefficiency, athletic performance eventually stagnates and even begins to decline. Age-related deterioration of performance is associated with insulin resistance. In fact, you might need that aggressive insulin spike from sugar when you take creatine only because you're already fighting insulin resistance, and persistent spiking will only worsen your condition. However, if you apply the proven insulin-efficiency-enhancing strategy of Ageless Performance instead of an insulin-secreting sugar load, your performance levels will be improved over the long term and without health consequences.

There is one time when these strategies are acceptable. These insulinogenic sports-nutrition strategies can facilitate nutrient absorption by cells and, if timed correctly, they'll support glycogen restoration of the body (i.e., the storage of energy). However, the right time to consume those high-glycemic, sugar-heavy, insulin-spiking sports supplements is immediately after a training session—and only then! We'll discuss these strategies in more detail later on.

Glycogen is the body's emergency source of stored carbohydrates. It accumulates primarily in the muscles, liver, and brain. The glycogen stockpiled intermuscularly is used as a readily available source of energy for physical work of the skeletal muscles. As much as liver stores are used to fuel liver activities, this glycogen is typically utilized to produce blood sugar in case levels drop too low to support the brain and other vital tissues. Since glycogen reserves are depleted during a bout of intense physical work, a sugar load from a meal is better tolerated by the body after exercise because it's used constructively to replenish intermuscular glycogen instead of accumulating in the blood to react uncontrollably. This regenerative process involves specialized enzymes called glycogen synthase, which actively pick up sugar from the blood to restore these stockpiles (1, 2).

The entire procedure helps to absorb the impact of high-glycemic-index meals; in fact, it actually buffers the insulinogenic effect of the sugar load, reducing the chemical strain on the body (3). By timing a sugary, high-glycemic meal appropriately, you can actually benefit the body instead of increasing its oxidative stress. But as with every other complex body system, glycogen-synthase activity depends on minerals and vitamins. If these mineral and vitamin co-factors and building blocks are deficient in your diet, your recovery from physical work, including sports, will be severely impaired. Minerals are essential to normal glucose regulation.

Supplementation with zinc, for example, can deliver insulinomimetic, or insulinlike, activity, and recent studies now demonstrate how this operates. Zinc supports glycogen-synthase activity through a complex network, and a shortage of the mineral simply reduces glycogen-restoration potential and sugar clearance from the blood (4). Magnesium is now recognized as a likely essential mineral for glycogen-synthase activity, as well (5). Minerals are crucial to glycogen repletion and therefore to optimal energy and power storage for sport. As we've seen time and again, complex biological human organisms require a comprehensive array of factors to drive metabolic function. Supply them all sufficiently and the body will perform according to design. Limit just one and the entire system begins to degrade very slowly. With the onset of this degeneration, pharmaceutical drug compensation might be required when all that's really needed is a more micronutrient-complete diet.

If creatine is part of your sports-nutrition program, consuming it immediately after a workout might alleviate the need for typical hyperinsulinogenic, or high-sugar/insulin-stimulating, formulations. Post-workout comsumption of creatine optimizes absorption potential to minimize the dose required for positive results. This strategy reduces the toxic potential of these sports products. Creatine, of course, is relatively nontoxic. What is poisonous is the added sugar.

Interestingly a recent study performed on rats at the University of Australia and released in April 2002 reveals that prolonged use of creatine in these animals did induce "abnormalities in pancreatic insulin secretion and changes in glucose homeostasis" (6). The doses used in the study were relatively hefty, and rats don't generally consume food that's rich in creatine, so this research might not be relevant to human applications. Nevertheless, as I do, you should avoid the sugar-loaded versions of creatine and, above all, make sure you supplement *after* a workout.

In fact, the post-exercise meal is recognized as critical to recovery from physical work, be it exercise or labor. Since muscles use their glycogen stores as fuel quite efficiently, maintaining these stockpiles is essential to performance potential whether you're a cyclist, runner, swimmer, bodybuilder, power lifter, soccer participant, or football player. This includes anyone who makes a living doing a physically demanding job. Again, research shows that the most effective means for replenishment of glycogen is consumption of the carbohydrate source immediately after the physical work is completed as opposed to several hours later. This is the same period when processed, high-glycemic-index food is better tolerated and can be safely eaten (7). Studies also demonstrate that protein in that same post-work meal further enhances glycogen restoration as well as muscle protein synthesis and tissue repair. This same research suggests that these strategies boost the potential of the subsequent work or workout session, as well, since the body has been fully reloaded for action once more (8).

UNDERSTANDING THE INDEX

Processed foods, being refined and devoid of fiber, tend to be higher in glycemic value (9, 10, 11). These foods should be avoided as much as possible and consumed only to help restore glycogen and tissue in the post-work opportunity or post-workout window. Eat these refined foods regularly and you're bound to accelerate the development of the insulin-resistant state, Type II diabetes, cholesterol problems, and serum-fat accumulation (12, 13). The low-glycemic-index diet is research-documented to reduce insulin secretions and induces a therapeutic effect on the condition of glucose intolerance/insulin resistance (14).

Exercise, even a daily brisk walk, plays a significant part in blood-sugar control. Not only does regular exercise stimulate blood-sugar clearance through the glycogen-synthase system, it actually promotes incorporation of glucose-transport sites in cell membranes. Studies show that the working body accommodates for its incremental energy requirement by recruiting more GLUT4 (one type of glucose transporter) within the cell membranes of the skeletal and heart muscles (15, 16). This actually means that glucose-transport systems are upgraded to a functional state by this process.

The Type II diabetic state is often characterized by a diminished quantity of GLUT4. Exercise helps reverse this condition and decrease the detrimental influence of the high-glycemic-index, processed diet North Americans have adopted as the norm. Our sedentary, computer-assisted lifestyles combined with our plastic foods are central to the pathology of our common epidemics. The preventive strategies, which include glycemic control, are summarized and incorporated into the final programs at the end of this book. Choosing to eat foods with lower glycemic values, say, below 60, promotes metabolic health. You'll get a small sample of these foods later in this chapter. A more complete list is included in Appendix A.

However, the glycemic index isn't as cut-and-dried as you might think. The glycemic value of a meal is actually a function of the entire mix and not any one food. Carrots and white potatoes, with a high rating of about 90, don't have the same insulinogenic impact when they're eaten with high-fiber, high-fat foods. Fiber and fat digest slowly and hold back the absorption potential that contributes to serum-glucose levels (17, 18). In addition, studies have indicated that monounsaturated fats, like the one found in olive oil, enhance blood-sugar tolerability by stimulating the secretion of a natural anti-diabetic hormone (glucagonlike peptide-1) within the body (19). Olive oil, added to a meal, helps buffer the negative influence of high-glycemic-index foods. My Heart Healthy Spread and Salad Dressing, whose recipes are found in Chapter 9, are a perfect fit for this strategy. Salmon-oil supplementation, in particular the DHA component of the oil, also supports healthy insulin function and enhances glucose tolerability. The right fats and fibers promote glucose control, and Ageless Performance is designed to deliver the appropriate fats and an abundance of healthy fiber.

Protein, as well, reduces the glycemic index of a meal by changing the pH in the gut. A lower pH (more acidic) slows the digestion of carbohydrates and therefore trims the glycemic index and insulinogenic potential of a meal (20). Carbohydrate-digesting enzymes (amylases) work best in an alkaline environment; they're inhibited by this lower pH.

You've likely experienced the sugar high that a processed, carbohydrate-only meal induces—one that's missing a protein source. If so, then you've likely felt the low that follows, which is caused by a decrease in blood sugar. Not too long after this lazy low, hunger pangs occur. If protein-laden nourishment is eaten with carbohydrate-rich food, you might not experience the hunger pangs that prompt you to eat too soon after a meal. The time between meals can be extended without loss of appetite control if a meal consists of high-biological-value protein combined with carbohydrates, especially if the latter is found in a low-glycemic-index food. Another factor that contributes to better blood-sugar and appetite control when dietary protein is consumed is the secretion of the hormone glucagon, which prevents blood sugar from falling too low as insulin pushes glucose out from the bloodstream into cells.

Dietary protein delivers a second beneficial characteristic to metabolic efficiency by inhibiting the effect that insulin has on arachidonic-acid production. Glucagon evokes a positive influence on fatty-acid metabolism, opposing the negative consequences of excessive insulin secretions. It also protects the insulin-secreting cells of the pancreas from nitric-oxide over-load, as recent studies have demonstrated. Ageless Performance bolsters insulin and blood-sugar health in many ways, and adequate dietary protein is a central component of the program.

Dieting strategies often involve fat elimination, and since most protein sources are relatively high in fat, it's common for protein intake to drop dramatically in a fat-reduced diet. The inevitable result of this strategy is an increased dietary carbohydrate intake to compensate for the required calories needed to get us through the day. Such protocols are perfect prescriptions for disease, and if this intake is processed and fiber-scant, the prognosis is likely to be even worse. These incomplete dietary habits send the appetite flailing out of control, making a restricted diet a hellish struggle. Such mental and emotional anguishes only add to the biochemical toxicity of the body.

GETTING INTO THE GLYCEMIC GROOVE

Ageless Performance isn't about severe restriction and elimination. The program doesn't require the complete exclusion of high-glycemic-index foods such as carrots, white pasta, white rice, turnips, beets, potatoes, many fruits, fruit juices, pastries, and breads. We can eat these foods, but only by correctly timing their consumption during the day. In addition, if serum-glucose regulation is already functioning normally, we'll have a *little* more freedom with high-glycemic-index foods. People battling insulin resistance or diabetes today, can take a little more fun-food freedom when correction is complete.

A food with a glycemic-index value of 100 is considered very high. Glucose is rated 100 and is used as a standard to measure the value of other foods. I consider any value over 67 to be high. A food with a rating of 60 or less is an acceptable low-glycemic-index food. A value less than 45 is considered very low.

Here are some specific examples of foods and their glycemic indexes. On the high side there are puffed rice (115+), Rice Krispies (110+), cornflakes (110+), dates (103), instant mashed potatoes (100+), maltodextrin (110), glucose (100, used as a standard), soda crackers (100), white bread (98), baked potatoes (95), apricots (94), raisins (93), carrots (90), whole-wheat bread (85, finely ground), boiled white rice (80), and ice cream (60 to 80, depending on fat content).

On the medium side there are rye pumpernickel bread (68), beets (65), yams (62), sweet potatoes (59), whole-wheat bread (57, stone ground), oranges (54), and green peas (50). And on the low side there are apples (49), whole-grain rye bread (42), navy beans (40), pinto beans (39), lentils (29), grapefruit (26), plums (24), cherries (23), and soybeans (20). A more complete list is available in Appendix A.

To prevent insulin resistance and diabetes from advancing prematurely, we need to stick to the foods in the medium and low categories as much as possible. When we consume foods from the high list, we have to combine them in the same meal with a much higher volume of low-category items. This strategy is critical to body-fat reduction and the prevention and reversal of insulin resistance and Type II diabetes. People contending with a diabetic state, cholesterol anomalies, hypertension, chronic inflammation, dementia and/or asthma, need to choose from the low-glycemic-index list for the larger portion of their diets until the problem is rectified or at least ameliorated.

The glycemic-index rating of foods on one list might differ slightly from another group, since many variables come into play. Don't get frustrated about the discrepancies that might exist from one professionals' list to another. We've read about many of these variability factors: variable fiber content, the pH of the food and the pH of the stomach at the time of assessment, the hidden protein content of the food, the nutrient status of the test subjects and their general state of insulin health, and the conditions in which the test was executed and the stress levels evoked by these conditions. Any or all of these factors can contribute to the different test results that account for the variations from one list to another. Aspects such as the degree of ripeness of fruits and some vegetables also dictate the level of glycemic or insulinogenic response. These issues can produce profound differences for one expert's results that aren't at all related to the findings another expert might tabulate.

In addition, foods can change dramatically when we alter them artificially. The sweetness of various fruits has been engineered to please our sugar-spoiled taste buds. This manipulation has transformed various genetic strains of apples, for example, to produce varieties that are sweeter. These modified apples contain so much more sugar that dental experts claim the consumption of them each day might actually promote caries. Worse, the same palatability factors will promote insulin resistance, accelerating the rate of biological aging and increasing the risk of disease.

Insulin resistance or pancreatic burnout isn't usually caused by the consumption of foods that have a high-glycemic-index rating in their natural state. Eating fruits and vegetables from the high category on a regular basis won't have the same detrimental effect as consuming processed, high-glycemic-index, nutrient-empty foods. Fruits and vegetables, even those with a high glycemic value, still deliver a healthy load of minerals and vitamins that support efficient metabolic function. However, once you've developed glucose intolerance or diabetes, even these natural, non-processed, high-glycemic-index foods will have a negative impact. The body just can't tolerate the mild strain once disease is active.

As we've seen, processed food is usually devoid of vital vitamins and minerals (chromium, zinc, and magnesium, for example), the co-factors that are essential for insulin production, efficiency, and other metabolic activities. Sulfur is another component lost during processing and it, too, is important for protein integrity and therefore insulin and receptor-site integrity. Many vitamins, including the Bs, are deactivated or removed from food during processing, and this also reduces our ability to metabolize carbohydrates, proteins, and fats. A processed food delivers a double whammy to the body—a sugar load that requires more insulin and a limitation of nutrients required for healthy insulin function—which compounds the overall problem and forces the body to pump out more insulin as compensation.

As fruit ripens, its sugar content can change to increase its glycemic-index value. Bananas are a good example. A green banana can have a glycemic index as low as 56 while a ripe one can reach as high as 90. Fruit juices usually have quite high glycemic ratings, and contrary to common belief, vegetable juices—carrot and beet in particular—do, too.

Juicing has become popular as advocates claim the vitamin, mineral, and phytonutrient levels are high in these extracts. And they're right: juicing is an excellent way to get a concentrated load of nutrients, but there are two factors about this practice that worry me. One is that these juices can also contain concentrates of the pesticide chemicals that were applied to cultivate the produce. As you'll see in the last chapter of this book, some of these pesticides actually raise the glycemic potential of food by stimulating the transport systems for glucose in the gut. This negative aspect can be limited by using organic produce. The other problem is the absence of vitally important fiber.

In their whole state, fruits and vegetables slowly release their carbohydrate content as the digestive process works through the fiber matrix to get to the carbohydrates. This slows the rate of carbohydrate digestion and absorption, reducing the glycemic-index value of the whole, intact food. Juicing removes this rate-reducing component and increases the glycemic score of the inherent carbohydrates. In addition, fiber provides a wide array of vital biochemicals such as lignins, phytic acid, pectins, amylopectins, and more. In the typical juicing process these beneficial constituents are eliminated, and gut bacteria, liver health, and immune-system potential can all be negatively affected.

However, juicing can be extremely beneficial during bouts with gastrointestinal disorders like peptic ulcers, colitis, Crohn's disease, or other inflammatory gastrointestinal disorders, including cancer. Selecting juices that don't have high-glycemic values is important. Combining a high-glycemic-index vegetable juice like carrot with a low one such as cabbage is also a good practice. In the case of gastrointestinal disease, especially therapeutic are the juices that contain an abundance of cabbage and broccoli in an amount surpassing a liter a day (21, 22). Delivering these phytonutrient benefits and the concentrated vitamins and minerals in this extracted form allows for nourishment to reach needy cells in the absence of fiber that might irritate an inflamed gastrointestinal tract. After disease goes into remission, however, this vital fiber must be reintroduced at a slow, incremental rate and, of course, an oral probiotic inoculation must be applied as outlined in previous chapters and described in more detail later in this book.

A WORD ABOUT SUGARS

In addition to the natural insulin-supportive co-factors (vitamins, minerals, and phytonutrients) supplied by a whole-carbohydrate source, the type of carbohydrate delivered by a food is a major element influencing the glycemic index. Sources of glucose, for example, usually have high-glycemic-index values. Grapes are naturally sweetened with glucose, and as noted previously, glucose is used to set the standard for the glycemic index. The value for pure glucose is 100. However, the glycemic-index rating for grapes, which are naturally sweetened with glucose, is about 45. Fiber and natural acids change the overall score of the grape's glucose content.

Dietary sugars of all types can only become biologically active as energy sources after they've been converted to glucose in our bodies, since our cells are designed to use glucose as carbohydrate energy sources *almost exclusively*. Food sources that are naturally elevated in glucose or have glucose added to them as sweetening agents generally have high-glycemic-index ratings.

Absorbed actively in the gut, glucose is assimilated through transport sites that function by way of a pump mechanism requiring ATP (energy molecule) and sodium (23, 24). This fast-pace absorption in addition to the fact that no metabolism is required to convert this carbohydrate into a usable source for cells contributes to the glycemic-index or serum-glucose spike from this sugar type and ultimately the consequential insulin elevation. We've seen in previous chapters how the body reacts to extremely high levels of blood sugar and insulin. These excessive levels are toxic and can be converted by the body into fat to alleviate the toxicity they present. If we keep pumping up that blood sugar and serum fat, our cholesterol and body-fat stores are sure to climb to unhealthy highs.

Glucose is referred to as a simple sugar or a monosaccharide, but not all single-molecule sugars have a high-glycemic-index value. Fructose, for example, is a monosaccharide, as well, but before it can influence blood-sugar levels it must be converted to glucose. This conversion delay, along with the relatively slower absorption of fructose from the gut, reduces the rate in which blood sugar rises as a consequence of fructose ingestion. Fructose is abundant in fruit and has a glycemic value of 23 as opposed to the 100 rating of glucose. Although fructose scores low on the glycemic index, it still delivers health consequences if overconsumed for prolonged periods. It induces hyperlipidemia or high blood fat (25).

The sweet tooth many of us have adopted is the problem, but it's a predicament that can be solved when we know which foods are safe. Once you have the list of foods you can eat, don't bring those that are harmful into your home. Leave them on the grocery-store shelf. That simple rule will help keep these addictive foods and early-onset insulin resistance out of your life.

A disaccharide has two simple sugars biochemically linked. Sucrose (table sugar) is a disaccharide and has a glycemic rating of about 65. Sucrose is made up of one molecule of fructose and another molecule of glucose. These molecules are tightly connected and must be separated before the glucose component of the sugar can enter the bloodstream for cellular uptake. In addition, the fructose component of sucrose must undergo that transformation to glucose before it can contribute to the glucose spike. Sucrose is still considered high on the glycemic index, and I don't have to tell you that it's toxic to the body in many ways. Recent studies have measured the free-radical load caused by sucrose consumption, and the conclusion is that even short-term use promotes significant oxidative stress on the heart and other tissues (26, 27). Once you understand the biochemical nature of sugar sources, you'll comprehend more about the varying glycemic-index values of foods.

NOT ALL CARBOHYDRATES ARE CREATED EQUAL

Starches are complex carbohydrates, but that doesn't mean they have low-glycemic ratings. Bread, for example, is made up of complex carbohydrates and, if added, some simple carbohydrates, as well. The breads we've adopted as common staples are high-glycemic-index foods. However, different breads display different glycemic-index values.

Most whole-wheat breads, believe it or not, are just slightly under 70, which isn't much different from the value of white bread. However, an extremely refined white bread can reach as high as 100 on the glycemic scale because the grains in it are usually ground down before being used. The finer the grinding, the higher the glycemic rating. Generally excessively refined breads or sugars, complex or not, are higher in glycemic-index value than less-refined ones, and if you think about the digestive process, this makes a lot of sense.

Grinding to a fine particle size increases the surface area of the food source and allows for more thorough enzyme digestion and rapid absorption. Whole-wheat bread that isn't ground so finely (stone-ground whole wheat, for example) can have a glycemic-index value of about 50 to 55. Whole-grain pumpernickel rye can even have a lower rating than stone-ground whole wheat. When whole-rye bread is made with no refined flours and no added molasses or sweetening agents, it's the bread to stick with if you must eat the stuff at all, since its glycemic-index value is between 40 and 50. My favorite bread contains whole, sprouted rye kernels with a bit of stone-ground whole-wheat flour devoid of added sugars and refined carbohydrates.

Dried-up rice puffs (the kind found in cereals or rice cakes) can exceed 100 on the glycemic-index scale. Yes, those rice cakes you might be munching on religiously aren't healthy foods! They'll just make weight loss more difficult unless the only time you eat them is right after an exercise session. A potato can have a glycemic-index value of more than 90, but with added fat such as in the common potato chip or french fry, the rating can drop to as low as 54 and 75 respectively.

Maltodextrin has made it into powdered-supplement drink mixes as a common carbohydrate source. It's essentially a glucose polymer, a chain of glucose units that delivers a concentrated carbohydrate load. In fact, so concentrated is this load that the glycemic index of maltodextrin is higher than that of glucose. Our digestive enzymes have easy access to the linear chain of glucose units in maltodextrin; digestion of maltodextrin is rapid as is absorption of the assimilated glucose units. Maltodextrin supplementation is definitely not conducive to healthy weight management, nor is it appropriate if chronic disease is a factor. The only time maltodextrin is recommended is immediately after intense physical exercise to help restore and build glycogen stores and muscle mass.

GAMBLING WITH GLYCERINE

Glycerine is another factor rarely recognized as a contributor to the glycemic index of food and, just like maltodextrin, it has made it into the nutraceutical industry in a big way. Ironically the increased use of glycerine or glycerol is in response to consumer demand for low-carbohydrate supplements. The call for low-carbohydrate supplements is justified in that the abundance of processed, high-glycemic-index foods is now recognized as a major cause of the common North American diseases. However, glycerine in place of carbohydrates isn't the solution, and those of you who are buying the low-carbohydrate claims for nutritional bars are literally eating up the glycemic blast from glycerine. The nutritional-bar industry is most guilty of this shell game that replaces carbohydrates with glycerine.

To produce a low-carbohydrate bar that's palatable and maintains a viable shelf life, glycerine must be included in the formulation, and usually the lower the carbohydrate content, the higher the glycerine level. A bar, for example, that has a higher protein level (the more recent protein bars in the health industry) tends to become hard and lose flavor in a shorter period of time than a bar with a lower protein content and a higher carbohydrate count. The typical high-protein, low-carbohydrate bar has a shorter shelf life, which presents a high risk of profit loss for manufacturers.

Glycerine, however, tends to bolster the moisture content of a nutritional bar while contributing to its sweetness. As much as 60% as sweet as cane sugar, glycerine has an energy or calorie potential almost 20% greater than a carbohydrate—4.57 versus 3.87 calories per gram respectively. A bar can contain more than 20 g of glycerine that might not ever make it into the carbohydrate calorie count of the product. However, glycerine *will* become a factor in the carbohydrate load and calorie deposition of your body. A bar that claims to have 160 calories but fails to disclose its glycerine content in the macronutrient profile is hiding an extra 100 calories!

The essence of this shell game is that glycerine is difficult to categorize as a macronutrient (fats, carbohydrates, proteins). Glycerine isn't a typical carbohydrate, it's not a fat, and it's not a protein. It's actually one component of the triacylglyceride (fat) molecule. In Canada and the United States, glycerine probably hasn't shown up in any of the macronutrient categories of the nutrition information on the wrappers of many nutritional bars, since Health Canada has only just recently forced manufacturers to include it in the carbohydrate listing.

In the past, manufacturers could label a bar with a carbohydrate content of 4 g and even 2 g and include a healthy dose of protein as high as 30 g per bar, but the 20 g or more of glycerine never made it into the count. If you're wondering why you can't shed those last few pounds, this might be the reason. The carbohydrate content is more likely to be 20 to 30 g per bar. Maltitol and xylitol are similar alcohol-sugars often included in such formulations to add palatability, but they, too, aren't included in the final carbohydrate value of the nutritional information. Bars with this sort of misleading labeling are still found in Canada and the United States as the governments try to phase them out. Keep in mind that glycerine adds to the glycemic potential of a food as well as to the carbohydrate count. The confusion arises because of the delayed increase in blood sugar caused by glycerine consumption, a characteristic of low-glycemic-index sugars. However, the load into the bloodstream accumulates rapidly later and the body eventually has to deal with it. Professionals are reluctant to assign a glycemic-index value to glycerine for this reason.

Make a note of the ingredients list of your favorite bar. Glycerine frequently has the highest concentration. It's usually the first thing on the list because each ingredient must be noted in descending order of concentration. However, the common trick used by manufacturers to deliver a different perception is to bundle up the protein sources such as casein, egg albumin, soy, and whey as one general category. When all of these protein sources are gathered together and placed in parentheses, they amount to a quantity greater than that of glycerine in the formulation. A term such as *ProGen*, used to name the blend of different protein sources in the nutritional information of a bar, is a made-up name that manufacturers often apply to suggest proprietary differentiation of their products. It doesn't have much meaning and is simply a marketing ploy to fool us into thinking a given manufacturer's protein source is special. Such a ruse is also a good way to push the protein category to the front of the ingredient list so that we think protein is the prevalent component. This might be the case when protein is combined into one category, but that doesn't change the fact that glycerine, a carbohydrate-like ingredient, is probably the ingredient with the highest concentration.

For example, here are the ingredients of a typical nutritional bar on the market: ProGen (casein, egg albumin, gelatin, soy protein isolate, whey protein isolate), glycerine, water, maltitol. If each of these protein ingredients were to be itemized according to their individual concentration level, they'd be scattered throughout the list. Glycerine would likely edge any one of these out with ease for first place. The ingredient list might look something like the following if it were designed correctly: glycerine, *casein*, fructose, *egg albumin*, *gelatin*, sorbitol, milk fat, soy lecithin, maltodextrin, *soy protein isolate*, natural and artificial flavors, water, *whey protein isolate*, maltitol. Whey protein would likely be way down the list for two reasons: its cost and the fact that too much whey in the formulation of bars usually reduces shelf life, softness, and palatability. Obviously the second version of the bar's ingredients is less appealing. However, it's the same bar except that the second list is the real reflection of the bar's ingredients in order of concentration. Manufacturers of powdered protein supplements play this same ingredient-shuffle game. Glycerine is a reasonable sweetener to employ if you want to hide the carbohydrate level of a protein powder. As soon as you see parentheses in the ingredient descriptions, assume the side-step shuffle has taken place.

Manufacturers don't normally warn that glycerine is *not* necessarily diabetic-friendly. Diabetics, unknowingly, consume these low-carbohydrate bars as do people who have chosen to limit the glycemic-index status and carbohydrates of their diet in an attempt to avoid the progression of insulin resistance, diabetes, weight gain, cardiovascular disease, inflammation, and other common ailments. The glycerine load makes the healthy goal more difficult to achieve, especially if the body has to face it regularly while disease is active. If glucose intolerance is a problem, glycerine loading isn't a great idea. Although studies show the sugar load into the bloodstream from oral glycerine to be delayed from the time of consumption, don't be fooled; it eventually contributes to blood sugar.

A very interesting study performed at Pantox Laboratories, San Diego, California, and reported in 2001 confirms just how glycerol is utilized in the body. The objective of this innovative group was to develop a strategy to promote a hypoglycemic state in the body that would cause cancer to starve. Most types of cancer can't survive in a hypoglycemic host, and since most tissues of the body can make normal use of glycerol and many cancers can't, glycerol might provide the perfect fuel to support the body during starvation of the disease. However, even after blocking the liver's ability to convert glycerol into glucose, it was found that other specialized enzymes in peripheral tissues of the body could also transform glycerol into glucose for their own use, thus contributing this production to blood sugar, as well.

Glycerine loading before exercise can sustain performance in many ways, but only if insulin activity is healthy. Glycerol or glycerine supplementation is a good way to hydrate and glycogen-load muscles. Endurance athletes, especially, will experience great results from these loading strategies, maintaining hydration and glycogen for better performance potential. But most important, the delayed gluconeogenic activity (production of glucose) induced by the oral load of glycerine delivers its energy source some time well into the physical activity when energy stores become depleted.

Many studies such as the one performed by Montner, et al, at the Department of Medicine, Veterans Affairs Medical Center, Albuquerque, New Mexico, verify that glycerol consumption (1.2 g per kilogram of body weight) prior to endurance activity can enhance hydration, lower the heart rate, and prolong endurance time. Other studies indicate that preloading can keep body temperature down during activity in extraordinarily warm environments, which makes glycerol a great supplement for endurance athletes.

Bodybuilders and power athletes can gain strength and size potential from glycerine or glycerol loading, as well. Glycerine supplementation can improve the effects of creatine, supporting cellular hydration for muscle size and strength. Studies have yet to prove the safety of glycerine indulgence by diabetics or for those of us who are aging, or more accurately, for those of us who have reached a biological state where insulin resistance has advanced. Moderation is my safety suggestion!

APPLYING FUNCTIONAL GLYCEMIC-INDEX-LOWERING STRATEGIES

Earlier we discussed the value of consuming the right fats and proteins with a carbohydrate meal to boost the body's tolerability of the carbohydrates. Enhancing the acidity (decreasing the pH) of a meal with lemon juice, vinegar, or other citrus or lower pH foods (acidic foods) will decrease glycemic potential (28, 29). Studies further demonstrate that eating a low-glycemic-index meal that's acid-enhanced for breakfast (bread containing lactic acid in this particular study) reduces the glycemic response of a high-glycemic-index meal eaten four hours later at lunch (30). Starting your day with low-glycemic-index meals is a good way to prevent the onset of that insulin/sugar roller-coaster ride.

Acetic acid (vinegar), consumed with a high-glycemic-index meal, improves tolerability. In other words, a vinegar-based dressing atop a salad of fibrous stems and leafy greens lowers the glycemic value of any meal you eat immediately afterward. Interestingly a 2002 rat study performed in Japan (31) reveals that acetic acid somehow stimulates glycogen-synthase activity (the enzyme involved in the restoration of the energy stores of muscles). The study suggests that the oral consumption of glucose with acetic acid accelerates glycogen repletion in skeletal muscles more readily than glucose can alone. This glycogen-synthase activity might be one way acetic acid enhances glucose clearance from blood, assisting insulin in its role. The pH reduction of the gut by vinegar (acetic acid), for example, to slow down carbohydrate-digesting enzymes is another glucose-control factor mentioned earlier.

The obvious strategy to apply for better blood-glucose control and insulin efficiency is to consume a green fibrous salad topped with flaxseed oil, lemon juice, vinegar, and even a bit of protein such as egg, tuna, or low-fat cottage cheese. Eat this mini-meal just before your main course.

Wait 10 minutes or so after this salad appetizer is consumed to give your stretch receptors a chance to relay the message that bulk has been received in the stomach, then proceed to your main meal. As a result of this strategy, you'll probably require much smaller portions in the main course, which is more likely to deliver more saturated fat and unnecessary calories. The salad itself can serve as a meal if the mixed vegetable content and protein supply is sufficient.

FOOD-COMBINING CAN LOWER THE INDEX

Combining high-glycemic-index carrots and white potatoes in a stir-fry that contains fibrous, low-glycemic broccoli, cauliflower, celery, and green peppers results in a much lower glycemic score for the combination than for the isolated carrots and white potatoes. Top a high-glycemic-index *small* bed of brown rice (rating of 70 to 80) with a *large* mound of a stir-fried variety of low-glycemic-index vegetables. A vegetable mixture consisting of combinations of cauliflower, broccoli, peas, Swiss chard, celery, beans, squash, and green peppers can have a glycemic value lower than 30. This vegetable medley decreases the glycemic potential of the rice or pasta on which it's served.

Typically a bed of rice or pasta is sprinkled with these vegetables. The healthy way to consume this sort of meal is to eat smaller volumes of the dense carbohydrate source (pasta, rice, or potatoes) and much larger volumes of the mixed low-glycemic-index, fibrous vegetables. I prefer the vegetable mix to be at least twice the volume of the pasta or rice in the meal. That's if I include a whole-grain pasta or rice at all.

Usually I skip the pasta or rice in the meal and instead include about two cups of mixed vegetables with my protein source—a broiled chicken breast, or poached, steamed, or broiled wild salmon, tuna, or halibut. The pasta or rice may be included in the post-workout meal more freely. If you do consume the more dense carbohydrate source, I recommend one of my common blends: one-third wild rice and two-thirds brown rice steamed together.

These simple strategies contribute to the metabolic correction detailed in previous chapters—insulin efficiency, glucose tolerance, and the improvement of that essential fatty-acid metabolism to produce healthier hormone balances. When you use these simple strategies, you'll quickly notice better fat loss and lean muscle tone without working any harder than you did before.

DIETARY PROTEIN IS VITAL

The protein component of a meal is crucial. Don't fall victim to the misconception that dietary protein is toxic to the body. It's only toxic to a body that can't tolerate it, one that's already poisoned. Ageless Performance is designed to increase protein tolerability by creating self-sufficiency—ammonia regulation and pH or acid/alkaline balance in the body. Protein is essential for life; you can't limit your intake because of some unfounded fear of toxicity. Incomplete and insufficient levels of dietary protein will result in compromised immune function.

Dietary protein doesn't contribute to disease. Poor-quality protein, however, can damage kidneys and create other problems in the body. Heat- and chemical-induced changes in processed dietary protein add to the indigestibility and poor absorption of a protein source and can harm organs and tissues. Processed protein meats are poor-quality protein. The high-quality protein sources listed in detail in Appendix C of this book won't evoke the toxic outcome you might think is possible. Whey protein isolates generally supply high-quality, undenatured protein that's easy to digest and absorb. That's why I advocate their regular use, especially in cases of disease or lifestyles in which physical and/or mental stress are extremely high.

The nature of Ageless Performance is such that the dietary component provides an abundance of fresh vegetables and whole grains. These foods help protect the body against acidosis and are an offset to the potentially acidifying dietary protein that you shouldn't limit (32). A restricted protein intake also induces acidosis of the body by pushing it into a catabolic state (33, 34). Catabolism is a form of protein breakdown in which the body begins to eat away at its own tissues, using them for fuel and immediate construction of vital tissues.

This catabolism, which can be induced by a deficiency in dietary protein, is equivalent to burning the wood that makes up your house to fuel your furnace. You might need the heat for immediate survival, but eventually you'll burn away enough of your home to leave you exposed to the elements, anyway. Supply enough protein and this type of catabolism won't take place.

A dietary deficiency of the balanced array of minerals can also result in acidosis (35). We discussed this complexity in Chapter 7. The common pre-competition diet for a bodybuilder involves high protein and often a limitation of whole foods (36). This sets up the ketogenic diet, which can also be toxic. The low/no-carbohydrate, ketogenic diet in itself can induce body catabolism and acidosis (37). Renal insufficiency can contribute to acidosis and requires that dietary protein intake be monitored (38). In these cases the quality of the protein intake must be even more meticulously regulated so that poor-quality protein isn't used and the kidneys' work is limited. The point of this protein-related discussion is to highlight the fact that many factors and not just protein intake contribute to acidosis, and compounding them often creates the problem. Our common Westernized diets deliver compounded acid-inducing influences. Poor-quality dietary protein in this biochemical environment can cause more inefficiency, but the solution isn't a reduced protein intake (39).

In earlier chapters I demonstrated how protein is critical to blood-sugar balance; similarly dietary equilibrium is critical to metabolic stability. Limit dietary protein and the glycemic index of meals will tend to rise and metabolic disarray is sure to develop. Meeting your daily requisite protein requirement is vital to overall health. However, this protein intake must be of the highest quality possible, so pay close attention to the list in Appendix C.

FOOD PREPARATION INFLUENCES THE INDEX

The glycemic index of foods can vary considerably thanks to preparation. As mentioned earlier, white potatoes when baked can have a glycemic index of more than 90, but french fries, which have much more fat due to deep-frying, have a rating closer to 75. Potato chips can have a value less than 60, but baked versions with lower fat content will likely rate higher. Of course, trans and saturated fats in these common processed snack foods can lead to even more serious health problems.

The same danger applies to low-fat versions of salad dressings, yogurt, sauces, and bread spreads. To compensate for the reduction in fat, starch is often added to low-fat dressings to maintain viscosity, mouth feel, and palatability. This addition raises the glycemic index of the dressing. Make sure you check the ingredient lists on salad dressings before you buy them. Compare the ingredient lists and carbohydrate contents on the labels of regular dressings to their low-fat alternatives. Make sure the serving sizes are also relatively the same because sometimes low-fat versions also provide macronutrient profiles for smaller serving sizes, which is downright deceitful.

THE INDEX AND EXERCISE

We've already discussed the timing of food and the glycemic influence on the body. A high-glycemic-index food can be consumed without the same negative impact after a period of exercise. Most of us choose to eat carbohydrate-rich foods just before exercise. That doesn't support health or performance. When you raise blood-sugar levels before exercise, your body will respond with an insulin secretion. Insulin is a hormone that pushes nutrients into your cells, storing them, limiting the availability of fats for oxidation during exercise, and more likely inducing hypoglycemia earlier during the training session (40).

Studies have shown that every meal that spikes blood-glucose levels can cause the body's stress hormones (catecholamines) to be secreted. The original spike increases catecholamine levels immediately (41). Then the sugar low that often occurs because of this extreme high causes more catecholamines to be released. If you throw exercise into this poorly designed formula, more stress is imposed on the body and a more rapid sugar depletion is induced. The result is an even more intense secretion of catecholamines, more catabolism of healthy tissue, and more disease.

In fact, studies as recent as 2002 confirm that the glucose load in the blood amplifies the cortisol secretions promoted by psychosocial stress as well as other strains such as smoking to compound the physiological consequences (42). Lower the glycemic index of your food intake and the stress that our fast-paced society has imposed on us can be better tolerated.

Carbohydrates should be avoided as much as 90 minutes prior to a workout in order to allow your body to burn fat during the exercise period. Contrary to what many people advocate, the carbohydrates eaten just before or after exercise aren't used as efficiently to fuel muscles the way stored glycogen is (43). Your body will replenish glycogen, both in the liver and muscles, as soon as it gets a supply of dietary carbohydrates. The sooner after work the better. Keep in mind that liver glycogen is essential for maximum health of this organ. If liver glycogen is depleted and this state persists, the organ's function can be severely compromised. This means impaired body detoxification, amino-acid synthesis, gluconeogenesis, hormone regulation, and an increased risk of disease (44, 45). Take advantage of that post-work (heavy labor) or post-workout window as much as possible to restore the nutrient status of the body.

Other studies have indicated that obese individuals have damaged glycogen-synthase systems (46, 47). This enzyme system, as we've seen, helps restore muscle glycogen after depletion has taken place. Independent research has shown that diabetics also have impaired glycogen-restoration systems (48). This impairment in both cases is due to insulin resistance. The problem with this situation is that the post-work/workout window isn't as effective in glycogen and muscle restoration. Furthermore, a post-work/workout, high-glycemic-index meal isn't as well tolerated under these circumstances and can give rise to hyperglycemia and hyperinsulinemia.

In other words, those suffering from these disorders can't splurge in a post-work/workout meal the way healthy individuals can on occasion. Diabetics can have a *small* treat after finishing the depleting physical work, but must employ greater discretion than someone with a fully functional glycogen-synthase system. This system is still functional in persons with these diseased states but at a compromised level. This highlights the importance of eating small, regular, low-glycemic-index meals to maintain nutrient and glycogen status of the body, especially if regular exercise is part of the lifestyle. However, as soon as an individual recovers from a state of insulin dysfunction, he or she, too, will be able to enjoy an *occasional bigger* treat after a workout without any ill effects. In fact, I use this post-workout meal to get my fill of a high-glycemic-index food, which I might desire *on occasion*, chocolate cake included!

In addition to rebuilding vitally important glycogen stores, this post-workout, high-glycemic-index carbohydrate helps reduce the levels of corticosteroid stress hormones that have likely been secreted by the body during the latter part of the exercise session. As serum glucose and glycogen are depleted in the latter part of the session, the body responds with fight-or-flight stress hormones. Studies demonstrate that healthy individuals usually reach a state of catabolism 40 minutes or so into a workout unless steroid drugs are involved (49).

By holding off on eating after intense physical work or a workout, these destructive hormones continue to circulate in the body for a prolonged period. A protein/carbohydrate supplement mix will bring this catabolism to a stop and get the recovery process started. I often use a whey protein isolate supplement combined with a small amount of maltodextrin or a ripe banana. At no other time in the day would I recommend using such a mixture. The nutritional bar is a good snack at this time, as well. The other meals of the day must consist of protein combined with low-glycemic-index carbohydrate sources.

If disease, including obesity, is a circumstance you're dealing with, your dietary carbohydrates must come from a variety of foods with a glycemic value lower than 60 and preferably no higher than 55 at all times until the disease is under control. Use the discussed glycemic-index-lowering strategies as much as possible.

Take the post-workout opportunity to consume the foods you desire. Again, I might occasionally eat a piece of cake or some ice cream with a small protein drink after a workout. More regularly I might consume a slice of bread, some pasta or rice, a banana, raisins, or a potato right after the run or workout. Don't get me wrong. I'm not suggesting you take the oppor-tunity for senseless junking out. We're talking about just an *occasional* treat and only a tidbit if you're fighting disease.

The post-workout window is also recognized as a short period in which the immune system has been suppressed, likely by cortisol secretions, especially those exuded during an intense workout. The body is more vulnerable to microbe infiltration at this time, and if contact with microbes takes place at this point, infection is much more probable than at any other moment in the day. This is the dynamic that gives rise to the cold and flu vulnerability common to competitive athletes.

Glutamine, added to the post-workout protein/carbohydrate mix, has been shown to further reduce cortisol secretions, reestablishing healthy immune function expeditiously (50, 51). This procedure includes the use of glutamine supplementation for recovery from trauma and surgery (52). My preferred glutamine source for these conditions, including the post-workout application, is the hard-to-find dipeptide (not at all the same as the common tripeptide, derived from wheat gluten) called alanyl-glutamine. This dipeptide (two amino acids linked together) combination delivers the two most abundant amino acids of lean tissue for speedy recovery—alanine and glutamine. Glutamine, as we've seen, acts as a significant cortisol blocker, and the gluconeogenic alanine promotes glucose production from the liver and delivers a small glucose spike. Alanine is also the second most abundant amino acid of the skeletal muscle mass and is required abundantly for complete tissue recovery. Finally the high concentration of glutamine (greater than in the common glutamine tripeptide described in previous chapters) feeds the immune system more completely. This dipeptide strategy can be used to block cortisol in the *absence* of a dietary carbohydrate in the post-workout meal to advance the more intense thermogenesis that a workout can initiate. You'll read more about this fat-burning trick in an upcoming chapter.

Ageless Performance is the perfect design for therapy, prevention, and powerful athletic performance. Apply it and experience the change of a lifetime. The glycemic index of food plays a central role in the program: keep it whole and low and you can eat abundantly without the caloric and metabolic consequences of the processed, refined diet.

13

DIETING DOESN'T WORK

The word *diet* has taken on a new meaning in English. Our evolved definition of diet is that of a calorie restriction of some sort, a program that involves *healthier* dietary measures when ironically the typically limiting diet is actually unhealthy. The scientific definition for diet has nothing to do with calorie or macronutrient restraint designed for managing body weight or other diseases. Diet simply means the "usual amount and variety of food consumed."

A diet can be restrictive or unlimited. Both extremes breed disease. Processed to the degree that it is, our North American diet is severely nutrient-deficient even with the usual volumes of food and calories we consume. The high calorie count creates a demand for more protective nutrients—the co-factors required for metabolism and antioxidants needed to neutralize the incremental free-radical load caused by the excessive calories. A reduction in a dietary intake that's already nutrient-compromised amplifies the festering that valueless food stews in our cells.

Nutrient restriction breeds the sort of dysfunction touched on throughout this book. Curb the required fats and disease is bound to develop. Limit the intake of protein and protective antioxidants and the risk of disease increases. That's why the common "dieting" practices are so unhealthy; they often contribute to nutrient deficiency, nutrient imbalance, and a diseased state. Vitamins, minerals, and antioxidants, as we've seen, interact in an intimate way with genes to regulate their activity. This nutrient-genomic programming is a biological operating system that depends on naturally occurring nutrients. Processed food is essentially a programming with a different language that can't operate this delicate genetic system. Additional restriction, by way of our extreme diets, are even further from our natural nutrient array and disrupt the genetic operating system more profoundly.

To mention all of the examples of gene modulation by nutrients that we know about would require a lengthy discussion. However, highlighting a few more instances easily demonstrates the value of unlimited nutrient density in our food supply. Vitamin A has been recently recognized as a regulator of the gene responsible for transcribing IGF-1 (1). In other words, low vitamin A status in the body results in a decline in the gene activity responsible for growth hormone production. Vitamin A induces various other genes such as those involved in intestinal health and it modulates the genes engaged in hepatic gluconeogenesis (2). A variety of amino acids modify genetic expression, as well (3, 4, 5), and selenium and zinc also affect gene modulation (6, 7).

The list of nutrients that can alter genetic expression goes on, but in addition to the many we know about, quite a few more are hidden in nature's cocktail. The more we alter the meticulous programming of the diet, the more crashes we'll experience in the operating genetic system. Processed food generates genetic distress. On the other hand, unlimited caloric consumption propagates free radicals, insulin overload, body-fat accumulation, and disease. A healthy diet is a carefully strategized, meticulously balanced program.

Weight management can be a complicated battle to plan against. However, with the right strategy it's not much of a contest at all. Ageless Performance is your answer to prevention and recovery from obesity. Instead of further limiting nutrient status of the body, the program provides an unlimited supply of building blocks and metabolic co-factors for tissues, gene regulation, and healthy hormone balance. Just as important, this nourishment is delivered with a relatively low calorie value.

The nutrient density of Ageless Performance helps meet nutrient demands to alleviate deficiency cravings, and the plentiful supply of balanced fats with all the navigational factors promotes healthy eicosanoid-hormone balance and cognitive well-being. The result is better biological feedback systems and self-awareness as well as a healthier emotional state.

Eicosanoid balance, as we've seen, sustains our natural fat-burning furnaces while the common restrictive diet interrupts this delicate chemistry, making weight management difficult. The poorly formulated diet disrupts the fat-burning furnaces, it pushes appetite out of control, and it makes dieting a hellish misery that kick-starts more disease-instigating emotional stress. Put plainly, Ageless Performance takes the war out of weight management.

Our bodies employ protection the second calorie and nutrient deprivation is introduced. They reduce basal metabolic rates to conserve energy (8). Add this metabolic shutdown to the loss of appetite control and every time we binge for a day or two we collect more body fat in a few days than we can shed in two weeks of restrictive dieting. Does that sound like something you might have experienced?

Calorie deprivation has significant health benefits, but not when it comes at the expense of nutrient deficit. Dietary calorie restriction without malnourishment in animals such as rats and rhesus monkeys is known to increase lifespan significantly (9, 10, 11, 12, 13, 14). These same studies demonstrate that even short-term calorie restriction can ameliorate insulin efficiency and blood-sugar control.

The reduction in hyperlipidemia (high blood fat) that calorie restriction promotes is only one way it advances glucose regulation. The animal studies demonstrate that skeletal muscle glucose transport is improved with the application of calorie deprivation even before body weight is decreased. It has been shown that calorie restriction without nutrient deprivation enhances cognitive function and mental and physical energy. The aforementioned studies also indicate that calorie deprivation can boost immune efficiency, but again this isn't possible if nutrient restriction accompanies calorie reduction.

Research has recently unveiled a deeper understanding of the chemistry of aging and how it relates to calorie consumption. As I've mentioned in previous chapters, the chemistry of inflammation is thought to be at the center of the aging process, a hypothesis supported by 2001 studies that demonstrate that calorie deprivation actually slows the age-related acceleration of cyclo oxygenase or cox activity (15, 16). This might be due to the fact that the metabolism or processing of calories gives rise to free radicals—more calories, more free radicals, and more tissue, DNA, mitochondrial, and general biological inflammation and damage.

Accelerated cox activity is responsible for the production of disease-instigating, inflammatory eicosanoid hormones such as excessive prostaglandin (PGE$_2$) production. Calorie deprivation has been shown to reduce age-related NF-kappa-B activity as well as decrease nitric-oxide synthase overactivity. As we've seen, free-radical load promotes NF-kappa-B activity, which subsequently stimulates gene activity and cox production. All of this results in more inflammation and advanced biological age. One of the studies mentioned above points out that a calorie-restricted diet supplemented with fish oils further down-regulates this biochemical action to reduce the age-related increase in inflammation and other diseases, including biological aging. Ageless Performance covers a lot of bases.

Most diets are nutrient-restricted from the start. As we've seen in previous chapters, our food supply today doesn't have the nutrient value it once had. Supplementation to raise nutrient density of nourishment is critically important to the long-term results of a weight-management program. This is especially so if we apply calorie-restrictive strategies. Ageless Performance is essentially a low-calorie, extremely nutrient-dense dietary program. It's not a *diet*; it's simply a lifelong commitment to eating well and nourishing the body without limitation.

That doesn't mean we have to avoid all the foods we desire. First of all, the craving for many high-glycemic-index, high-fat foods will diminish once Ageless Performance is initiated. Eating less-than-whole foods on occasion isn't a predicament when the metabolic rate operates healthily. And when timing strategies, as discussed in the previous chapter, are implemented the situation becomes even less problematic. As complex as many of the discussed concepts might seem, they're incorporated into an easy-to-apply program in Chapter 15. Follow the instructions there and all of these biochemical corrections will begin to take place without further thought.

FATTY-ACID IMBALANCE AND FAD DIETS

Most of the numerous diets available facilitate short-term weight loss. They're severely calorie-restricted, which means, of course, that weight loss is inevitable. However, a protein-deficient diet results in muscle catabolism, while a carbohydrate-restricted one brings on glycogen depletion and can induce muscle loss, particularly if it's applied poorly and especially if physical activity is extreme. Obviously lean tissue and glycogen depletions will result in disease.

The metabolism or cellular processing of essential fats is critically dependent on many nutrients, and if just one is limited, the entire path is thrown off-kilter. The imbalance results in metabolic havoc and cell death, which translates into weight loss but not the kind you want. The true gauge of healthy weight loss is the test for body-mass proportions along with the measure for general weight. This involves calculating lean and fat body mass concurrently to determine which is being burned away. In fact, the more aggressive fat-reduction plans strip away much more of these precious lean tissues and vital elements; in other words, the faster the weight loss, the quicker these essential elements slip away. Generally a reduction of fat that approximates two pounds per week is safe. However, don't look at the weight scale every few days, since even small alterations in body status of water, glycogen, and gastrointestinal fill can result in daily changes of two to four pounds, up or down, independent of fat loss. Again the proportional measure of lean to fat mass is the most accurate method to assess progress.

The body-mass proportions of a successful or healthy fat-reduction endeavor will change, maintaining a relatively similar lean-muscle mass but reducing fat mass significantly. The best-case scenario for the muscle-wasted, sedentary individual is a gain in lean muscle while fat loss is experienced. Obviously a common weight scale isn't a useful tool for assessing the success rate of any program, since muscle weighs significantly more than fat. By embarking on an exercise program and a proper diet, you could lose a lot of fat and gain a very small volume of muscle with no change on the weight scale. Fat is much less dense than muscle. Ageless Performance is structured to maintain lean mass, while it blocks the eicosanoid hormones that interfere with natural thermogenesis. You'll quite likely gain lean weight quickly with the application of Ageless Performance while losing fat, especially if muscle mass has atrophied to dangerously low levels before the program is applied. A mirror is a better assessment tool than a common scale. The body shape alters profoundly with incremental muscle and a loss of fat even if a weight-scale measure doesn't change at all.

The lean mass of the body supports the biological systems in many crucial ways, supplying glutamine and branched-chain amino acids as backup nourishment for the brain, gastrointestinal tract, and the immune system during times of emergency. Poorly strategized dieting often results in glutamine deficiency, and the outcome, lean-muscle loss, can be quite severe, especially in the elderly and if disease is already present (17, 18, 19). Lose muscle and you forfeit the emergency backup system for immune fuel.

Studies reveal that the glutamine status of the body is related to glutathione standing, and a dietary deficiency of the former can result in a cellular depletion of the latter. The consequences are immune dysfunction, uncontrolled oxidative stress, and a severely increased danger of disease. Maintaining a healthy dietary supply and muscle storage of glutamine is important. In short, a healthy muscle mass is the basis of general metabolic vigor and emergency life support for the body. That's one way resistance (weight-training) exercise promotes long-term resilience to disease and helps ensure robust muscle mass. Regular exercise also promotes the health of bones, mental faculties, and insulin as well as cardiovascular well-being.

A glutamine-rich diet bolsters protein synthesis and recovery from all kinds of disease: infection, inflammation, gastrointestinal disorders, and free-radical damage (20, 21, 22, 23). Dietary glutamine deficiency amid physiological or mental stress can result in lean-mass depletion. You might have experienced this phenomenon yourself or noticed the muscle loss in others who have faced trauma or surgery. No matter how well these individuals nourished themselves before or immediately after the traumatic experience, lean-muscle degradation was inevitable and muscle regeneration ensued slowly for the first week of recovery. Lean-muscle-sourced glutamine and branched chain amino acids are extracted from muscle during these periods as an immediate source of fuel for the immune system and tissues in need of recovery.

Facing this traumatic situation with an already compromised lean mass makes coping and recovery even more difficult, and being prepared is the best defense. That's what makes Ageless Performance the perfect match for fitness, prevention, and fat loss. It causes the body to burn away unnecessary pounds naturally while maintaining maximum lean mass.

Regular activity, especially that of weight training even twice weekly, helps preserve lean-muscle tissue, but only if all of the required nutrients are available for restoration of spent tissue. Most restrictive dieting endeavors are coupled with exercise to facilitate calorie expenditure and promote faster weight loss. Nutrient restriction amid increased physical work presents an obvious problem. Muscle is metabolically active. The loss of this tissue is inevitable if nutrient deprivation accompanies excess calorie expenditure. This reduction in active tissue makes fat loss more difficult, and if you play sports of any kind, the stripping away of lean muscle is certain to compromise your game.

Dietary protein is an important factor for muscle maintenance and growth from training. Whey protein isolate supplementation that's next to zero percent lactose and fat is my preferred choice of lean-muscle and immune-system building blocks. There's one source I trust as a staple in my diet because my independent research reveals it has consistent quality assurance. Not a brand name, it's a raw material that our team at Biologic Nutritional Research Inc. works into many industry fromulations. For those who are interested, I discuss this very clean, pure raw material on our Web site (*www.biologicnr.com*), and many of the retail brands applying this base material are also presented for consumers.

Biologic Nutritional Research Inc. has recently employed a health-industry policing program that involves testing retail nutritional products. Not only do we test at our own research center, but we have independent laboratories pick these products from store shelves to assess them for accuracy of label claim. Proceeds from our literary work such as those from this book pay for the cost of analyzing these products in order to provide consumers with a list of nutritional products that pass the independent tests. The Biologic LIST (Label Integrity Standard Test) program is designed for use by consumers and health-care professionals to choose efficacious, safe, and true products. Our Web site presents this community service.

YO-YO DIETING

Let's face it, fluctuating body weight isn't healthy. A temporary state of deprivation might transform the way we look for a short period, but lost weight is usually regained unless the program incorporates easy-to-apply lifestyle changes. Most diets result in the same outcome: fast-paced, indiscriminate weight loss followed by a reward system that sends us back to the original problem—carbohydrate addiction. The outcome is the yo-yo effect, which entails weight loss, weight gain and, inevitably, more anguish.

Exponents of this kind of diet say, "Cut back to one meal per day to really shed the pounds!" But one meal a day can't supply the nutrients required to meet demands; our nutrient absorption sites just aren't able to absorb the necessary nutrition from only one daily opportunity. The metabolic reduction that results from this single meal is the body's attempt to reserve calories, since it thinks it's facing a period of food scarcity. Ageless Performance involves the consumption of four and even six small meals daily. These multiple daily meals improve metabolic rate.

As discussed in the previous chapter, dietary fats are most commonly eliminated in the fat-loss diet, since they deliver more than two times the calories of both carbohydrates and protein. It might seem to make more sense to cut back dietary fat because each gram delivers nine calories while protein and carbohydrates each deliver four calories per gram. However, we've previously discussed the consequences of limited dietary essential fatty acids: poor energy levels, hunger pangs for endorphin-secreting fats, cellular havoc, hormone imbalance, and disease, including obesity. Since animal protein sources usually contain more fat than vegetation, animal protein sources become restricted in this kind of diet. The lack of protein in the common hyper-restricted diet presents two other serious problems: it contributes to the degradation of lean muscle and compromises immune-system activity. The simple addition of protein supplementation to the weight-management program helps manage appetite and stimulate thermogenesis.

Limitations in dietary protein and fat, as I've already mentioned, also result in an increase in the glycemic index of the diet, which makes fat accumulation difficult to control. The common processed North American diet is a bomb that can detonate into disease, and indiscriminate yo-yo dieting increases the firepower of the explosive and further sensitizes the trigger mechanism. By limiting essential fats and other nutrients crucial to metabolic navigation, the fat proportions of cells can become imbalanced. Eicosanoid-hormone balance is then thrown into disease-instigating proportion in which arachidonic-acid-derived hormones can be overproduced.

The deadliness of this metabolic bomb is further enhanced when we give in to uncontrollable cravings. Surrendering to appetite can result in the abundant consumption of junk food for a day or two or even a week before we return to a restrictive diet. The binge will likely involve the consumption of processed, trans-fat-loaded food. As such essential-fat-deprived cells can become inundated with a surge of trans fats that can be used to fill in the gaps left by the missing correct fats from the preceding restriction. After the gorging, the cravings will set in again because the uncontrolled plastic food failed to deliver the right fats for healthy cell turnover.

Dietary fat limitations, as we've already seen, prompt desires for an endorphin rush and inspire an unforgiving need for essential building blocks. Stick to a poorly designed diet and you'll eventually require that addictive rush. Exercise also induces endorphin secretions in the brain and relieves the craving for fat. Regular exercise and regular essential-fat supplementation eliminate this unhealthy need to binge on fatty foods. Ageless Performance fulfills the requisite fat requirements to eradicate these cravings and maintains healthy cellular-fat proportions while activating the fat-burning thermogenic system—natural weight management made easy.

We saw in Chapter 11 how the metabolic pathway gives rise to the prostaglandin (PGE$_2$) production that's responsible for shutting down thermogenesis. Calorie deprivation amid nutrient density, however, blocks these prostaglandins, too. The Ageless Performance strategy focuses on this hormone system to free the thermogenic fat-burner from multiple inhibitory factors. Even with a couple of days of fatty-food binging, the healthy metabolic momentum created by weeks of Ageless Performance can't be derailed. Ageless Performance isn't about deprivation; on the contrary, it entails intense nutrient density without limitation.

THE ATKINS DIET

As we've all seen, diets come and go and come again. Most fat-loss strategies deliver horrific consequences, but amazingly they're kept alive by people desperately seeking magical solutions. Most diets result in weight loss because they lack calories but also deplete the body of glycogen, water, and muscle. You probably know many of these nutrient-deficient prescriptions for disaster: the grapefruit-and-water diet; the banana-and-water diet; the crème-and-protein-diet; the high-carbohydrate, low-to-no-fat diet; the liquids-only diet; the one-meal-per-day diet; the fruit-only diet; the lemon/water fasting; the high-protein, high-fat diet; the no-carbohydrate diet.

One diet that really scares me, though, is the high-protein, high-fat, no-carbohydrate one popularized by the late Dr. Robert C. Atkins, which has been widely marketed and media-hyped. To my astonishment, this outlandish program has been universally accepted as safe. The Atkins Diet involves the consumption of as much protein from red-meat sources with as much animal fat as desired. I'm a proponent of abundant dietary fat, but not just any old fat. As we've seen, there are some fats we need to avoid and others we should consume abundantly.

The Atkins Diet is ketogenic. Few people know what they're actually doing to their biochemistry by struggling through such a regimen. Within the liver two molecules of acetyl coenzyme A (acetyl COA) are combined to yield ketone bodies—acetoacetic acid, beta-hydroxybutyric acid, and acetone, which are ultimately produced as a result of ketogenesis. Acetyl COA can be obtained from dietary fats, dietary protein, or body tissues.

When dietary carbohydrates are depleted, the body quickly uses up its stored glycogen levels. Athletes or those in pursuit of quick weight loss learn to use ketone sticks (which measure ketone body levels in urine) to determine whether ketosis (the abnormal increase of ketone bodies in the body) has been induced by a low- to zero-carbohydrate diet. Once the ketogenic state is reached, however, most of these athletes know to back away from the carbohydrate restriction and increase dietary carbohydrates to a level that prevents muscle catabolism and ketosis from persisting. It takes about 50 to 70 g (one potato, two apples, or two bananas) of carbohydrates daily to prevent ketosis for the average person.

The popular ketogenic Atkins Diet involves the indiscriminate consumption of deep-fried and pan-fried globs of animal fat. This high-fat, high-protein, low- or no-carbohydrate program promotes the production of ketone bodies. Cells in muscles and other tissues have the ability to employ these substances as a source of energy. When dietary carbohydrates are severely limited, ketone bodies can be produced in greater quantities than the body can use for energy. The Atkins Diet involves severe carbohydrate limitation.

When dietary protein and fat are too high, ketone bodies *can't* be oxidized in the body fast enough to remove the potential danger they pose. The body expels excessive ketone bodies in the urine and through the lungs. In fact, you can often smell acetone on the breath of an individual who's been in ketosis for some time. Ketone bodies can also be detected on the breath of a diabetic when he or she fails to metabolize carbohydrates efficiently due to inefficient or insufficient insulin secretions.

The Atkins Diet promotes the abundant consumption of beef and dairy fats, which contain a great deal of arachidonic acid. Overconsumption of these arachidonic-acid-laden sources multiplies the risk of biochemical imbalances that are at the root of a multitude of epidemics, including obesity. That's especially so when a diet such as the Atkins one is devoid of vegetables, whole grains, and legumes that would otherwise supply antioxidants, vitamins, and fuel for a starving body and friendly intestinal bacteria. The change in colon pH that this diet encourages is a perfect environment for pathogenic bacteria to disrupt friendly bacterial health, increasing the danger of colon cancer (24, 25). Not only does the lack of fiber in this diet contribute to the incidence of colon cancer, the high degree of dietary saturated fat does, as well. The indiscriminate fat consumption advocated by the Atkins Diet can also facilitate cardiovascular problems and interrupt insulin function. Furthermore, abundant red-meat consumption can cause colon cancer through factors independent of fat content (26). With a near-zero intake of dietary carbohydrates, this diet creates a temporary depletion of hepatic glycogen. Glycogen is the liver's main fuel for detoxification and metabolic activity. Exhaust this energy source and you're in trouble.

The ketogenic state induced by the Atkins Diet and others like it alters the pH (acid/base balance) of the blood and body to induce more metabolic havoc (27, 28). The body functions in a pH range that's quite narrow. Mild deviations result in profound metabolic impairment. Interestingly the ketogenic diet doesn't change the pH of the brain. Carbohydrate-restricted diets like the one expounded by Dr. Atkins have been in use since the 1920s to help treat epileptic children with great success (29, 30, 31). The ketogenic diet somehow reduces seizure activity, but scientists still don't know why. And ketogenic diets have been shown through some unknown mechanism to boost brain ATP, as well (32).

However, a ketogenic diet must be carefully monitored in these therapeutic applications to help manage the potential acidosis of the body. As the body fights to maintain its functional acid-alkaline balance, nutrient stores, such as calcium and phosphorus from bone mass, might be taxed. Furthermore, cases of renal stone development, gastritis, ulcerative colitis, alteration of mentation, and hyperlipidemia have been reported with the administration of a ketogenic diet. Of course, with professional monitoring the risk of these side effects can be minimized (33). The dangers might be a good trade-off when considering the implications of an uncontrollable epileptic condition, especially when it's severe. Still, for basic weight management a ketogenic diet isn't advisable. The risks aren't lower than those posed by excess body fat.

If an epileptic condition presents significant danger in your life, sure, the ketogenic diet is likely a reasonable choice, but I still believe that ketogenesis might not have anything to do, or at least all to do, with the beneficial effect of the typical ketogenic diet on an epileptic condition. Keep in mind that the biochemical process by which ketogenesis seems to eliminate or reduce seizure activity isn't known. Many studies demonstrate that polyunsaturated fatty-acid supplementation with linoleic and alpha linolenic acid, as well as with the fish-oil-derived DHA and EPA, also promotes brain health and inhibits epileptic seizures (34, 35, 36, 37, 38). The typical ketogenic diet involves greater intakes of fats, primarily animal ones, that have high essential-fat content as well as healthy EPA and DHA levels. It also entails the consumption of a lot of vegetable oils that consist of a bounty of linoleic and alpha linolenic acids.

Could it be that the method of therapeutic activity for the anti-epileptic ketogenic diet is simply through its rich supply of the essential and other health-promoting polyunsaturated, omega-3 fats that in the absence of dietary carbohydrates and reduced insulin activity leaves more fats for the brain to take up? Likely so. It's at least one major contributing factor. I'm confident that the high polyunsaturated-fat version of Ageless Performance will prove to be a significant therapy for epileptic seizures the way ketogenic diets have but without the side effects and with a broader array of health benefits. Studies may ensue in the near future.

In addition to increased cardiovascular risk from the abundant dietary saturated fat, the dearth of vegetation and whole grains in the ketogenic Atkins-type diet results in a lack of the vitamin co-factors required to metabolize homocysteine. The accumulation of homocysteine occurs due to inefficient methionine metabolism. Red meats are rich in methionine. Eat them lavishly with few or no vegetables and you'll likely run into trouble. A shortage of vitamins B_6 and B_{12}, folic acid, and methyldonors (such as SAMe and trimethylglycine) can increase the incidence of homocysteine-related problems. Homocysteine buildup has been implicated in cardiovascular disease, cerebrovascular problems, inflammation, chronic fatigue, and cognitive and other brain disorders. The Atkins Diet can create a predisposition for these common risks with the silent killer, cardiovascular disease, creeping up to get you without previous warning.

Although Ageless Performance focuses on limiting dietary carbohydrates, the objective is far from elimination. As part of the program, low-glycemic-index carbohydrates are consumed abundantly to fuel the brain and body without imposing an extreme insulinogenic influence, and ketogenesis doesn't enter the picture. In the stressed ketogenic state, weight reduction can be significant (as much as 10 to 15 pounds in a week or two); however, most of the weight lost in the first phase of the Atkins Diet is water, glycogen, and muscle, not fat (39).

Although the Atkins Diet weight loss is attributed to the depletion of the body's carbohydrate (glycogen) stores, most people are fooled into thinking this is a healthy outcome. Earlier I explained the carbohydrate-depletion tricks for making weight classes at bodybuilding shows. Low or zero carbohydrate diets cause glycogen to be lost in the body rapidly. This also causes water to leave the body very quickly. The result is significant: immediate weight loss might exceed 10 pounds, though fat won't nexessarily be reduced. Wrestlers use the same techniques to make weight classes, and a 1993 review in the *International Journal of Sports Medicine* indicates that the weight losses in these cases aren't necessarily fat, either; worse, the metabolic impairment these practices induce can make fat loss even harder to achieve in future attempts (40).

Ageless Performance makes weight management easy and without compromise. In fact, the reason weight management is so efficient with Ageless Performance is because it empowers the built-in biological systems to work in your favor. This includes the potent fat-burning thermogenic system and the restoration and maintenance of calorie-burning, lean-muscle tissue. Ageless Performance gets your body working for you instead of making you struggle and overexercise against a dysfunctional metabolism.

EXERCISE IS MUCH MORE THAN CALORIE EXPENDITURE

The value of exercise to a preventive or anti-aging program is paramount. Exercise helps normalize blood pressure and lipid profiles, and it enhances heart condition, lung capacity, blood flow, insulin health, and thermogenic activity. With exercise calories are expended to allow greater caloric intake for the purpose of improved nutrient ingestion, ultimately allowing more leeway when it comes to desired high-glycemic-index and fatty foods.

Physical activity, like the previously mentioned resistance work, is crucial to the maintenance of lean muscle, as well (41). Age-related muscle loss, as we've seen, is caused by a number of factors: insulin resistance, a lack of nutrient building blocks and co-factors from the diet, and an elevation in NF-kappa-B. Ageless Performance addresses all these problems. A deficiency of exercise or general physical activity also plays a significant role in age-related muscle atrophy. The reintroduction of physical activity into the routines of the elderly has been shown to enhance general joint flexibility and muscle strength, but that isn't possible unless adequate nourishment is provided by the diet at the same time (42). Antioxidant needs increase with the onset of a more active lifestyle, and Ageless Performance accommodates for this demand, too. Still, the calorie contribution is maintained low, making exercise/training results even better—more muscle and less body fat.

If physical work is intense and prolonged enough to deplete energy stores and induce catecholamine secretions such as epinephrine and corticosteroids, more tissue damage by free-radical assault will result. The strategies of Ageless Performance counter this problem, as well. Exercise stimulates the production and activity of the uncoupling proteins in brown adipose fat. More accurately, free fatty acids enter the bloodstream in large amounts due to exercise, inducing uncoupling protein activity and accelerating the thermogenic process. (43, 44). Since free-fatty-acid elevation is recognized as the cause for exercise-induced thermogenesis, higher-than-normal, post-workout, free-fatty-acid levels in blood must be maintained for as long as possible in order for maximum thermogenic potential to be experienced. Keep in mind that this thermogenic calorie expenditure is independent and additional to the work-induced ATP/calorie outlay. Thermogenic-related calorie losses can continue indefinitely long after exercise is terminated.

However, once free-fatty-acid levels are cleared from the blood, thermogenic-activation potential is lost. The immediate introduction of high-glycemic-index food after exercise puts out the thermogenic fire by raising insulin levels. Insulin, remember, sweeps substrates like glucose, amino acids, and free fatty acids from the blood and into storage. For this reason, to optimize fat-loss endeavors, you should wait 20 to 30 minutes after exercise before high-glycemic-index foods are consumed. That goes against what I've said in previous discussions. Of course, as we've seen, this delay strategy increases the exposure to cortisol (a stress hormone produced during prolonged exercise) and reduces the potential for muscle and glycogen restoration. To counter this problem I run for 30 minutes or so in the morning and then work out in the late afternoon with weights for about 30 to 40 minutes. I try not to exceed 40 minutes per session. Sometimes I exercise in the morning and run in the afternoon. One of these sessions is followed by supplementation of glutamine and branched-chain amino acid, while holding off for 20 to 30 minutes on the post-workout or post-run carbohydrate-loaded meal/supplement drink.

Glutamine (3 to 5 g), alpha ketoglutaric acid (2 g), and a mix of branched-chain amino acids (2 g) block cortisol secretions and promote protein synthesis to boost immune function and immediate tissue recovery, including muscle anabolism. Two to three grams of hydroxymethylbutyrate

(HMB) is another great addition to the blend. Taking this multiple-amino-acid combination immediately after a workout supports health and maximizes fat loss by allowing serum fatty acids to maintain thermogenesis in the on position. However, maximum glycogen stores, muscle building, and strength aren't possible applying this regimen all the time. Once the targeted fat mass is reached, though, go back to consuming high-glycemic-index carbohydrates and high-biological-value protein immediately after the training session to optimize strength and muscle results. Getting all of these strategies into your program will result in profound changes in your metabolic status quickly.

There are three metabolic types: mesomorphic, endomorphic, and ectomorphic. All of us can exhibit characteristics of each of these categories. In fact, most of us go through life experiencing varying degrees of all three at different times or stages. But we do have the ability to turn an endomorphic state (a slower metabolism that tends to put on fat easily) into a mesomorphic and even an ectomorphic type. I've done it myself and have seen remarkable changes in others who have accomplished the same.

These metabolism-related terms merely relate to the layers of the embryos from which we were all formed. The endoderm, for instance, is the innermost layer of the embryo and gives rise to the gastrointestinal tract, lungs, and other internal organs. The endomorphic individual is said to have a body type characterized predominantly by the abdomen and *softer* tissue distribution, resulting in lower lean mass and higher fat mass. The mesomorphic body type has a more muscular, stockier body that primarily derives from the mesodermal (middle) layer of the embryo. Finally the ectomorph displays a skinnier, relatively lankier body type that exhibits less muscle and less fat. This individual develops body structure largely from the ectodermal (outermost) layer of the embryo.

There is some value to these descriptions, but the various body types are also a result of environmental influences, including diet and workload. Such factors acting upon genes give rise to the predominance of tissue type developed in an individual. Although there's some degree of genetic limitation, you can shift your body type with relative ease. Another considerable influence that molds us into certain body types is what we're led to believe about ourselves—mind over matter. If you're told by someone you deem credible that you're an endomorphic type who will put on fat and have difficulty losing it, you'll live up to that characterization. Don't believe it, don't be imprinted by others and, more important, don't saddle yourself with a self-imposed boundary. Your limitations are only as true as you allow them to be. Believe you possess restrictions and you'll burden yourself with them. Believe you can change the way you are and you will. You can make substantial alterations in who you are the second you have faith in yourself, even when it comes to body-typing.

When I was 12 years old, I looked and felt much like a mesomorph. From 13 to 17 I had the appearance of an ectomorph as fitness became a bigger part of my life. Obviously a growth spurt, which is typical at this stage of life for most people, contributed to such physical changes. Then when weight training became my focal activity in my mid-teens and a more mature body began to fill in with muscle, I started to look like a mesomorph again. These are the transitions most of us experience.

As we age and our fitness levels decline, we tend to move toward the endomorphic body type, or if you're an ectomorph during young adulthood you may seem to become more like a mesomorph. But that doesn't have to happen. These changes are a function of biological aging and metabolic deterioration. I've frequently seen adults shift from endomorphic body types to physiques that have the appearance and functions of the mesomorph and even the ectomorph. The predominant tissue type that we develop or transform into depends on how we want our genes to be influenced. Each of us is composed of all of these tissue types—choose the one you want your body to characterize. It's up to you to make the revolution happen, and with Ageless Performance that's easy to achieve. Believe in your potential and extract it from within. You can do it!

14

STATE OF MIND MATTERS

Taste buds, olfactory receptors, eyes, and ears are sensory receptacles composed of highly specialized networks of nutrients that come from our food, liquid, and the air we breathe. These molecular networks form transmission conduits from our sense receptors to our brains. Not surprisingly, a compromised diet gives rise to compromised tissues, and that includes the neural network and our sense of perception.

The transmission and interpretation from sensation depend on how well this network is composed. It relies on the availability of essential nutrition, which involves far more than merely meeting caloric demand. We've seen how easy it is to meet caloric needs and how often we don't achieve nutrient demands. In order for the neural network, and the conscious awareness it's intimately related to, to manifest a healthy state, each and every micro- and macronutrient must be made available in unlimited supply.

If at any point, from perception chemistry to the neural conduits and all the way to the composition of the brain, this system is nutrient-deficient or interrupted by toxicity like chemical poisons and oxidation, sensation interpretation and conscious awareness are also disrupted. Conscious thought is a matter of chemistry that must be made available from our nutrient stores. Subconscious thought is also a matter of chemical composition that requires nutrient building blocks and co-factors for manifestation. Poor biochemical makeup results in a suboptimal conscious state that's more likely to initiate a negative mental attitude—a seed for disease.

Keep in mind that the chemistry we're talking about is composed of atoms that consist of 99%+ empty space, which means they're ultimately bioenergy. At another level of the same concept the condition of consciousness is highly dependent on the bioenergetic state of being, which in turn relies heavily on the quality of nutrient bioenergies. Whole food contributes to whole and healthy consciousness; bioenergetically altered food, that is, food that's processed, gives rise to a modified state of consciousness. Altered subconscious states devastate our entire beings and guide us down destructive paths so slowly that we rarely realize the significance of these deviations until one day we identify that we're not where we want to be in life. Disease is often a result of such mental and emotional unrest, and it's often the factor that forces us to identify the need for change.

A more complete nutritional state of the body allows for better awareness and the ability to recognize a need for change before that state of emergency—disease—is reached. Without complete nutrition our perception chemistries are unable to function optimally and our conscious presentations of ourselves and of the universe can't be clearly articulated or envisioned. In these compromised states our places in the universal scheme are unclear as are our positions in a more proximate society. Incomplete nourishment impedes the ability to interact and function in the world. The body and mind rely on complete nutrition that was specially designed by a distinct evolutionary path. *Natural* food supply fulfills this evolutionary design; *human-altered* nourishment doesn't. As much as nutrient imbalances and limitations interfere with the biochemical function of the body and the mind independently, they also influence the dynamic interaction between them. What affects the body has an impact on the mind and vice versa.

When altered nourishment is incorporated into perception chemistry, it interferes with the senses and with the conscious interpretation of sensation. Since this foreign chemistry makes up the neural conduits to and from conscious awareness, the state of mind and the condition of the body can't help but be detrimentally influenced. As the mind experiences a distorted state of reality due to this contamination, the body manifests disease. As physical disease becomes intense, the mind is infused with more negative sensory chemistry, propelling the cycle out of control and into metabolic arrhythmia and a multiple-disease status. The experience of life can only be as complete as our nutritional condition and as incomplete as our nutritional situation.

We depend on our five senses for interaction and development in the world. Whole, natural nourishment is a critical factor that links perception chemistry to the natural environment. Synthetic chemicals that weren't part of our evolutionary designs are incorporated into our bodies, altering the energy patterns of our essences. In other words, artificial chemistry transforms our perceptive and conscious states much as drugs do. Sound a bit farfetched? It's not. Synthetic chemicals interfere with the natural flow of bioenergy. They're "grammatically" incorrect for nature's biochemical "speech," and these extra-universal substances interrupt the cosmic message when they're used to form the communication conduits (neural or other) or language of consciousness.

Don't discount this unconventional presentation of artificial chemistry; it's a deep reality that makes a lot of sense. Artificial sweeteners and fats join the myriad of other synthetic chemicals in our world, each adding a small contribution. Together they make a significant impact on our emotional or mental states and ultimately seed physical disease. This shift in perception and consciousness is rarely identified. Unlike the profound transformation caused by drugs such as alcohol, marijuana, cocaine, and even tobacco, the changes induced by this artificial chemistry are usually subtle. In fact, a great deal of recreational drug use shadows any of these subtle alterations, making their identifications impossible by the substance abuser and giving rise to numerous questions. Do these nutrient imbalances and limitations and bioenergy modifications promote the addictive behavior of a substance abuser? Is the substance abuse a required masking agent for the subconscious and physical misfiring caused by a combination of nutrient imbalance, artificial chemistry, and lifelong emotional duress? Is the emotional duress a function of the nutritional and artificial chemistry status? Is the nutritional status a function of the emotional state? In fact, the answer to all of the aforementioned is likely yes to one degree or another. What's also valid is that any change in perception and mind will promote physical disease, even perception shifts as subtle as those imposed by synthetics such as artificial sweeteners.

Since there's no absolute escape from the interference of foreign chemicals, we have to do everything in our power to neutralize it. The first step is to reduce the number of factors contributing to the toxic alien chemistry.

This requires that natural whole nourishment be supplied in abundance by our diets while processed and artificial foods and additives are eliminated or at least restricted. The next step is to heighten the antioxidant status of the body through supplementation. Antioxidants are vital factors that counteract the oxidative effects of this harmful chemistry, ensuring that the body functions free of interference and disease while making certain the operation of the mind isn't interrupted by artificial bioenergy.

Our genetic designs (the composition of our DNAS) evolved over millions of years based on the influences of natural whole food. Our master codes depend on the complementary nutrient triggers and modulators they were designed to work intimately with. Today genetic programming still depends on this nutritional modulation. Genetic programming wasn't formulated amid the toxic free-radical load we're bathed in currently, either, so it can't survive efficiently without our conscious participation. Our genes don't have the accommodative codes for the extra antioxidant protection we need to endure disease-free in this cesspool. As a result, we require higher levels of antioxidant protection from dietary sources today than we did years ago. To compound the problem, an aging body produces compromised levels of endogenous antioxidants, allowing this excessive environmental free-radical interference to impair an unprotected state of being with greater ease over time. In order for perception of any type to operate according to our gene-programmed realities, we have to combat this free-radical attack by neutralizing it with an abundance of supplemental antioxidants, and the older we get the more important these supplements become to both mental and physical health.

Since this perception chemistry is formulated by genetic programming, it's our genes that encode our interpretation of the world, the multitude of sensations we experience, and even everything we can't sense. Ageless Performance maximizes gene expression and thwarts foreign toxicity to clear perception, transmission of sensation, and conscious awareness of the environment and ourselves. This, in turn, helps us maintain better physical and mental health as well as optimal performance potential.

We assume that some things and some abilities don't exist because we can't feel them tactilely. Intuition is the sixth sense that few of us employ. It, too, depends on clear perception, transmission, and interpretation.

And, like the other senses, it relies on a consistent supply of whole, unprocessed food or bioenergy. Although we don't need this less tangible sixth sense today for survival, it's deeply embedded in us in anticipation of new levels of human evolution. This powerful tool can be developed to guide us through life from another dimension of reality, but only if we learn to use it and only if we maintain a healthy, clear, bioenergetic state. We can't see or measure this sense, so most of us don't believe in it. However, we can't really see or measure the energy of our other senses except through our own interpretations. Our sixth sense isn't much different We can learn to develop this sixth sense the same way those who lose their sight often cultivate better touch, taste, hearing, and smell to help decipher the world.

Think about it: a person blind from birth lives in the world but experiences it much differently. Color isn't a comprehensible concept for this person. How can you describe light or color to someone who's never seen them? Does the inability to perceive color or light mean they don't exist? Of course not. All it suggests is that color doesn't exist in the world of that blind person. Unlike the blind person, we can see that the world is colorful and beautifully lit, but unlike the blind person, our appreciation for the smells and textures around us might not be so deep.

The same thing pertains to the intuitive sense. Until we've identified with the experience we can't comprehend the nature of the sense and the conscious message that derives from it. Actually we've all felt various degrees and types of intuitive messages throughout our lives but often don't know what they really are. Although we're not likely to increase intuitive sensory perception to the point where we can rely on it exclusively during our lifetimes, we can improve this ability by amplifying the message. We shouldn't discount this gift until we've applied it. It's the most powerful sense humanity will have in the future—so potent, in fact, that even minute degrees of this potential can propel us into new states of being today.

Since this intuitive perception is so underdeveloped in most of us, every effort must be made to nourish the conduit and eliminate as much interruption as possible. The weak signals from this sense can be magnified in this way. Second, we must focus and listen intently for the faint signals and try to amplify them further through meditation, which calms the interference and brings the intuitive message to the surface with clarity. Sound corny? Don't dismiss it out of hand because, if you do, you'll miss out on the most significant life force you have.

Ageless Performance is designed to clean up the airways, clearing the mind and focusing it in the process. Consequently all forms of perception become more vivid. With a little help from regular meditation the intuitive perception can be enhanced to provide a new sense of being, a new feeling of confidence, and a reliable navigation beacon in life.

DIRECTING DESTINY

Whether they're the right paths or not, the courses we take are the ones we've chosen. If we're not satisfied with the state of physical or mental health we find ourselves in, it's up to *us* to change direction. Altering our personal paths can be as easy as breaking away from the same routes we venture on day in and day out to and from our jobs. The automatic courses we take to our places of employment are ones that we can detour from with little effort. We merely tend to choose habitual patterns. Change starts with a decision to make a different choice. The choice is up to us individually; take the first step in a different direction, then the next step until you're farther and farther away from the wrong course and embarked on the correct personal journey. The alternative is to stick with a habit, even though it may feel wrong and numb the senses to the outcome or mute the intuitive message that warns like a persistent aching to change.

However, the new directions we choose will be futile unless we're aware of all the factors that have prompted a decision to implement change. This level of awareness requires that all perceptive abilities are functioning at full capacity, including the intuitive guide. Our personal navigators signal like relentless beacons. When we can't focus on these signals or heed them, that means the conduit has been impaired. Impairment may be caused by poor nutritional state, emotional or mental instability, and even physical disease. Still, even in a state of disruption, the signals can get through faintly. But even when they do, many of us dismiss them and bury them deeper, sometimes retrospectively acknowledging that we felt something odd but failing to heed the intuitive warnings.

Life's successes, whatever they are for you, are guided by these warnings. Neglect them, fail to allow them into your life, and you'll never find your personal way. Following the paths of others won't take you down your unique road, either. If you're healthy and down-to-earth enough to interpret these messages from within correctly, you'll be propelled along a course where things seem to happen in your favor. Travel someone else's path and you'll experience resistance in your life because you're not supposed to be there.

In this day and age it's likely you've already applied healthy measures of one type or another. However, the adoption of healthy practices amid a variety of unhealthy habits can render your efforts futile. The same nutritional strategies we've seen throughout this book contribute to the well-being of the mind and the perception chemistry it relies on, and that includes the clarification of the intuitive navigational sense. Human resilience is formidable; misuse, overuse, and abuse are rarely considered harmful until evidenced by disease. Remember, you can *choose* to change your ways before disease develops.

If you're fighting disease today, you've likely had numerous warnings and ample time to avoid the inevitable. Too often we fail to identify the nature of these omens and bury them deep—out of sight, out of mind. The problem is that these interments fester in the subconscious where they act negatively on your personal and professional lives and your well-being.

Health deteriorates slowly. It usually takes years for disease to develop to the point where symptoms become apparent. Too frequently we bury ourselves in denial with the help of substance abuse, workaholism, or other obsessive behavior, and it takes an undisturbed, completely nourished mind to recognize the subtle signs that something is wrong. A lot of courage is needed to make bold changes, but when you've developed a reliable sense of intuition, you'll feel confident about your decision. This inner health—and the self-confidence it breeds—relies immensely on proper nourishment.

Your sensibility is accessible only to you. Only you can know your direction in life. But you can't proceed along your personal path without honing in on your internal beacon. The task of supplying the right nutrients to accomplish this is yours. The job of alleviating emotional disturbance is yours, too. Your body and mind will tell you when you've journeyed down the wrong road, when your nutritional condition is deficient, and when your emotional state is undermining your well-being. It's up to you to focus your healthy mind, listen to the messages, and react positively— proactively. This is a critical component of disease prevention and crucial to personal and professional success.

The miracles that lie deep within you can't be deployed without complete nutrition. They can also be prompted by instructions from a healthy mind that has a clear conduit to the body. If you believe that negative thoughts and toxic emotions can manifest an adverse physical outcome, then you won't have any trouble accepting that a positive mental influence can bring about a positive physical result, as well. The human brain is thought to be more developed than that of any other animal, yet most of us are lucky if we use 5% of the potential that vibrates between our ears. The time has come for you to tap into this amazing potential and make the health of your brain and mind a central focus for prevention, healing, and athletic performance.

Ageless Performance is structured to support maximum cognitive health because the state of mind sets the pace for physical well-being. Remember when someone you know "lost" his or her mind? How quickly did his or her state of physical health degrade? The person's physical health likely declined significantly after a loss of mental capacity. Patients with mental disorders usually have a higher incidence of physical disease, especially if the former problem is the kind that induces a state of confusion, anguish, anger, anxiety, or depression (1, 2, 3, 4).

A healthy mindset isn't something that just happens. Some of us have to work harder than others to maintain this positive state. Unfortunately many of us fall into chronic depression, but even with clinically depressed patients there are things that can be done at least partially. Exercise and diet are crucial in the management of this condition, and so is meditation.

Studies have shown that cardiovascular health is significantly affected by mental state, and depression amplifies the danger to the heart (5). Cardiovascular patients are at greater risk of mortality if a depressed condition persists through the recovery period. In fact, the possibility of sudden death increases for these patients when depression enters the picture (6).

For those people battling depression, drugs can't be their only crutches if they care about long-term health. The common tricyclic antidepressant drugs have recently been identified as factors that multiply the risk of breast cancer and non-Hodgkin's lymphoma. Further investigation has revealed a likely genotoxic effect by tricyclic antidepressants, inducing some sort of gene mutation (7, 8, 9). Ageless Performance applied diligently can help wean such people off potentially hazardous synthetic drugs, *but only with a doctor's approval and guidance*. By using the program's alternative strategies, drug requirements may drop, reducing the associated risks. Eventually, when biochemical balance is established, drugs might not be needed at all.

MIND-BUILDING

Mind-building is just like bodybuilding. Practicing meditation techniques for decades, masters of this realm dive deeper into the mind than most of us can ever imagine. Having practiced for more than a decade, I, too, realize that infinity exists deep within us. In this peaceful place the mind is freed from flesh and blood. Once relieved from the tangled web of what should be, what should have been, what others expect, what needs to be, and what is right or wrong, the influence of the mind on the body can't be negative. It just is. To practice meditation daily is to build a stronger, sharper, more focused mind to support a sturdy, vibrant, and resilient body.

If you live life without a break from daily skirmishes, you'll never hear the cry for help your cells, body, and soul might be broadcasting to your consciousness. A properly tuned mind not only recognizes the warnings from within, it also sends out life preservation and life recovery to the cells in need. An unhealthy mind can't bring the warnings to the surface and instead transmits distress signals of its own that become etched in the cells.

After practicing mind-building for a while, you, too, will be able to reach sanctuary and remain there in peace for 15 minutes a day before executing the second phase of the meditation program. The second phase of the program

I like to use is visualization of recovery, maintenance, and/or performance. The first phase is less mind-active while the second is proactive—mind over matter, mind to matter. By regularly practicing and perfecting this technique, the mind eventually becomes sharper and more receptive to all of the senses, including intuition.

Successful athletes learn to use this powerful tool to accomplish what others fail to see possible in themselves. A seasoned businessperson crafts a plan of action with market studies, costs, revenue projections, profits, and a clearly defined method of execution. In order to achieve a personal or professional goal it has to be seen clearly and a plan needs to be implemented with conviction. Visualization puts the goal in sight and keeps it there.

The mind and body work much the same way. The difference is that cells are already preprogrammed with miraculous metabolic systems that can manifest a visualized outcome. The planning is already there in the form of genetic instruction, and the tools are inherent, as well; all that has to be done is to define clearly what the outcome from that instruction and activity must be. In other words, we have healing and recovery potential already built into our genetic programming. Our minds can mediate the process by instructing and directing these systems to the sites where their activity is required.

See the vision with clarity, believe in its achievement each and every day, and your body will employ its generative biochemical cascade. These miracles are just waiting for the development of healthy conduits through correct nutrition and positive instruction by a focused mind.

Ask successful athletes about their meditation techniques. You'll discover that some of them don't even realize they meditate or visualize a preferred outcome. It's likely viewed as regular or even ritual mental preparation for their training or competition. That's how I began my meditation. Athletes use their mental powers to prepare for physical performance, recover from daily training, and build their bodies, minds, and spirits to levels of majestic harmony. True genetic potential is experienced only when this harmony is established. Whatever it's called, it's the typical mind-over-matter doctrine and, I assure you, it's a critical part of any successful athlete's training.

Athlete or not, meditation and visualization *must* be part of our lives.

They're powerful facilitators of healing and prevention. If you can't believe the mind is a potent method of healing, prevention, and self-realization, this itself might be one of the biggest hurdles you'll need to overcome. Ageless Performance helps you realize your mind's potential and trust your intuitive sense.

THE BODY COMMUNICATES IN SIGNS

We're all exposed to so-called stressors, but it's the way we perceive them or allow them to influence us emotionally that ultimately determines whether or not they're experienced as negative, neutral, or positive biochemistry. The most stressful thing we can do in life is to try to conform to someone else's expectations. Stick to your core and you'll find most of the answers you need in life within yourself.

If you believe the feelings we experience don't have a physical outcome, think again. These feelings are caused by chemicals that have as much if not more of an impact from the inside of our bodies as physical contact has from the outside. The very fact that we *feel* is evidence enough that feelings manifest physical change. Let's face it. The wrath of emotional assault on the body causes anxiety to squeeze the breath out of us, anguish and worry to twist our stomachs, and anger to raise pressure in our heads to excruciating levels. Emotions mold both the chemical and physical states.

Meditation clears the mind of interference and launches us on the path to better mental focus, initiating a sort of emotional reset. It facilitates the reception of those subtle intuitive messages and helps us to interpret them as well as to determine the needs of our bodies. Meditation instills emotional and mental stability so that we can identify with greater ease the subtle signs, but there are more overt symptoms that often beset us when we fail to register the fainter indications. These bolder symptoms are obvious: sleeplessness, lethargy, mysterious pains, acute or chronic inflammation, recurring indigestion or constipation, stomach acid reflux, low or high blood pressure, tachycardia, anxiety, loss of appetite, frequent colds and flu, anemia, chronic edema, prolonged post-training soreness, frequent physical injury, constant unexplainable bleeding, carbohydrate and fat cravings, obesity, stiff muscles, head tension, unconscious frowning, teeth grinding, night sweats, heart palpitations, bloating, diarrhea, and inexplicable weight loss.

Some of the above symptoms are common occurrences that many of us experience without concern, but they're actually signs of wear and tear, dysfunction, disorder, subconscious distress, and even possible disease if they persist. With clear awareness and action upon interpretation of the subtle messages that precede these more dangerous symptoms, the development of disease can be intercepted long before it's had a chance to take us down.

PSYCHONEURAL HEALING

An important part of Ageless Performance involves the tuning of the mind to drive the natural healing process, the inherent protective shield, and elite athletic performance. Meditating once or twice doesn't extract the potential. It requires persistence and practice, just as it takes many years of application to become a good professional hockey player. The human nervous system, as we know it, is organized into different functional systems: (a) the central nervous system, which consists of the brain and spinal cord; (b) the peripheral nervous system, which transmits neural impulses from the central nervous system to the effector and receptor sites; and (c) direct neuropeptide communication in which the central nervous system communicates directly with the organs of the body via neuropeptides (short chains of amino acids).

Disease breeds anxiety, despair, grief, denial, and anger, and these emotions interfere with the healing process. Neuropeptides communicate directly with peripheral systems, including the immune and organ systems. Emotions or mental stimuli can beat drugs and nutrients to the punch when it comes to recovery or performance.

Conventional medicine now more readily accepts multiple alternative approaches, which include herbal and homeopathic remedies, nutritional prevention programs, and even meditation, visualization, and relaxation therapies. It's a common misunderstanding to believe that drugs and exogenous therapies employ healing when, in fact, the body repairs itself with the assistance of these chemicals. Antibiotics, for example, bring infection to a controllable level so that the body can deploy its intrinsic forces and resume the healing process. Vaccines simply empower the immune system to protect the body. However, our inadvertent dependence on these drugs has actually turned them against us. Our reluctance to facilitate internal healing and our penchant for relying exclusively on antibiotics have resulted in the development of strains of bacteria that are more devastating and deadlier than ever.

Today's treatment or assault on cancer is a primitive concept. Radiation and chemotherapy indiscriminately attack all living tissues, hoping to kill the cancer before destroying the host. Future therapies will involve arming the target-specific immune system of the host with the tools it needs to remove diseased tissue. Meditation and visualization aid this process.

The most potent therapy is the application of nutraceutical and psychoneuro *prevention* to lessen the risk of disease, and nutraceutical and psychoneuro *therapy* to assist recovery. The *last* functional choice to resort to if absolutely necessary for disease recovery is the nutraceutical and psychoneuro therapy accompanied by pharmaceuticals. Such a program might reduce the level of foreign chemical drugs required, and it will help address the biochemical cause of disease for long-term recovery while combating the negative side effects typically associated with pharmaceuticals.

You might not have the education to prescribe a complementary remedy, but you can choose to place your faith in the professional who does. Without an understanding of how diet and nutrition influence humans, health-care education is incomplete. In taking on the responsibility of health care, a professional in this field must also accept the need to upgrade his or her knowledge base with the advent of new discoveries. Today's health professional *must* be well versed in both naturopathy and conventional medicine. It's a tall order, but it's today's reality.

The faith you place in your health-care practitioner also influences your potential for recovery. Believe in this person and your chances for recuperation are greater, but if you question the professional opinion and the therapy, the likelihood of total improvement is reduced. Ask as many questions as it takes to gain the faith you need to allow your inherent miracle to be deployed without interruption. If you're not convinced, your intrinsic healing process can't work in synergy with your health-care professional's application. In fact, it might even oppose the therapy. Psychoneuro activity is powerful stuff; learn to use it to your advantage every time you can. Find every reason you can to believe in your choice and it will work for you with much greater efficiency.

Psychoneuro immunology is a rapidly growing mind-body science. The Imperial Cancer Research Fund laboratory takes a "new approach to cancer treatment." It's brought together "scientists, clinicians, peptide technology, and biotechnology to investigate a new concept at the Clinical Oncology Unit." The organization claims to have found that "molecules called neuropeptides are potent growth factors that can dock on the receptor sites of cancer cells and deliver signals that make cells multiply out of control. Cancer cells can even manufacture these growth factors themselves, accelerating the multiplying process still further."

These researchers claim to have identified a group of antagonists that actually block these growth factors. The research is still in its infancy and the experimental trials are still investigative. The researchers hope to combine this therapy with conventional chemotherapy in the near future, and once completely developed this immune-driven strategy might possibly be a treatment for some forms of cancer.

Neuropeptides were important in my bodybuilding career. I actually imagined the recovery and growth of each body part that was trained earlier that day and watched my body shift into the shape my mind's eye set as a goal. The vision eventually became so clear that it was as though I'd glimpsed it before, and without even realizing it I slowly but surely tailored my physique to reflect this fantastic insight. I saw, I believed, and I made it happen. You can do the same for sport, for prevention, and for therapy.

UNLEASHING THE POWER

Western Gym in Vancouver was a temple and a fellowship with a way of its own. It was the hard-core fitness center where I spent most of my competitive training years. The atmosphere was thick with the sounds of clashing metal plates and the thundering echo of heavy weights pounding black-matted floors. The support by cheering members of the fellowship was muffled by the grunting of lifters pushing "poundages" typically associated with forklift limits. Western Gym was a unique environment. Energy oozed from the place, attracting people from the busy street like a magnet. The windowless pit resonated with chants of encouragement and roars of conquest, making it sound and feel like a medieval place of torture.

Amid this explosive ambience the momentum toward my dream ran its course at warp speed. The energy possessed by a group of people pushing for the same goal is a phenomenal force, and the success experienced by numerous members of this group wasn't coincidental. Western Gym bred many of the top power lifters and bodybuilders in Canada for two reasons: first, only those with this extreme goal remained in the intense environment and those who survived it had iron wills; and second, the electric atmosphere stimulated psychneuro recovery and performance.

On many occasions I lifted serious poundages: squatting 715 pounds for reps of three, shoulder-pressing 365 pounds for multiple repetitions, and bench-pressing with 495 pounds. In fact, these were loads that national power lifters were lucky to be able to lift in competition at that time. Preparing the mind for the 715-pound squat was an amazing process. I'd begin my ritual sit in front of a towering squat cage that held a power bar with seven 45-pound plates and a 10-pounder, with a heavy-duty clamp on each side. Other gym members would crowd around the rack, postponing their own workouts to support my effort. The room around me would become fuzzy, with only the squat rack and bar visible in my dreamlike concentration. Within seconds my heart rate would accelerate; a few moments more and power would be transferred to my legs.

My mind's eye would witness the squat several times before the attempt, and in each instance the vision would be clearer, the lift easier. At that point, outside myself, I'd know I was ready to lift. It would seem as if I actually watched the lift from another plane of existence, with the crowd's muffled chants barely recognizable. All sense of logic and reason would be removed from the situation to enable me to step under a bar that held more than two feet of iron plate on each side, lift it onto an almost bare shoulder, and feel the thick metal Olympic bar bow from the load.

Some people might say I was out of my mind to attempt such a feat, but it was more like *out of body*, a technique that worked for me!

Power athletes commonly employ this type of preparation for a lift or other physical feats and take for granted the potential of the skill they've developed. Most people can't fathom or relate to this experience. It takes years of practice to develop such a mind-body connection, but once it's achieved the applications for this capacity are endless. However, athletes who have fine-tuned this incredible tool too often fail to apply its full potential to athletics let alone activities outside sport.

BELIEVE TO ACHIEVE

In my bodybuilding days I believed with conviction that by focusing my mind on each organ or gland I could produce adrenaline emissions, testosterone secretions, and endorphins to prepare for extraordinary power output and recovery. The belief that my mind could stimulate this activity on command eventually gave me the ability to do so. I saw a whirling ball of glittering particles, glowing with positive energy as it orbited my brain. When the glowing mass gained momentum, it picked up more of these glittering particles, which represented neuropeptides and stimulating neurotransmitters. Leaving a trailing tail like that of a comet, the ball of positive psychoneuro energy was hurled repeatedly through an animated conduit to reach the target in my body in need of stimulation.

Soon I could actually feel my heart rate and blood pressure rise and my body pulse with energy. In time my body responded more promptly and profoundly to my commands. The energy from within was accompanied by the outside energy from my peers, and my body was transformed each time into something I couldn't identify. My body would power the lift in my absence! Without this preparation I could barely haul the same loaded bar off the rack.

My daily weight-training regimen developed this mind-body connection more effectively with each session. I tapped into this inner power a few times per day, each occasion making the connection clearer. While some of the "lighter" training days needed little concentration, the "heavy" ones required a deeper dive to access the power source.

I used a similar technique to induce recovery from a workout. In my mind's eye I developed the same power surge of neuropeptides, boosting hormone secretions and assisting the delivery of nutrients to tissues that needed them, with my goal of stronger and bigger muscle mass as constant reference points. As much as I believed that my mind contributed to the extraordinary results I was experiencing as a bodybuilder, I wasn't aware of the true potential this exceptional gift could provide until I was challenged by the next test.

TRIAL OF A LIFETIME

While nearing the peak of my bodybuilding career, after winning my class title, the overall title, and the best poser award at the Western Canadian Bodybuilding Championships, I was diagnosed with severe ulcerative colitis. Extensive tests of blood samples and tissue biopsies confirmed the diagnosis. Before I knew it I was in a hospital bed, anemic and barely able to stand. Twenty days later I was wheeled out of the hospital weighing about 170 pounds from a prediagnosis weight of approximately 225. I was informed that I should prepare myself for surgery and that my bodybuilding career was over.

The physical pain paled in comparison to the psychological demolition. My dreams shattered and my life about to change forever, I bounced through a perpetual cycle of anger, pity, denial, and depression. Just as I seemed to get better, I had a turn for the worse and was back in a state of depression and self-pity, a process that continued for several weeks as my condition progressively deteriorated.

It wasn't until I accepted the illness and took on the responsibility for recovery that everything changed. First, a transformation in my mindset eliminated negative emotional distress. After that I increased my education on the medication I was taking to research a deeper understanding of the biochemical influences. Soon I learned that one of the major contributing factors to my depression, anger, and even homicidal and suicidal thoughts was the dreaded corticosteroid therapy.

The emotional and psychological manifestations associated with corticosteroid therapy are quite serious and might contribute to the physical side effects as well as to the perpetuation of the primary disease. The psychic derangements listed in *The Compendium of Pharmaceuticals and Specialties* that are associated with the administration of prednisone (a commonly prescribed corticosteroid-type drug) are as follows: "euphoria, insomnia, mood swings, personality changes, severe depression...psychotic manifestations...also existing emotional and psychotic tendencies may be aggravated."

Patients are rarely advised of these side effects but must be aware of them in order to anticipate emotional changes. With an understanding of the origin of emotional outbursts and mood swings, we're better equipped to deal with them. I tried many times to get off the drug slowly, but the inflammatory condition raged out of control even more each time. Having accumulated extensive biochemical and nutritional education, I was quick to comprehend the biochemistry of the drugs that were prescribed. The more I uncovered, the more I realized I had to wean myself off prednisone, but it took a clever strategy and a lot of patience to do so.

The fact that prednisone and other corticosteroid therapies often impart psychosomatic side effects makes meditation, visualization, and readjustment of mindset critical to a healthy outcome. This mindset must be addressed by concurrent administration of nutraceuticals that support better mental health and combat any other side effects of the drugs. The essential and other omega fats, along with the nutrient navigational factors of Ageless Performance, are a perfect complement to such pharmaceutical therapies. In fact, much of Ageless Performance's design was inspired by my study of these pharmaceuticals.

A major advantage I had during this period was a deep knowledge of the eicosanoid-hormone science with a performance objective that I was researching at the university. My illness set the stage for a sudden shift in my research directive. Survival is a powerful motivator. Another advantage I didn't know I possessed at the time was that my mind-body connection was already strong and functional far beyond the abilities of the average individual. In other words, I had a head start. When I applied the potential of meditation and visualization, there was no learning or building curve and recovery ensued almost immediately.

Finally, in order to take myself off prednisone expeditiously, adrenal support had to be administered before, during, and for some time after the therapy. How do you apply this preventive measure before the administration of a drug if you don't know you're going to be taking it? Very simple. It's part of the preventive strategy incorporated into Ageless Performance. The only addition that has to be made while on these adrenal-depleting drugs is licorice root and panax ginseng extracts. The other important factors, including substantial doses of vitamin C, are already part of Ageless Performance. Adrenal support is critical to longevity regardless of state of health or fitness.

Many of these nutraceutical (nutritional) requirements are available through a database on the Biologic Nutritional Research Inc. Web site (*www.biologicnr.com*) for professionals and consumers to access free of charge. It's a service I've identified to be essential for optimal health care. In addition these databases deliver information on pharmaceutical drug–nutraceutical interactions to help professionals and consumers create efficacious and safe complementary strategies.

Essential fatty-acid and fish-source omega-3 fat supplementation suddenly became the central facet of my therapeutic program. I was deep into the research, with the scientific evidence piling up so high that I was convinced I was on the correct biochemical path. This belief encouraged new hope that in turn sparked recovery. After implementing the program for three or four weeks, I felt better. In fact, 10 weeks after leaving the hospital I was back in the gym training lightly with no intention of pursuing my bodybuilding dream anytime soon. However, soon after I employed the facilitative co-factors for the metabolism of essential fats, recuperation progressed quickly. Ageless Performance, as I've already mentioned, was developed through these trials and tribulations.

Every day during that period I employed pervasive visualization. Before this my application of visualization was strictly used for bodybuilding, power, and athletic performance. Again my whirling ball of healing neuropeptides swarmed cells to stimulate their natural ability to heal. I imagined my immune system marching troops of phagocytic cells to the site, removing cells damaged beyond repair. Each day the construction site was easier to imagine and each day the tissue looked healthier.

This program took me from a state of mental and physical breakdown to a condition of self-sufficiency. I soon achieved a recovery that allowed me to compete and win the IFBB North American Bodybuilding Championships. Much more than that, I was able to accomplish slowly but surely a complete recuperation from a disease that medical professionals said was lifelong. Only a few years after diagnosis and a prognosis that was grim, I was back to above-average health with no sign of disease. Doctors were confused and amazed at the same time. Today, more than 10 years later, I still possess top physical and mental health. This is the kind of miracle that resides within everyone, the sort of miracle that waits for the right formula to activate it. Ageless Performance will nurture this potential to fruition just as it has for me and many others.

You don't have to have a medical or physiology degree to use the afore-mentioned visualization strategy. Nor do you need to know precisely how these tissues and systems interact or look. You can make up your own animated version of recovery. Better yet, study a few physiology texts to gain an idea of how the endocrine, digestive, cardiovascular, and other systems appear and relate. Use these references to visualize your own functional version. Employ a daily routine in which the mind sends out positive instruction and energy. However, you do have to utilize this process daily and take a mentally active role. By "mentally active" I mean there must be an effort to remove everything unrelated from your mind during the meditation and you must attempt to activate your internal systems. This activation requires extreme mental focus and energy. Use this practice for sport but employ it daily to maintain general biological recovery and a healthy body and mind. But be warned: if you only implement your inner powers for sport the way I did for many years, you'll create physical and mental imbalances.

GETTING INTO MEDITATION

Find a room in your home that's quiet and free of traffic. Let everyone in your house know you don't want to be disturbed for 15 to 30 minutes. Take five to 10 minutes to remove all thoughts from your mind. Once you're able to dive deep into that dark place free of physical and mental impositions, you're ready for the next phase. It might be hard to find this depth at first, but it will get easier.

As thoughts enter your mind, allow them to go away. Don't get frustrated if you find it difficult to expel all thought from your mind. Eventually you'll have a blank screen, and when you do, maintain your attention on the darkness, the vastness, the emptiness. Don't fight intrusive thoughts, just allow them to come and go and try to stay with the emptiness as much as possible. Some people employ mantras to focus their minds; others prefer to concentrate on each breath as it travels through the body. Use whatever method serves you best.

Maintaining blankness is the most difficult task. You'll find that you can go farther and farther into the vastness as you get better at meditation, but it takes time to be able to stay with the darkness. As your ability to delve deeper improves, so does your general mental and emotional stability and focus. Be aware that even as you improve, some mediations will be better concentrated than others. Days when you just can't focus will be positive experiences, as well, because they'll tell you how each thing in your life is influencing your ability to focus. Process the message and make the appropriate changes! These lifestyle changes in response to this deep awareness are the most powerful preventive factors you can implement.

Once you've had ample time to stay with the peaceful darkness, say, seven to 15 minutes, you can move on to the active phase—visualization. Again, don't be upset if your quiet time is interrupted many times by unavoidable thought. Just let the thoughts come and go passively.

VISUALIZING RECOVERY

Now it's time to guide your immune system, neuropeptides, and nutrient building blocks and fuels to the site of construction where you can supervise recovery. If your image is made unclear by other thoughts that enter the picture, just continue to concentrate on the important task at hand and don't fret about secondary thoughts.

When I was a practicing bodybuilder, I visualized my goal whether it was muscle mass for upcoming shows or benchmarks I set for lifts. Each time I saw myself work and build toward these targets. It only took 15 to 30 minutes each day. During my competitive years, if time permitted, I'd meditate or visualize before my workout and as soon as I could afterward. Again, while in bed before sleeping, I'd visualize recovery and muscle building. Now once per day is enough for me. Some people, though, meditate several times daily.

If you include visualization and meditation as part of your recovery strategy from disease without having used them previously, results might not be significant until you've practiced the techniques for a while. As soon as you begin to attain some goals, however, your belief in the system will drive exponential recovery.

Ageless Performance must be employed in its entirety to ensure that recovery from disease is expeditious and complete and that the most powerful prevention is achieved. You'll experience good results—more energy, stable energy levels, leaner measures, and even prevention to a degree— if you follow the diet and forgo the supplementation and visualization. However, if you're looking for phenomenal therapeutic, preventive, and athletic potential, you need to include the supplemental portion of Ageless Performance. The icing on the cake is the concurrent application of meditation and visualization to speed up the incorporation of vital nutrients into healthy, powerful tissue. *Minding* your health will change your life forever. The choice to apply this gift is now yours.

PART III

GETTING WITH THE PROGRAM

15

APPLYING AGELESS PERFORMANCE

Ageless Performance has four facets. In order of priority they are: (1) Solid Ground Foundation—Dietary Component; (2) Nutraceutical Supplementation—Supplement Component; (3) Psychoneuro Induction—Meditation and Visualization or Spiritual Component; and (4) Exercise/Active Lifestyle—Regular Exercise or Other Activity.

The four goal-specific programs in this chapter include the recommendations for:

- Healthy, Fit, and Active Athletes Seeking Performance Improvement
- Muscle-Building/Power Athletes
- Diabetes, Insulin Resistance, and Weight Management/Obesity
- Cardiovascular Disease, Asthma, Inflammation, Biological Aging, and Cognitive and Intestinal Disorders

Don't skip content to jump to your category of interest, because as we progress through each program you'll learn more about your personal needs and the relationship between all of the nutrients discussed earlier. The information from one category will contribute to knowledge of the next. The different categories can also be merged to address multiple needs and goals concurrently. Let's begin!

RECOMMENDATIONS
for Healthy, Fit, and Active Athletes Seeking Performance Improvement

People who have demanding, labor-intensive jobs, who work five days a week, and who run or weight-train regularly (three to five days per week) require higher nutrient intakes than more sedentary individuals. With a greater energy expenditure, a higher nutrient intake must be consumed, but determining this requirement by mere calorie calculation only sets the foundation for more disarray. The more common way to establish a daily allotment of nourishment is the estimation of necessary caloric intake to accommodate for lifestyle—and metabolism-specific expenditure by the body. From this master value nutrient requirements such as protein, fat, and carbohydrate intake are often calculated using strict mathematical guidelines. But this method makes no sense at all. The empty calories that processed foods deliver breed more nutrient deficiency in the body. Processed nourishment can cause malnutrition as essential nutrient co-factors are depleted from the body's stores during metabolism. This calorie-centered belief system is way off the mark when it comes to biological needs.

Individuals who are extremely active, of course, need more calories. And if they're fighting disease, they require even more calories for the struggle. However, fuel demands metabolic co-factors for metabolism. The immune system needs all kinds of vitamin and mineral co-factors that aren't accounted for in the typical estimation of calorie intake. The increased requirement for antioxidants and specialized polyunsaturated fats, which an incremental physical and immune-system activity promotes, isn't provided by the common calorie.

White processed bread, rice, and pasta deliver carbohydrates, minuscule quantities of protein and, of course, calories. If this is your choice to supply the calorie increment during stressful periods, you'll further diminish your body's metabolic sparks. Although you might seem to recover from your disease or workout-induced physical degradation with a blind increment of caloric intake, the nutrient deficit will continue to fester in an alternate metabolic system. Eventually the shortage will resurface as the same disease or another unless it's replenished in the form of essential nutrients.

Health-care professionals often speak about the need for increased caloric intake to accommodate for incremental immune-system activity during a battle with disease. Frequently medium-chain triglycerides (MCTS) are recommended as easy-to-assimilate fat calories that can make up requisite energy needs. Here again the concept is completely absurd, yet it's a common strategy used by uninformed professionals—common because most medical people don't have a clue about the nutritional needs of the very biological system they're treating.

Although the extra calories required to fuel the body are easily made up with the consumption of MCT oils (nine calories per gram), the co-factors that are *essential* for MCT metabolism aren't supplied by these relatively empty calories unless a multi-vitamin, multi-mineral formulation is concurrently administered. These calories lack protein crucial for tissue recovery and immune-system immunoglobulin and antibody production. The immune system retrieves its protein building blocks from the diet, but if calories devoid of sufficient immune-specific fuels are relied on to power the body, protein-containing tissue such as muscle mass is catabolized (broken down) to supply the irreplaceable amino-acid building blocks for immunity to be employed. In essence tissues are literally eaten up to provide immune function.

If we were to depend on valueless calories to furnish incremental energy requirements created by work, nutrient status throughout the body would absorb the dietary deficit of vitamin and mineral co-factors, giving rise eventually to a predisposition for disease. When muscle recovery is needed due to extreme activity, whether by exercise or other work, the immune system and muscles compete for a limited supply of protein building blocks. In this case both immunity and muscle recovery are compromised. Athletic performance, in this state, is suboptimal as is immune capacity, and for this reason such athletes fall victim to the common cold and flu regularly. Supply these amino-acid building blocks through sufficient dietary protein and all of the co-dependent systems will receive their requisite fuels and building blocks.

With incremental physical and mental work, dietary calories must be increased, but the additional calories have to be a function of the primary requirement. The primary requirement is an incremental need for essential nutrition, and in this case many nutrients that we might not normally consider critical become so, such as glutamine, alpha lipoic acid, and acetyl l-carnitine. Protein intake must be escalated, essential fat must be boosted, and the intake of whole, fresh carbohydrate sources must be increased. All of these increments contribute to a jump in caloric intake, but again these calories are merely a consequence of augmented nutrient density.

The determination of nutritional requirements for Ageless Performance is assessed first by calculating protein needs. The program for an active individual includes a higher protein and carbohydrate intake than that necessary for a less active person. By calculation this amounts to an intake of about 1 to 1.2 g of protein per gram of lean body weight per day. Lean body weight is a lot different from total body weight, even if you consider yourself fit. The former can be arrived at by having a bio-impedance mass-proportion assessment made or by utilizing more accurate infrared inductance technology. Density testing by water displacement is the most accurate gauge of lean-mass proportion of the body, but it's the least likely to be available to the public. Your local fitness center will have one method available or will know where an assessment can be procured.

Health-care professionals are beginning to recognize the value of body-mass-proportion assessment as opposed to the overall body mass or weight that a typical scale measures. However, if you wish to employ a macronutrient co-factor value suitable for most individuals without measuring lean body mass precisely, use the protein co-factor (PC) of 1—1 g of protein per pound of total body weight per day. This method works for those who don't have extremely excessive body-fat masses (under 20%).

If your body weight is 170 pounds and this Active category is where you best fit, your protein intake for the day should be 170 g (Active PC = 1 g of protein times 170 pounds = 170 g of protein per day). Keep in mind that this daily protein total is for *active* individuals who are turning tissues and nutrients over at a faster rate than sedentary folk. The total protein is best consumed over five meals so that the body can absorb the quantity efficiently. In this case, four meals, as opposed to five, are less likely to deliver the total absorbable protein requirement for the day, since the average maximum absorption potential of protein per meal might be as much as 40 g for men and 30 g or less for women.

That means you can't double up a protein count for a meal if you miss one. The solution to the meal-frequency problem is the use of protein-supplement beverage mixes between food meals—primarily whey protein isolates. If food is used exclusively—devoid of supplementation—to make up the daily protein intake, the consequential caloric ingestion and an abundance of the wrong fats from high-protein foods could be problematic. By including whey supplements in the diet, three complete food meals can be bolstered by two protein drinks (separate times) daily to meet demands with nominal caloric contribution. This protein-supplementation strategy is more realistic in terms of convenience, as well. You wouldn't want to prepare five or six meals each day, would you? Keep in mind that protein drinks must be accompanied by polyunsaturated fats (flax and/or fish oils). The absorption of many nutrients is enhanced by dietary protein, which means supplementing nutraceuticals (multi-vitamin/mineral/phytonutrient) with protein drinks isn't a bad idea.

The only time protein-absorption potential will exceed the 40 g average per meal for men and 30 g average for women is immediately after exercise. This window of opportunity (one to three hours after exercise) must always be used to consume more protein and carbohydrates than would be eaten in the typical meal of the day, hence facilitating both glycogen and tissue recovery from the training load. As much as 50 to 55 g of protein for men and 40 g for women in this post-workout meal or drink is sufficient and safe, and the whey protein isolate drink will be more efficiently absorbed. Often, for my post-workout drink, I consume whey protein isolate in orange juice with a blend of frozen berries and a banana, one of the few occasions I mix whey protein in anything other than water.

Carbohydrate consumption can be doubled for a meal during this post-workout window of opportunity. Taking advantage of the post-workout period is important in order for work-induced catabolism of tissue to be limited, muscle and liver glycogen recovery to ensue to completion, and tissue recovery to be as whole as possible. With this total recuperation, the next training session is more likely to be supported by a full load of fuel, provided healthy dietary habits are continued after the post-workout loading. If glycogen stores are fully restored and tissue anabolism is completed from training session to training session, performance potential can accumulate instead of a situation that leads to plateau or decline. In addition, these restorative strategies will decrease the risk of disease, which will inevitably escalate if intense physical work persists amid nutrient scarcity.

The recommendation for a very active individual is to accompany the total protein requirement for the day with a carbohydrate intake that's about 175% of the protein consumption, say, 298 g daily for a 170-pound individual. The Active carbohydrate co-factor (cc) is therefore 1.75 g of carbohydrates per gram of daily protein required (Active cc = 1.75 g of carbohydrates times 170 g of total protein required = 298 g of dietary carbohydrates per day).

THE RIGHT CARBOHYDRATE SOURCES AND THEIR CORRECT PROPORTIONS

Each meal requires about 40 to 50 g of carbohydrates. With four meals per day in addition to the super-carbohydrate-loaded post-workout meal, the total of 298 g is easy to meet. Half or just over half (20 to 25 g per meal) of the carbohydrate total for each meal can be provided by a denser carbohydrate source such as whole-grain bread (stone ground), white potato (after a workout only), whole-wheat pasta, kamut, couscous, or whole brown rice.

About a half cup of cooked brown rice supplies 25 g of relatively high-glycemic-index, dense carbohydrates. The high-glycemic-index carbohydrate sources are best saved for eating immediately after training unless energy expenditure is extreme, requiring extensive carbohydrate consumption throughout the day. Even in the latter case, low-glycemic-index, micronutrient-dense carbohydrate sources are usually called for—in other words, whole foods.

Keep in mind that the post-workout window can stay open for as much as three or more hours for individuals involved in extremely intense (super sets for an hour or so) and/or prolonged two- to four-hour sessions of physical activity (endurance training, for example). This three-hour window allows a person to eat two super-loaded carbohydrate meals separated by approximately two to two and a half hours. In fact, in extreme cases such as marathon, distance cycling, and triathlon training, doubling up (two super-loaded consecutive meals within three hours) the post-workout repletion strategy for glycogen reloading is *essential* if complete glycogen recovery is to take place. The first meal must be consumed immediately upon completion of the exercise.

Again, for most other daily meals the low-glycemic-index, dense carbohydrate sources (brown rice, whole-grain pasta, whole-kernel rye bread) makes up just over half of the carbohydrate portion of a meal (20 to 25 g). The rest of the required carbohydrate content for a meal (15 to 20 g) is supplied by even lower glycemic-index vegetable sources such as a mix or one of the following: chicory greens, leeks, broccoli, cauliflower, cabbage, yams, zucchini, squash, green beans, and other legumes. Another way to design a healthy low-glycemic-index meal is to include soups that contain various combinations of the aforementioned vegetables.

Note that the volume of typical low-glycemic-value vegetables required to deliver 15 to 20 g of carbohydrates is quite large: about two cups of vegetable-carbohydrate volume compared to less than half a cup of a dense source such as rice for a similar carbohydrate macronutrient contribution—a half cup of white rice equals 25 g of carbohydrates; a half cup of brown rice equals 25 g of carbohydrates (includes nondigestible fiber); a half cup of broccoli equals 7 g of carbohydrates (includes an abundance of nondigestible fiber); and 1.5 cups of broccoli equals 21 g of carbohydrates.

Eating the volume of food this strategy delivers isn't easy, and that's the amazing thing about this design: low-glycemic-index vegetables are filling. The volume you can consume is huge if you desire abundance. Just eat what you can, getting enough of each food group but keeping the proportions of the design consistent to instill hormone balance and nutrient density within the body. Remember, these foods induce hormonal cascades and these hormone proportions are a direct function of the macronutrient ratio within a meal. Stick to the program design and all of the biological systems will flow healthily, providing optimal hormone balance and maximum restorative and performance potential.

The large servings of low-glycemic-index, high-fiber vegetables serve many purposes in this program. Fiber hasn't been discussed in detail in this book so far, yet it plays a considerable role in human health from many perspectives. It imparts a variety of beneficial nutrients that can be directly utilized by the body or employed by gut bacteria to produce critical metabolites. Some of the constituents of fiber are lignins, phytates, pectins, gums, mucilages, cellulose, and hemicellulose. The processed, fiber-reduced, fast-food diet often lacks these vitally precious constituents. Here's what you're missing when you eliminate them from your diet:

- Fiber fills the gut to enhance satiety of the meal.
- The friendly bacterial byproducts of fiber metabolism (short-chained fatty acids) fuel liver and immune function as well as cardiac and skeletal muscle.
- Bacterial metabolites produced from these fiber components maintain an acidic environment in the colon to keep pathogens and disease at bay, including cancer.
- Fiber constituents also retain sugar in the gut lumen to slow the release of sugar into the bloodstream, lowering the glycemic index of a meal.
- Dietary fiber retains toxins so they aren't absorbed into the body.
- A large portion of fiber is nondigestible, so it doesn't make it into the body, failing to contribute to biologically active calories.
- Fiber sources are loaded with natural vitamins, minerals, and antioxidants.
- An array of healthy fiber sources fuels and supports friendly bacteria; maintains healthy colon activity beyond the benefit of healthy pH; physically cleans the gastrointestinal tract; bolsters biological pH balance in the body; helps control blood pressure through bacterial byproduct assimilation; lowers cholesterol by binding it to carry it out of the body as well as chemically influencing the liver to slow production; and provides fuel for the mucosal cells to proliferate (i.e., fuels cells of the gut lining so they can grow, multiply, and recover).

Our bodies have a vital dependence on natural fiber, which does far more than promote regular bowel movement. Using processed artificial fiber won't help you any better than processed food that's devoid of fiber does. Our evolution-based biology depends on a wide range of natural fibers that have dictated our biological design. A variety of whole foods delivers what we need. The fiber load received with the proper diet increases the demand for water. Some fibers absorb water to maintain better gut flow. Clean, purified water must be consumed abundantly throughout the day.

Fiber content significantly alters the bioavailable calorie count of a meal. Dietary fiber also influences the total calories of a meal by way of fat and other nutrient retention in the gut, including sugar, as mentioned above. By slowing the digestion and absorption of these major calorie-contributing macronutrients and binding them, the total calorie absorption into the body from a meal is down-regulated by dietary fiber—different than you might calculate from tabulated values.

If we determine the total caloric intake from a meal that incorporates this high intake of natural fiber through whole foods, we find that the actual absorption might not be as high as our estimation would indicate. The higher satiety level this fiber-rich food produces also reduces the volume of food we consume per sitting to, once again, lower caloric intake. When nutrient density is elevated, such as the case with this greater natural fiber intake from whole foods, calories needn't be extensive and the body can function much more efficiently to perform at a higher level. Further enhance this nutrient density with a specialized supplementation program and better appetite control and lower calorie consumption will be instilled.

Anti-aging programs center on such calorie-restriction strategies. Many bodybuilders, for example, think they have to consume 5,000 and even as much as 7,000 or 9,000 calories each day to build or maintain their hard-earned, extraordinarily massive lean tissue. It's true that a lot of calories are required to sustain this bio-mass if nutrient density is scant, but if nutrient density is boosted the body's efficiency level will increase, as well. Furthermore, with fewer calories the body is taxed less and fewer free radicals will interfere with metabolic function. With this application, body-fat levels will drop and lean muscle can actually be built with less food volume. The result of applying this strategy is leaner measures, more muscle, less muscle fatigue and soreness, better energy and stamina, and lower risk of disease. This is Ageless Performance at work!

I have a very active lifestyle, working out with weights 30 to 45 minutes five to six times weekly and running 30 to 45 minutes five to six times weekly (15 to 25 miles weekly). Frequently I include an additional 30- to

40-minute late-night walk with my dogs. I rarely exceed 2,250 calories for the day and am often well under this value. These calories support an active body weighing 168 to 170 pounds, with a body-fat mass ranging between 8% to 9%. My macronutrient intake looks like this: 190 to 204 g of protein daily—PC = 1.2; 230 to 250 g of carbohydrates daily; 35 to 45 g of a quality blend of fats.

My regimen is a hybrid of the Active and the Bodybuilding/Power Program displayed in the next goal-specific discussion. I've also incorporated a more aggressive anti-aging nutraceutical component. You might require the development of your own hybrid program to fit your unique metabolic demands and personal goals. Although the calories seem low for my level of activity, the actual bioavailable calorie total of the daily intake is even lower than the calculated values indicate due to the higher-than-average fiber content of the meals.

Extreme endurance sports increase the demands for carbohydrates above the values recommended in this category. If you're participating in marathon- or triathlon-type activity, you'll have to boost carbohydrates for the day significantly from the tabulated recommendations found later in this chapter. However, don't increase your carbohydrates from your regular volumes before trying this new protein-rich approach, since a greater amount of protein and the fat that comes with it will elevate your energy intake to levels that might be acceptable.

The body can use protein as a backup source of energy if carbohydrates (stores and dietary sources) run out. Begin with the recommended (formula-calculated or table-reference) carbohydrate intake and, if required, slowly up your dietary carbohydrates to find your required plateau by trial and error. For ease, use the pertinent tables in this chapter to find your starting point and then make the alterations necessary to personalize the plan.

If you're a proponent of conventional endurance nutrition, which involves inadvertent megaloads of dietary carbohydrates with no consideration for protein and vitamin and mineral co-factors, then you haven't yet reached your full potential in sport. Higher dietary protein intakes will better support lean-muscle-mass recovery from physical work and, therefore, recovery potential from your training. This will provide strength for endurance activity, and if you think muscle strength isn't conducive to endurance sport, you'll lose out to someone who does. Note, however, that these extreme macronutrient strategies are designed for athletes training a maximum of one and a half to two hours daily.

Individuals who work over the two-hour mark have atypical training habits and will need atypical carbohydrate consumption. Again, you'll have to find your personal requirement based on your distinct metabolism and personal activity level. With a four-hour-per-day training schedule, you might require as much as 1,000 g of dietary carbohydrate in addition to the protein and healthy fats supplied by Ageless Performance.

A cautionary warning, though: extreme-exercise rigors and the consequential carbohydrate requirements will take a significant toll on the body. Such programs will degrade the state of health by overwhelming the body with oxidative stress from the extra calories and the extraordinary physical work. I understand the competitive psyche; I've been there. But in this psychological state health isn't usually the primary consideration; winning is. Ageless Performance will escort you down this competitive path with a winning formula that will also preserve as much of your health as possible under the straining conditions.

If you're in this Active category, applying the supplemental portion of the program is an absolute must. The nutraceutical design will facilitate healthy gene activity to enhance recovery and performance potential. The supplemental portion of the program is critical, as well, to the maintenance of immune function and protection from the exceptional level of free-radical stress this level of activity imposes.

Experts claim that exercise sessions lasting more than 40 minutes will overwhelm the antioxidant capacity of the body and induce excessive cortisol secretions (1). Obviously the intensity of the exercise will be a major factor of influence, with a greater level reducing your allowed exercise period before free-radical overload is reached. The additional macronutrients and calories (from carbohydrate sources) required because of the extreme work will also contribute to the oxidative toll of the body. Antioxidant supplementation is crucial in order to ensure health and maximum performance.

EYEBALL-ESTIMATING A MEAL

Calculating your nutrient requirements for each meal might be a little unrealistic for you. If so, use the eyeball-estimation method. This technique for determining a meal's macronutrient proportions necessitates dividing the dinner plate in two. Fill one half of a plate with a vegetable medley or single vegetable from the list described earlier in this chapter. The other half of the plate will be divided again in half. Half of this second half will be filled with a dense carbohydrate source such as rice or potato. I often mix brown rice (70%) with wild rice (30%) to make a wholesome dense carbohydrate source. The other half of the second half will consist of a quality protein source chosen from the list in Appendix C.

It's crucial that an athlete meet the necessary protein requirement each day. Check Appendix C to get an idea of the protein count inherent in the common protein sources and the average volume needed to meet the daily requirement. Stick to the higher biological value (BV) sources, those exceeding a measure of 75. Biological value is the worth assigned to a protein source, reflecting the body's ability to digest, absorb, and use it for tissue, hormone, biochemical, and metabolic functions. The higher the BV, the more easily and more efficiently the body can use the protein source for recovery and maintenance. The size of a plate is an obvious factor contributing to total caloric/nutrient intake; using this estimation method maintains healthy proportions of the food groups regardless of the size of a serving plate. Meal proportion, remember, dictates the essence of the hormonal cascade.

If you employ this estimation method, be sure of the correct protein volume required for the meal in relation to your body weight in order to set a standard for the plate size you'll rely on in the future. Once you acquire a relative idea of protein requirements by volume, you won't have to refer to a nutritional almanac or the appendices of this book anymore. Using the same or similar plate size day in and day out, you'll be able to calculate the volume correctly for each meal.

The volume and total weight of one protein source delivering 20 g of protein might not precisely match that of another food providing the same quantity of protein. The fat, carbohydrate content, and hydration level of the protein food dictate how dense the protein content of the source is.

Three ounces of salmon, for example, might impart 17 g of protein (farm salmon generally supplies less protein and more fat). Three ounces of white meat chicken deliver more than 20 g of protein, while three ounces of dark meat chicken provide about 17 g of protein and a little more fat.

The extreme athlete's goal might call for some of the vegetable allowance on the divided plate to be replaced with denser carbohydrate sources if the daily carbohydrate requirement must be higher. If fatigue sets in prematurely during training and glycogen loads deplete severely, dietary carbohydrate intake likely needs to be increased. If you've been in the game for a while, you'll know when you should boost your carbohydrate intake from the starting point (the tabulated suggestion). Glycogen depletion is characteristic of that flat muscle tone—a muscle belly that lacks robustness, muscle weakness, and general lethargy. If this condition prevails, up the daily carbohydrates by increasing the intake of denser ones such as rice, pasta, kamut, and potatoes.

Lower glycemic-index choices of dense carbohydrate sources are better for carbohydrate repletion throughout the day, i.e., yam, sweet potato, oatmeal, aboveground vegetables, and legumes. If and when needed to boost glycogen status of the body, include carbohydrate sources with higher glycemic indexes and greater density in daytime meals, i.e., brown rice, whole-wheat pasta, stone-ground bread, white and yellow potatoes. Again, the post-training meal will always include a more abundant serving of these higher glycemic, denser carbohydrate choices.

For those people battling disease of any kind, the high-density carbohydrate sources must come from choices that rate below 60—the lower the better. This strategy will deliver a healthy supply of carbohydrates at a safe pace that's more easily tolerated by the likely disturbed insulin/glucagon axis of the body. These carbohydrate sources have lower glycemic indexes (GI = below 60) but still fairly high densities and can be used as post-training glycogen loaders for this challenged group. Refer to Appendix A.

Sedentary folk fighting diseases should be restricted to carbohydrate selections with much lower glycemic indexes and, if at all possible, should *only* consume high-density, low-glycemic-index carbohydrate sources (yam, sweet potato) every second day and in small volumes. The best strategy for the sedentary individual struggling with disease is to consume low-glycemic-index, low-density carbohydrates as energy sources (GI = below 60), excluding any other carbohydrate sources from the diet until recovery is well under way.

SAMPLE OF HIGH-DENSITY AND LOW-DENSITY CARBOHYDRATE SOURCES

High Density	Glycemic Index (GI)
Maltodextrin	110
Millet	95–100
White Potato	88–93
Sweet Corn	65–80
Whole-Wheat Pasta	67–70
Couscous	66–69
Whole Brown Rice	55–65
Yam	55–60
Bulgur	55–60
Sweet Potato	53–57
Oatmeal	48–52
Rye Kernels	45–50
Whole-Rye Bread	45–50
Barley	27–33

Low Density	Glycemic Index (GI)
Pinto Bean	33–38
Lentil	33–38
Black Bean	30–35
Soybean	17–25
Tomato	15–20
Squash	12–15
Lettuce	12–15
Pepper	12–15
Zucchini	12–15

These macronutrient proportions, the protein and carbohydrate levels in the meal, will be consistent for three or four meals of the day. They'll quickly add up to meet your needs. If more carbohydrates are required due to extreme energy expenditure, your supplemented protein (protein drinks or other protein snacks between meals) will have to be accompanied by dietary carbohydrates. Planning to cook extra quantities of a healthy carbohydrate source when preparing a meal will allow for the availability of healthy carbohydrate sources for snacking such as yams, sweet potatoes, oatmeal, beans, and whole-grain rye bread. These proactive strategies will support healthier eating habits when you're looking for a convenient carbohydrate snack.

Snack on fruit between meals, as well, if dietary carbohydrates must be raised to a higher level than average. Keep in mind that these suggestions are for relatively active individuals. Recommended fruit snacks include blueberries, strawberries, blackberries, and raspberries. These berries have low glycemic indexes and provide a concentrated supply of powerful protective antioxidants. Semi-ripe bananas work well also. My favorites are cantaloupe and watermelon when they're seasonally available and not too ripe. Watermelon can have a relatively low glycemic index if it hasn't ripened too much. The fruit delivers an abundance of water and electrolytes, as well. What follows is a short list of healthy fruit choices that contain carbohydrates.

Healthy Fruit Snacks	Glycemic Index
Banana (just turning yellow from green)	50–60
Apple	40–50
Orange	40–50
Watermelon (medium maturity)	35–55
Peach	32–40
Pear	32–40
Grapefruit	23–26
Raspberry	15–20
Blackberry	15–20
Strawberry	15–20
Blueberry	15–20

The extreme demands faced by the triathlon athlete, for example, might require that the adjustment of the plate proportions reach equal portions for each group of food (one-third high-glycemic-index, dense carbohydrate source [brown rice], one-third low-glycemic-index vegetable carbohydrates [cauliflower and broccoli], and one-third protein source). Still, the protein intake must be at the requisite volume for each meal. A 170-pound individual will require 35 to 40 g of protein per meal. A 150-pound athlete will require 30 to 35 g of protein per meal—four to five full, complete meals a day to be accompanied by carbohydrate snacking. A less-active individual will likely perform well without these additional carbohydrate accommodations.

Here are a few reference points for the volume of protein required for the Active Athlete category: seven ounces (half a cup plus) of salmon delivers about 40 g of protein; six ounces (almost a half cup) of tuna provides about 40 g of protein; seven ounces (a half cup plus) of halibut has about 41 g of protein; one large egg supplies about 7 g of protein; six ounces (almost half a cup) of white meat chicken contributes 40 g of protein; and one cup of low-fat cottage cheese furnishes about 30 g of protein.

Low-fat, plain yogurt makes a reasonable snack. However, its carbohydrate content puts it in the category of carbohydrate/protein snack as opposed to an exclusive protein snack. Supplementing a yogurt snack with dry-curd cottage cheese to boost its protein potential is a good idea. I often mix two or three tablespoons of dry-curd cottage cheese into a three-quarter-cup serving of low-fat yogurt, then add some berries. Frequently I stir a heaping tablespoon or two of high-quality whey protein isolate powder (plain and unflavored) into a bit of low-fat, fruit-flavored yogurt (100 ml or so) and a larger portion of low-fat, plain yogurt (an additional 200 to 250 ml), which makes a great high-quality, protein-rich snack. Dry-curd cottage cheese can be added to this yogurt blend instead of, or in addition to, the whey protein isolate powder to enrich this protein source. This strategy raises the protein-to-carbohydrate ratio of the yogurt and promotes healthier, noninflammatory or even anti-inflammatory autocrine-hormone cascades from the mini-meal. Throw in a dash of flaxseed oil to further augment the nutrient value of this snack. Use it as a healthy dessert alternative by incorporating a higher fruit yogurt (preblended-type) component if you desire.

When it comes to eggs as a source of protein, I recommend using one yolk for every three whites. This procedure maintains a healthy amino-acid and fat profile for the white-and-yolk combination. Since an egg white contains about 3 g of protein, an egg meal for me usually consists of two whole eggs and four additional whites, which delivers about 24 to 26 g of protein. But this is a bit on the short side for my total meal requirement. Add a half cup of low-fat or dry-curd cottage cheese to four egg whites and two whole eggs to create a high-quality, reasonably low-fat protein blend—a 40 g total that fulfills the meal requirement. This egg/cottage cheese protein blend can be made into an omelet, accompanied by a slice or two of whole, sprouted, rye-kernel bread, providing a good breakfast or lunch.

Usually I supplement my daily protein intake with two and sometimes three whey protein drinks consumed halfway between meals just to make up my required personal protein total. My program consists of three food meals and two to three protein drinks daily—a high protein intake to account for the demands created by my extra physical work.

The protein in legumes isn't as dense as you might think, and the quality isn't high enough to sustain optimal biological function even when combined with the complementary amino acids from cereals. Mixing legume protein with cereal protein completes the amino-acid profile and supports health, but this common protein complement doesn't deliver optimal immune function or maximum human performance. If athletic performance is an important personal goal, quality protein such as one of or combinations of low-fat cheese, egg, chicken, fish, and whey protein supplementation must make up the protein selection for at least three meals during the day.

If immune function has been a significant lifelong problem, anti-aging is your goal, and/or regular athletic performance is called for in your lifestyle, you must reassess your protein requirements. Regardless of your personal goal, my recommendation is that you consume one serving of a whey protein isolate supplement at least once every day. This will facilitate efficient immune function, lean-mass maintenance, and metabolic health, including insulin efficiency and healthy fat metabolism.

SOY VERSUS WHEY PROTEIN

Soy protein supplementation is just as popular as whey. However, these two sources supply very different properties and dissimilar biological support. Soy is rich in isoflavones, lignins, phytic acid, and biologically therapeutic saponins. These active constituents help down-regulate LDL (bad) cholesterol, up-regulate HDL (good) cholesterol, and promote blood-vessel health to reduce the risk of clots and atherosclerosis (2, 3, 4). Soy isoflavones protect breast, endometrial, and prostate tissue from disease, even cancer. They've been shown to protect and help build bone density, reduce the severity of menopausal symptoms and post-menstrual syndrome, and even safeguard neural tissue and cognition (5, 6, 7).

However, soy as a protein source for lean-muscle tissue recovery and direct immune support might not be as great as that of whey, which delivers a much higher quality amino-acid profile. My recommendation for women is to combine a quality, water-processed soy protein supplement (one-third) with whey (two-thirds) for a daily drink. Water-extraction methods retain the isoflavone content and activity in the soy isolate supplement. These water-extracted sources are the healthier choices. I consume approximately three to four servings of soy protein isolate supplementation each week in addition to the soy curd I eat in an occasional meal. I recommend that men consider eating isoflavone-rich soy protein sources two times per week minimum.

HOW MUCH PROTEIN IS TOO MUCH?

Dietary protein isn't normally toxic unless your lifestyle is already poisonous. The body has built-in systems designed to metabolize dietary protein and neutralize byproducts of this metabolism. However, these systems can't function if the diet and the body are already toxic. Protein is essential for life. Quality protein that's efficiently digested, absorbed, and utilized promotes a more efficient metabolism.

Consuming a lower BV protein requires more work for the metabolism and taxes the body more than a higher BV protein does. A protein source has a low BV when it rates less than 77; a BV of 77 or higher is reasonably good for tissue recovery and immune support. Again, the higher the better. Whey protein isolates can have a BV as much as 159, while soy protein supplement powders rate about 74. The benefits of soy mostly come from factors other than its protein content, though some specialized amino-acid activity for soy has been reported such as that provided by the high arginine content (8, 9).

Protein toxicity is a function of metabolic health, the pH (acid/alkaline balance) of the diet, and the type of protein used. If health is poor, dietary protein quality must be maximized in order to reduce the stress on the body when the protein is digested, absorbed, utilized, and metabolized. Active people need to eat more protein than the average individual. This requires the higher protein content to be clean and easily utilized, which means that a higher BV protein source is necessary. If you aren't concerned about maximum performance, the quality of your protein source can slide a little; however, if it drops too low, immune function will be compromised as previously described.

The acid/alkaline balance of the body is supported by the copious amounts of low-glycemic-index vegetables found in the Ageless Performance strategy. Appendix D is a depiction of the alkalinizing foods and the acidifying foods. Generally the processed North American diet leads to acidosis of the body. Therefore, we must actively lean toward choosing alkalinizing foods to combat this toxicity.

If you're fighting disease or are extremely active, you'll have to fuel your body with a higher level of alkalinizing foods to prevent acidosis from leaching nutrients. If you consume an abundance of protein, you must also eat an abundance of green and colorful vegetables to promote healthy protein metabolism, to limit homocysteine and ammonia accumulation, and to offset potential protein-induced acidosis. You needn't worry about adding additional dietary and supplemental factors to compensate for these toxicity issues; the preventive, pH-balancing components are built right into the Ageless Performance design.

The quantity and quality of protein that Ageless Performance calls for won't be toxic to your system. Dietary protein is essential to your health; you can't live without it and it must be consumed adequately each day without concern for toxicity. Protein toxicity won't be a problem if you employ Ageless Performance in its entirety.

A reminder: the totals below are to be eaten over four to five meals daily. Again, the macronutrient totals in the table below won't work for individuals who exceed two hours of endurance training each day. For these extreme training schedules a higher volume of dense carbohydrate sources must be ingested throughout the day. The quantity required depends on several factors: lean body weight, metabolic rate, duration of training, and aerobic/anaerobic nature of the activity.

The post-workout application can amount to about 30% of the day's total carbohydrate intake. For a 140-pound individual this can easily amount to 73 g (70 to 75 g) of carbohydrates after the training session (one and a half cups of cooked brown rice). Of course, this carbohydrate content will be combined with a protein source regardless of the sport or physical work.

Summary of the Athlete's/Active Individual's Requirements Using Relatable Examples

Body Weight in Pounds	Protein from High BV Sources	Total Daily Carbohydrates	Carbohydrates from Dense Sources (Brown Rice, Whole-Wheat Pasta)	Carbohydrates from Low-Glycemic Vegetable Sources	Post-Workout Carbohydrates
200	200 g per day (men: 40 g per meal)	350 g per day	men: 20 to 25g per meal (approximately a half cup cooked)	men: 15 to 20 g per meal (approximately 2 cups steamed)	100 g
180	180 g per day (men: 35 to 40 g per meal; women: 25 to 30 g per meal)	315 g per day	men: 20 to 25 g per meal (approximately a half cup); women: 20 g per meal (approximately one-third-plus cup)	men: 15 to 20 g per meal (approximately 2 cups); women: 15 g per meal (approximately 1.5 cups)	95 g
160	160 g per day (men: 30 to 35 g per meal; women: 25 to 30 g per meal)	280 g per day	men: 15 to 20 g per meal (approximately less than a half cup); women:15 to 20 g per meal (approximately one-third-plus cup)	men: 15 to 20 g per meal (approximately less than 2 cups); women: 15 g per meal (approximately 1.5 cups)	85 g
140	140 g per day (men: 30 to 35 g per meal; women: 25 to 30 g per meal)	245 g per day	men: 20 to 25 g per meal (approximately a half cup); women:15 to 20 g per meal (approximately one-third cup)	men: 15 to 20 g per meal (approximately less than 2 cups); women: 15 g per meal (approximately 1.5 cups)	75 g
120	120 g per day (men: 30 to 35 g per meal; women: 25 to 30 g per meal)	210 g per day	men: 20 to 25 g per meal (approximately a half cup); women: 15 g per meal (approximately one-third cup)	men: 15 to 20 g per meal (approximately less than 2 cups); women: 15 g per meal (approximately 1 cup)	60 g
100	100 g per day (women: 25 to 30 g per meal)	175 g per day	women: 15 g per meal (approximately one-third cup)	women: 10 to 15 g per meal (approximately 1 cup plus)	52 g

RECOMMENDATIONS
for Muscle-Building/Power Athletes

The bodybuilder's training program promotes the breakdown of more muscle fiber than that experienced by the endurance athlete and at a much deeper tissue level, as well. The nature of the intense resistance training performed by the power or bodybuilder athlete is such that it strains the muscle tissue with greater intensity to induce deeply penetrating muscle-fiber damage— the heavier the training the greater the micro-damage.

The body builds this stress-damaged muscle to be bigger and stronger than before the resistance training, *but only if the building blocks for this renovation are available in unlimited supply*. The building blocks come from the diet. This phenomenon can result in the sort of metamorphosis you might have recognized in someone who's been training regularly with weights. However, the transformation is slow and the muscle growth isn't that impressive unless you haven't seen the individual for a long time as he or she amasses the incremental muscle fiber by fiber.

The muscle-fiber construction is ongoing but so gradual that the individual involved in the training rarely sees any significant change. In fact, a good result from a well-planned, regular weight-training program might amount to a 15-pound total muscle gain within one full year of training. It doesn't sound like much, but it's quite significant. Weight gains that exceed this typical rate often include an increase in body fat, as well. Another explanation for gains that surpass this muscling rate is "muscle memory," experienced by individuals who have resumed weight training after taking time off. Muscle memory contributes to a quicker pace to achieve the result attained prior to taking time off from training.

The other factor that might accelerate the rate of muscle anabolism is the use of steroids (anabolic steroid drugs or testosterone analogue drugs) which, as we all know, have consequences. Despite the biological motive and facilitation to build muscle mass and strength by the body, this genetically inherent coping mechanism relies on the availability of nutrient building blocks and co-factors the way any other biological system we've discussed does. Limited nutrition results in limited gains and limited coping potential. If an individual has difficulty increasing muscle, it's probably because he or she isn't meeting the demand for protein, carbohydrates, essential fats, vitamins, and/or minerals. Even if that person megaloads the protein intake, muscle gains will be restricted to the availability of the co-factors protein metabolism depends on. Genetic potential can be severely hindered by a limited diet. If the diet is processed, the body hasn't reached its full potential. If you think your genetic potential to develop muscle is restricted in comparison to that of someone who's progressing faster than you, think again after assessing your diet, which involves a lot more than just your daily protein intake.

A slight limitation in the B vitamins required for protein metabolism, for example, will limit protein availability as though the protein itself were in short supply in the diet. My guess is that people working the gym scene want every bit of lean muscle and power gain possible for the arduous time and effort they invest in the gym.

My research, as well as my personal and consulting experience, tell me that a co-factor of 1.2 g of protein per day per pound of body weight will serve an athlete well as long as the body-fat mass doesn't exceed 20%. A 170-pound bodybuilder or power lifter must consume about 200 (195 to 205) g of protein daily divided into five or six sittings (combination of protein drinks and meals). The bodybuilder and power athlete's protein co-factor (PC) is 1.2: 1.2 g of protein x 170 pounds = 204 g of protein per day per pound of body weight.

Eating all this protein from food alone would likely result in overconsumption of calories and an excessive intake of arachidonic acid, the fat that's loaded into beef and whole dairy protein sources. Protein supplementation with a whey isolate is crucial to muscle gain without an increase in body fat. Since I have access to many types of protein sources at the raw-material stage, I've had the privilege of scientifically assaying and personally using various types of whey isolates before any ingredients are added to create the flavored and *nutrient-enhanced* products on retail shelves. If you're a manufacturer of such products, you'll agree, after applying my suggested raw-material source, that it's by far among the best whey materials on the market today. And if you're an elite athlete and are in tune with your physique, you'll realize within a few days of using it how different it really is. Check the Biologic Nutritional Research Inc. Web site (*www.biologicnr.com*) for details on how to get this approved source.

In order for maximum muscle and strength gains to occur with minimum fat accumulation amid little or no cardiovascular training, carbohydrate intake for the day should only amount to about 150% of the protein consumed. The active carbohydrate co-factor (cc) for this category is therefore 1.5: 1.5 g of carbohydrates per gram of daily protein required, which means that the bodybuilder/power athlete cc is 1.5 g of carbohydrates x 204 g of total protein required = 306 g of dietary carbohydrates per day.

My recommendation is to include one form of regular cardiovascular exercise to establish a balanced program. Muscle-building athletes who think cardiovascular training degrades muscle are wrong. A little cardio work helps remove lactic acid and normalize blood and muscle pH to enhance recovery as long as the work is done slowly. Twenty minutes three times per week will suffice if the calorie-restrictive, nutrient-dense Ageless Performance program is adhered to. This will facilitate recovery, build cardiovascular health, and keep the fat mass at a healthy minimum.

The table on page 386 doesn't include recommendations regarding the proportions of high-density versus low-density carbohydrate sources. Refer to the table in the previous section for those proportions. The table in this section includes the suggested carbohydrate and protein intakes for a post-workout meal or snack, while the table in the previous section doesn't. However, the post-workout recommendations found here must be applied to the preceding Active Athlete category, as well. Use both tables to establish nutrient needs and timing.

Keep in mind the importance of post-workout protein consumption for muscle reconstruction. This meal is critical to the rebuilding phase of tissue (10). The bodybuilder/power athlete who includes some regular cardio-vascular training can apply the carbohydrate proportions and quantities displayed in the previous section's table. In the absence of cardiovascular training, the cc of 1.5 might work better for lean-measure maintenance.

A large portion of the daily carbohydrate total (30% or so) must be ingested in the post-workout window to maximize glycogen restoration, lean-muscle recovery, and preparation for the next training session. This portion can be consumed over two meals within two to three hours if the training sessions are intense and long enough. The remainder of the carbohydrate requirement for the day can consist of meals that include a combination of the low-glycemic-index vegetables described for the Active Athlete program.

This vegetable medley can be combined with small amounts of a denser carbohydrate source whose quantity can be determined by personal energy requirements. Again, each person is responsible for identifying his or her functional proportion of low-glycemic, fiber-rich vegetables to a denser carbohydrate source for daily carbohydrate intake, using the tables to understand the protocols and find a starting point.

Don't fall victim to the extreme 2 g of protein per pound of body weight per day. This is only required if carbohydrate levels drop to extreme lows. Dietary carbohydrates spare dietary protein for maintenance and tissue recovery (11, 12). A limitation in dietary carbohydrates causes some of the dietary protein to be used as an energy source, which is costly for two reasons: it taxes the body and it makes food bills expensive.

Always stick to the protein intake indicated in the table below whether you need to lose fat or not. With your starting point identified, you can

Summary of the Bodybuilder's Requirement Using Relatable Examples

Body Weight in Pounds	Protein (Total per Day from High BV Sources)	Carbohydrates (Total per Day)	Protein/Carbohydrates Immediately After Workout; Protein from High BV Sources; Carbohydrates from High-Glycemic-Index Sources (30% of Daily Total)
240	280 g per day (men: 40 g per meal)	420 g per day	Protein: 65 g; carbohydrates: 125 g (2.5 cups of cooked rice fill the carbohydrate demand)
220	260 g per day (men: 35 to 40 g per meal; women: 25 to 30 g per meal)	390 g per day	Protein: 60 g; carbohydrates: 120 g (3 large ripe bananas fill the carbohydrate demand)
200	240 g per day (men: 30 to 35 g per meal; women: 25 to 30 g per meal)	360 g per day	Protein: 55 g; carbohydrates: 108 g (2 cups of macaroni fill the carbohydrate demand)
180	215 g per day (men: 30 to 35 g per meal; women: 25 to 30 g per meal)	320 g per day	Protein: 50 g; carbohydrates: 95 g (95 g of maltodextrin [glucose polymer] fill the demand)
160	190 g per day (men: 30 to 35 g per meal; women: 25 to 30 g per meal)	285 g per day	Protein: 50 g; carbohydrates: 85 g (2 large ripe bananas fill the carbohydrate demand)
140	170 g per day (men: 30 to 35 g per meal; women: 25 to 30 g per meal)	255 g per day	Protein: 50 g; carbohydrates: 75 g (7 rice cakes fill the carbohydrate demand)
120	140 g per day (men: 30 to 35 g per meal; women: 25 to 30 g per meal)	210 g per day	Protein: 40 g; carbohydrates: 60 g (1 cup plus of cooked white rice fills the carbohydrate demand)
100	120 g per day (men: 30 to 35 g per meal; women: 25 to 30 g per meal)	180 g per day	Protein: 40 g; carbohydrates: 55 g (5 rice cakes fill the carbohydrate demand)

begin to ingest your necessary carbohydrates from dense sources mixed with an abundance of vegetable sources. To shed fat drop your dense carbohydrate source slightly (refer to the table of carbohydrate densities on page 376) and raise the quantity of fiber-rich vegetable carbohydrates. You'll find that the low-glycemic-index vegetable carbohydrate sources fill the stomach faster. But you might want to increase the amount of cardio work you're doing and decrease rest between weight-resistance sets, as well, if fat loss is desired.

Here's a good reference to keep in mind as a quick glycemic-index evaluation: vegetables growing above the ground tend to have a lower value (squash, zucchini, beans [legumes], eggplant, leafy greens, chicory greens, broccoli, cauliflower, cabbage) than those that grow below (potatoes, parsnips, turnips, beets, carrots). Regulating the proportion of low-glycemic-index vegetables to high-glycemic carbohydrate sources in a meal is a great way to manage body fat without restricting food volume. I use it myself; two of my daily meals consist of the vegetable medley or a large quantity of a single, low-glycemic-index vegetable alongside a protein source. I don't usually include denser carbohydrates for these two meals. A third meal might consist of whole-grain rye bread with an egg/cottage cheese mix (breakfast or lunch), with two subsequent meals featuring a variable whey protein beverage. A third whey protein drink might be required to meet my protein demands. Fruit for snacking fits into the program well. Limit fruit snacking if fat loss is desired while applying this program.

If I require a larger volume of dense carbohydrates because I need more food for energy and glycogen loading, I reduce the vegetable portion and add a denser carbohydrate source (sweet potato, yam, or some brown rice) for a day or two or as long as I need. If I seem to be gaining a little fat, I reverse the process by reducing the quantity of dense carbohydrates and boosting fiber-rich (nondigestible-carbohydrate-source) vegetables. Eventually you'll find the balance that maintains your preferred body-fat mass. Keep in mind that you are not likely to store body fat from a meal until approximately 72 hours after it's consumed. It takes that long to process the dietary calories into adipose fat. The excess body weight experienced the day after a binge is likely due to water retention caused by a *salty* meal. Here's what the applied program might look like.

AGELESS PERFORMANCE REGIMEN: ACTIVE INDIVIDUAL—160 TO 170 POUNDS

6:45 a.m.—Breakfast 1

Whey protein beverage: 30 g scoop of whey protein isolate; half teaspoon of ornithine alpha-ketoglutarate (OKG); half teaspoon of psyllium husk (stirred into six to eight ounces of purified water).

You can also mix your protein and any other nutraceutical additions in a blender with fresh or frozen berries, or a semi-ripe fresh or frozen banana. Blending with the low-glycemic-index frozen berries is my preferred fruit blend if a smoothie-type texture is desired. This keeps the glycemic value of the drink low, and the frozen fruit gives the drink a thick, frothy texture. Furthermore, it's a good strategy to apply for the post-workout drink and a good method to increase satiety. If a higher glycemic index can be tolerated, use half water and half orange juice as the liquid base. Be careful, though: the volume quickly adds up to a large shake. Drink lots of purified water throughout the day.

Other supplements: multi-vitamin/mineral; salmon oil: 2,000 to 3,000 mg; flax oil: 2,000 to 4,000 mg; alpha lipoic acid (R+): 100 mg.

One cup of organic, freshly ground coffee.

7:30 a.m.—Run or brisk walk for 30 to 45 minutes

8:30 a.m.—Breakfast 2

Drink lots of purified water.

One to two slices of whole-rye bread or rye blend (ingredients of the latter can read something like this: whole-kernel rye or sprouted rye kernel, pure water, whole-meal rye, whole-meal wheat, oat flakes, barley flakes, linseed, non-iodized salt, sesame, yeast).

Two whole eggs plus four egg whites (you can use these eggs to make an omelet, with the small addition of dry-curd cottage cheese to supplement the protein count for the meal—add the curd right into the omelet before cooking).

Supplements: CoQ10: 15 mg; vitamin C: 1,000 mg; flax oil: 2,000 to 4,000 mg; curcumin (95% curcuminoids): 500 mg; bromelain: 500 mg; GTF chromium: 200 mcg.

Antioxidant booster formula: one caplet might deliver 7,000 to 8,000 IU beta-carotene, 150 to 200 mg vitamin C, 100 IU of vitamin E, 50 to 75 mcg of selenium (ACES is a common fundamental antioxidant combination containing vitamins A, C, and E, and selenium; this formula tops off the multi-vitamin/mineral's antioxidant levels).

10:00 a.m.—Snack 1

Apple and/or orange or other low-glycemic-index fruit: pear, peach, grapefruit, etc.

Drink lots of purified water.

11:30 a.m.—Lunch

One whole chicken breast.

One to two cups of steamed or lightly stir-fried vegetable medley (this meal would have been left over from the night before when extra was purposely planned for and packaged for the next day's lunch; may or may not include a denser carbohydrate source such as brown rice or whole-wheat pasta in a small quantity [one-half to one cup]).

Supplements: multi-vitamin/mineral caplet; CoQ10: 15 mg; vitamin E: 200 IU; curcumin (95% curcuminoids): 700 mg; bromelain: 700 mg; alpha lipoic acid (R+): 100 to 200 mg; GTF chromium: 200 mcg; grapeseed extract: 100 mg.

2:30 p.m.—Snack 2

One serving (30 g) whey protein drink (plain) without the additions of the first drink (this makes for a more convenient drink in the workplace; whey isolate preferred to concentrate).

Supplements: flax oil: 3,000 mg (gel capsules for convenience); salmon oil: 3,000 to 6,000 mg (gel capsules); grapeseed extract: 100 mg; antioxidant booster: one tablet/caplet; vitamin C: 2,000 mg.

4:00 p.m.—Snack 3

Apple and/or orange or other low-glycemic-index fruit: pear, peach, grapefruit, etc.

Lots of purified water.

5:00 p.m.—Snack 4

Pre-workout protein drink if workout is to be implemented before dinner (whey isolate preferred). This would be my protocol.

6:30 p.m.—Dinner

Five to seven ounces of halibut steak or tuna or chicken.

Different vegetable medley (maybe this one is steamed as opposed to the other stir-fried version).

Tossed salad with the Heart Healthy Dressing (recipe detailed in Chapter 9).

One glass of wine (optional).

Lots of purified water.

Supplements: multi-vitamin/mineral caplet; curcumin (95% curcuminoids): 500 mg; bromelain: 500 mg; alpha lipoic acid (R+): 100 to 200 mg; GTF chromium: 200 mcg; grapeseed extract: 100 mg; calcium/magnesium: 250 mg/250 mg (one to two tablets supplying these elemental levels); salmon oil: 2,000 mg; flax oil: 2,000 mg.

A late-night snack might consist of a protein source only. No carbohydrate sources are to be eaten past 7:30 p.m., since dietary carbohydrates consumed late in the evening can contribute more easily to fat deposition and ultimately lead to insulin impairment over long-term practice. As previously stressed, it's very important to avoid progressed insulin resistance if optimal health and performance are to be ensured over time. Maintenance of healthy insulin activity longer in life also preserves the operation of naturally secreted growth hormone (GH) and insulinlike growth factor (IGF) in the body (13).

Diabetes and insulin resistance impair the GH-IGF system, and this in turn impedes, during sleep, immune-system deployment and general metabolic and biological recovery from physical and mental strain. Preserve insulin health at all costs for as long as you can in life. Insulin health is the crux of optimal health and the platform for maximum performance. Guard it with Ageless Performance. If your muscle-building training schedule includes more cardiovascular/endurance training than average, you'll have to try to plan your day to get your carbohydrate fill before 7:30 p.m. That might be tough and, if so, just consume sources in the evening that are as low as possible in the glycemic index.

At bedtime take 15 to 30 g of a whey protein (plain), adding a few grams of glutamine and OKG. In addition, 1 to 3 mg of melatonin and 2 to 3 g of salmon oil can supplement the bedtime drink. Melatonin is a potent antioxidant that jump-starts circadian rhythm for healthy hormone cascade (14). It's a powerful neutralizer of the hydroxyl free radical and an enhancer of vitamins C and E and glutathione activity (15).

The hydroxyl free radical is responsible for much of the damage sustained by the pineal gland. This is the gland that synchronizes hormone activity with the day/night cycles of the planet, producing melatonin. Support of longevity depends on protection of this gland early in life before it's propelled into dysfunction. This preemptive safeguarding allows it to manufacture its natural flow of melatonin, and orally supplied melatonin does the trick by blocking the destructive cycle from escalating exponentially. Upon being assailed by hydroxyl radicals, the compromised melatonin secretion by the injured pineal gland allows the free radical to proliferate unchallenged. The result is even more harm to the pineal gland, which expedites hormone imbalance and biological aging. Starting melatonin supplementation by age 30 to 35 slows this degeneration and might add years to your life, or at least quality to your senior years.

Melatonin supplementation also improves insulin efficiency and preserves healthy delta-6-desaturase activity—the enzyme involved in fatty-acid metabolism into eicosanoid-hormone status (16). Recommended melatonin supplementation is 1 mg for every decade past 25 years of age. Experts say melatonin levels shouldn't exceed 3 mg daily.

Arginine supplementation is something else I often include at bedtime. Nitric-oxide production is supported by arginine for cardiovascular health, and don't worry, in combination with all of the regulatory synergies of Ageless Performance, it's safe. Arginine also promotes that pumped feeling during training and delivers sexual stamina for men, as well. Take 1 to 3 g of arginine before bedtime, but gradually work up the intake, since aggressive dosing can result in a bit of diarrhea. This arginine supplementation is powerful for many forms of performance if done correctly.

We've touched on nitric-oxide production in the body and the value of its regulation to prevent free-radical damage that can be generated from uncontrolled activity. Ageless Performance will prove to be a powerful regulator of nitric oxide while the additional arginine supplementation can help boost nitric-oxide levels where needed, but only if the target systems have optimally functional enzyme activity (nitric-oxide synthase is the enzyme).

To stimulate nitric-oxide-enzyme activity in the tissues that need to perform better, simply piling in the arginine might not deliver the results you're looking for unless you trigger the enzyme with specialized herbs. Many of our common herbs, as we'll see in more detail and with scientific references in the next chapter, have been recently shown to display this target-specific enhancement of nitric-oxide-synthase activity. Grapeseed extract, for example, will stimulate the enzymes in the blood vessels, promoting more efficient nitric-oxide production in these tissues from arginine. The results are blood-pressure reduction and better peripheral blood flow. Combining the nitric-oxide precursor arginine with grapeseed-extract supplementation compounds results.

The same is true with Tribulus terrestris supplementation. The natural herb Tribulus initiates nitric-oxide-synthase activity in the penis, elevating nitric-oxide levels in this tissue. That's one major way it works as a libido enhancer. The results are better blood flow and more efficient, fuller, and even prolonged erectile function. Tribulus has been used for some time as a sexual aid for men and women. However, now there's a more accurate understanding of its method of activity, demonstrating that it has even greater potential. Take a 2 to 3 g arginine load—the nitric-oxide precursor—two times daily in conjunction with 400 to 500 mg of Tribulus terrestris (40% plus furostenol levels) twice daily, and if everything else is working correctly, you'll feel as if you're a teenager again in a few days (the next day for most people). Viagra works in a similar fashion through a different biochemical system—by prolonging and elevating nitric-oxide levels in the penis. The natural way might not function as quickly as Viagra for most individuals, but it delivers great results and doesn't pose the same risks.

The above nutritional program amounts to the following daily macronutrient and caloric values for a 165- to 170-pound active individual.

Macro-Profile	Total Grams	Calories	% Calories
Protein	166	664	35%
Fat	32	288	15%
Carbohydrate	240	960	50%
Total	494	1912	100%

This low-calorie, high-nutrient-density program is designed to keep body fat and biological age to a minimum. If more sustenance is required in the day, a can of tuna with my Heart Healthy Salad Dressing (see Chapter 9) is a tasty snack. The Heart Healthy Dressing adds life to canned tuna by way of flavor and essential fatty acids that were likely destroyed during processing. Fresh tuna is the preferred choice.

Additional protein and carbohydrate snacks might be required in the day by men with relatively higher lean-body-mass proportions. Low-fat cottage cheese, dry-curd cottage cheese, low-fat yogurt, extra whey protein supplementation, and tuna (preferably fresh) are my preferred healthy "fast-food" choices. Performance-enhancing drugs such as anabolic steroids will boost the ability of the body to absorb and assimilate protein, necessitating an increase in the daily requirement for dietary protein. Although the use of steroids isn't advocated, the caution to consume more protein is important in order to prevent degradation of other tissues if this risky route is taken.

The above nutrient-intake program resembles my own except I usually include a short weight-training workout in the early evening. The intensified demands this training session creates have to be countered with the inclusion of an additional whey protein drink just before the workout at about 5:30 p.m. and with another protein-plus-carbohydrate-source beverage *immediately* after the workout. A meal can follow this post-workout repletion drink (highly bioavailable/absorbable food) after an hour has passed.

My personal regimen also includes higher doses of the nutraceuticals in this Ageless Performance program. As well, I take various nutraceuticals that aren't in the program I've outlined already. These include SAMe, acetyl l-carnitine, Tribulus terrestris, saw palmetto, pygeum extract, panax ginseng, folic acid, acidophilus- and bifidus-friendly bacteria, MSM, FOS, and extra

B-vitamin-complex support with a three-week cycle of ASA (20 to 40 mg daily) every other month.

If you stick to the fundamental plan, however, it will be comprehensive enough to accomplish your goal. The additions I feature in my personal program are simply recommended inclusions for those who wish to apply a *very* aggressive anti-aging strategy. Some of these nutraceuticals will also be necessary for more difficult cases of disease. I'll specify which ones in upcoming pages.

If a resistance-training session is included several times per week, at least one extra protein-rich meal *must* be added to the daily total shown above. Additional supplementation to consider for the day (including the resistance-training workout): 30 g of whey protein (plain) in water only, with 3 g each of salmon and flax oils (This protein drink is displayed at 5:00 p.m. in the program on page 390.). It's a good idea to repeat this protein supplementation immediately after the workout. If this is cost-prohibitive or an overload of calories, cut this before-and-after strategy to one-half to one-third of a serving. With these additions to the program, the totals for the day can exceed those detailed in the following table for a 165- to 170-pound bodybuilding/power athlete.

Macro-Profile	Total Grams	Calories	% Calories
Protein	200	800	34%
Fat	37	315	14%
Carbohydrate	302	1208	52%
Total	529	2323	100%

I might replace some of the dinner's vegetable carbohydrate source with a denser one like brown rice, since this meal is post-workout (see the previous sample regimen). An alternative to the denser carbohydrate alteration when the workout precedes this meal might be a treat with a small serving of ice cream for dessert, but only as part of the post-workout meal on occasion. You don't have to be restrictive all the time. In addition, the last protein drink of the day (before bedtime) when weight training is included regularly might consist of more than a half serving to enhance the daily total if it's required. That doesn't mean the extra protein is needed *only* on training days. This is a misconception I often encounter. The body's recovery process proceeds at a slug's pace, but indefinitely each day. The diet must supply the extra protein and co-factors *every day* in order to support this ongoing recovery. In fact, the off days are when most recovery takes place, since energy and nutrient resources are focused exclusively on this endeavor.

Committing to Ageless Performance doesn't mean you have to struggle against the desire for a tasty treat for the rest of your life. If you decide to indulge, just return to the healthy program afterward. As I've previously mentioned, the metabolic momentum established by the program will prevent a minor detour from making a major dent in the healthy metabolic flow. And your cravings for calorie-dense junk food will likely diminish when you've been on this nutrient-dense program for a while.

In the calculation in which total body weight is multiplied by the protein co-factor (1.2 g of protein per pound of body weight, for example) to determine the daily protein requirement of the active individual, the fact that women carry, on average, a slightly lower lean-muscle to fat-mass proportion than men hasn't been accommodated for. An adjustment for this fact would result in a slight reduction of the daily protein requirement per pound of total body weight for women.

However, we're dealing with active individuals who have greater-than-average leaner masses, and that includes a likely larger lean- to fat-mass proportion for these women, as well. Despite slight gender-related differences, we'll use the same protein requirements for women as for men, since they may vary only slightly in this category.

REDUCING BODY FAT WHILE BUILDING MUSCLE

During fat-loss programs, if fat loss exceeds two to three pounds per week, an extra snack such as the protein sources (tuna, cottage cheese) and/or carbohydrate sources such as low-glycemic-index fruit can be included to meet the demand. A two- to three-pound weekly loss is almost impossible to assess accurately without body-mass-proportion assessment, since slight changes in body water, electrolytes, and food in gastrointestinal transition can change daily to contribute significantly to weight changes.

The only way to determine whether weight loss is water, muscle, glycogen, or fat is to do a bio-impedance mass proportion test. Better yet use infrared inductance technology.

As I've disclosed, you'll have to reduce your total dietary carbohydrate levels and/or carbohydrate source proportions from the displayed benchmarks if fat loss is required. Don't ever reduce your total daily carbohydrate intake below 50 g; 50 g per day will prevent the onset of ketosis and, as we've seen, you don't want to stay in ketosis, especially if you're exercising regularly.

Since I tend to limit the level of dense carbohydrates in my diet, I occasionally reach a state of glycogen depletion, especially if I'm participating in more cardiovascular training than my regular program. When and if I do increase my energy output, I also boost my carbohydrate intake. Even so, there are many occasions when I'm caught short of daily carbohydrates and become glycogen-depleted and lethargic.

The simple solution is to increase daily carbohydrate intake for two to three days with an additional 100 to 200 g daily to help with the repletion of glycogen stores and then proceed with the original plan. To accomplish this feat I consume more dense carbohydrate sources such as yams, sweet potatoes, and oatmeal. I also include whole-wheat pasta, white potatoes, and whole brown rice if I need even more dietary carbohydrates. Snacking on fruit facilitates the carbohydrate load, as well.

It's a good idea to plan ahead. Load glycogen stores for a period starting a few days before an event you know will exceed your typical energy requirements. If you have a weekend tournament coming up or an out-of-the ordinary planned cross-country bicycle ride with a group of friends, take a few days to load carbohydrates so as not to plunge to destructive lows during the activity. This will also make your event more endurable and pleasurable. Don't forget the extra water requirement with the dietary carbohydrate increment and during that entire loading period. Remember: after the event, when glycogen stores diminish, replete with dietary carbohydrates and clean water as quickly as possible; liver glycogen stores *must* be maintained in order to support optimal health.

CREATINE SUPPLEMENTATION AND OTHER PERFORMANCE STRATEGIES

There's no doubt that creatine works. It delivers tremendous ergogenic potential and builds muscle mass fast. However, the majority of the immediate gains are attributed to intramuscular water retention due to cross-sectional muscle-fiber enlargement and changes in osmotic gradients that creatine induces (17, 18). This intracellular water retention is lost when creatine administration ceases. Creatine, though, also indirectly supports protein synthesis by enhancing ATP status and protein assimilation and delivering anti-catabolic activity (19). The supplement supports ATP status in the brain, as well. Recent studies performed with rats showed that creatine augmentation promotes neuron protein synthesis and energy production to protect neurons from cell death (20). Used in moderation and with correct cycling it isn't toxic unless previous liver and kidney diseases exist (21, 22). However, diabetics shouldn't use creatine.

With the Ageless Performance foundation in place, creatine will enhance strength and muscle size as never before, and the results are substantial within weeks. Essential and other omega-3 fats facilitate creatine transport, utilization, and recovery potential. The insulin efficiency that Ageless Performance provides further enhances creatine's potential. Optimal function of creatine depends on the availability of other nutrients that Ageless Performance offers.

Creatine improves protein anabolism; therefore sufficient protein must be made available in order to maximize the tissue-building potential creatine imparts. This construction requires higher levels of the B vitamins, vitamin C, minerals, and the special fats that are central to Ageless Performance. Antioxidants, too, must be adequately available to foster peak recovery and growth potential. Creatine advances muscle strength at a much greater pace than it does for tendons and other connective tissue. That means you should be careful when pushing performance limits while on creatine or other ergogenic substances. Muscle is more vascular than connective tissue and receives nutrients more abundantly, allowing it to recover faster. Creatine supplementation has been shown in scientific reports as recent as January 2002 to deliver effective antioxidant activity, significantly quelling peroxynitrite, superoxide, and other tissue-destructive free radicals. Since these antioxidants can impair muscle performance, this is likely one way creatine boosts work capacity and inhibits tissue damage (23).

For the best outcome from a creatine cycle, apply Ageless Performance in its entirety, beginning the creatine cycle no sooner than three weeks after the program has been initiated. This will give your nutrient stores a head start to prepare for the creatine and workload to come. With this complete strategy in place, the results from creatine administration will outweigh any suboptimal gains from previous applications. Other additions to an aggressive performance-enhancing program are glutamine (3 to 7 g daily) and okg (3 to 4 g daily), taken with protein drinks as previously outlined. Arginine cycling works well also. Supplementation of arginine, as described earlier, also supports maximum growth hormone (gh) secretions by actually causing the body to override its gh regulatory/inhibitory processes (24). The natural feedback mechanisms that inhibit gh production when levels reach the highest point are overridden by arginine's influence to make the body produce more of the hormone.

Don't take the above to mean that gh can be raised far beyond normal baseline levels. Eventually the body catches up to manage this system and usually fairly immediately. My strategy ensures that maximum gh production ensues for optimal immune-system and anabolic drive if all the other related systems are functional. Maximum potential of the human body is a formidable state that few people achieve. If you reach it, you'll perform athletically beyond your expectations.

Glutamine supports gh output, protein synthesis, and nitrogen retention when taken as detailed in the sample program (25, 26). Supplementation of glutamine is critical for individuals under physical and emotional stress, including trauma, and should definitely be part of a pre- and post-surgical nutritional protocol. It's highly recommended as an anti-catabolic agent for people who have to administer corticosteroid therapy. I prefer the use of glutamine dipeptides (alanyl-glutamine and glycyl-glutamine) as oral sources. They're more stable than free-form glutamine and deliver a much higher concentration than the more common, cheaper tripeptide types derived from wheat gluten hydrolysis (27).

Studies demonstrate that this new method of glutamine delivery improves nitrogen retention and immunity and survival from illness without the potential of toxic ammonia. Glutamine is known to contribute to ammonia accumulation in the body when overconsumed. This effect is combated by OKG supplementation, which further enhances the glutamine and arginine status of the body while it protects against potential ammonia toxicity. By scavenging ammonia, OKG gives rise to glutamine and arginine in the process and provides fuels and building blocks for extremely healthy immune function (28). This glutamine- and arginine-enhancing potential delivers incremental GH support, as well.

I recommend the following additions to the Ageless Performance program for maximum performance potential: potassium phosphate for stamina enhancement (1 to 2 g daily) and hydroxymethylbutyrate (HMB) for endurance and better tissue-recovery potential (2 to 4 g daily). Potassium phosphate works synergistically with creatine to buffer muscle pH, and HMB improves physical performance as it enhances tissue recovery via muscle-building and endurance potential through, in part, lactate regulation. Furthermore, HMB mediates a healthier inflammatory response and bolsters immune-system efficiency (29, 30).

Ribose, which supports myocardial ATP availability and is great for endurance-type activity, is another important program inclusion. It's been used with great success in the treatment of ischemic heart disease without side effects (31).

There is some controversy about glutamine. Studies show that glutamine peptides do deliver a bioavailable source of glutamine, but only about 25% to 27% of their weight is glutamine. If a serving size of glutamine peptides is 3 g, it only provides 750 mg of glutamine (25% of 3 g). Few companies, if any, disclose these facts on product labels. Free-form glutamine supplies almost 100% of the amino acid. As a result, I prefer to employ a combination of the two. I find the results are much better with the blend than for either one independently. However, I only use the previous blend if I can't get my hands on the hard-to-find dipeptides of glutamine, alanyl- or glycyl-glutamine.

In fact, research shows that cancer-related malaise and muscle-wasting can be successfully fought with the supplementation of HMB, arginine, and glutamine and/or OKG. The results achieved among cancer patients administered this combination convey irrefutably that the concoction retards muscle degradation and promotes protein synthesis to increase lean mass (32, 33).

Applying the entire Ageless Performance strategy can cost an arm and a leg, especially if every enhancer is utilized at once. Don't bother jumping to creatine formulations for sport, though, unless Ageless Performance is in place. This includes the dietary and supplemental foundations; results won't be optimal and they'll be completely wiped out after creatine dispensation ceases.

You might make mediocre water gains by ingesting creatine amid poor nutritional intake. However, all of this positive weight will be lost when creatine administration is stopped. By employing the complete program, more muscle is actually built, and when creatine supplementation is terminated there's a much better chance of retaining the muscle tissue as long as training persists with the same intensity and nourishment supports muscle maintenance.

For muscle mass and strength endeavors, use the typical saturation phase with a creatine monohydrate. The creatine label will detail this protocol. Typically saturation involves higher, body-weight-dependent doses daily for four to five days. Follow this saturation period with the lower maintenance doses outlined on the product label.

Endurance athletes should forgo the saturation phase and use smaller maintenance doses to reduce the risk of too much weight gain; alternatively they can ingest the creatine citrate form. Long-term gains from creatine aren't as significant for short cycles, even though the majority of the improvement is made in the first month of use. I prefer cycling 12 to 13 weeks on and 10 weeks off, and I don't touch glucose- or maltodextrin-spiked products. These high-glycemic-index formulations might enhance creatine absorption, but at the risk of contributing to insulin resistance. The only time this insulin-spiking strategy is better tolerated by the body is immediately after a workout when most of the high-glycemic-index carbohydrates can be employed to restore expended muscle and liver glycogen.

Some people believe long-term use of creatine supplementation is safe. Case studies reveal that individuals have been employing the substance for several years without a break and with no side effects. However, I suggest cycling it or taking (as I do) 2 to 3 g (half a teaspoon) daily in a protein drink. Even with these small doses of creatine I tend to feel a bit water-retentive/edemic when I stay on it for too long.

Methoxyisoflavone entered the sports-nutrition marketplace some time ago and slowly faded, but it's still around. The problem is the cost involved when using it correctly. Common doses are set at 200 to 300 mg, and even at those low levels it's extremely expensive. Studies show that methoxyisoflavone displays antiaromatase activity (34), which blocks testosterone conversion to estrogen, *potentially* increasing the half-life of the former in the bloodstream. Ecdysterone is a phytosteroid often utilized with methoxyisoflavone. The phytosteroid isn't like testosterone at all, but it does appear to enhance insulin function and protein synthesis (35).

I've used methoxyisoflavone in combination with ecdysterone, and like most people, I've experienced...nothing. Then I upped my daily dose to 800 mg of each for three weeks. Still nothing! A few months later I started on 1,500 mg each of methoxyisoflavone and ecdysterone and within four days—*bam!* The increments in lean-muscle size and strength were significant, and the workout pump and recovery were much better. In fact, the increase measure by bio-impedance is so impressive and so quick to be achieved that it can't be attributed to muscle synthesis and must be due to glycogen retention or osmotic differences such as those caused by creatine. Of course, a testosterone increment will induce similar effects, which *could* be a factor, as well. I'm not completely sold on the science regarding ecdysterone, though there is some research to bolster it, but the personal experiences are definitely irrefutable. The science supporting ecdysterone may be contradictory, but that underpinning 5-methyl-7-methoxyisoflavone is more convincing.

In the next chapter we'll see how to employ the full potential of this testosterone increment by freeing it from its binding proteins to unleash the testosterone activity. This binding protein deactivates the circulating testosterone. Keep in mind that this report of personal success with methoxyisoflavone is definitely not scientific, but I've been in bodybuilding for 20 years and can't even begin to count how many products I've tried during that time. I know methoxyisoflavone works, but it's dependent on nutrient availability. Speed up muscle synthesis and you have to boost nutrient intake to support the anabolic construction. However, to make this strategy succeed you've got to take about 10 mg per pound of body weight of each flavone (methoxyisoflavone and ecdysterone) per day, and that's not cheap! It's up to you to weigh the pros and the *costs*.

RECOMMENDATIONS
for Diabetes, Insulin Resistance, and Weight Management/Obesity

The meal plan required to assist recovery from disease differs only slightly from the athlete's program. However, the nutraceutical-supplement component remains relatively the same for both; the prioritized summary tables for Ageless Performance near the end of this chapter can serve as common guides. Consideration of the condition-specific programs in the next chapter as additions to the Ageless Performance nutritional supplement foundation is strongly suggested for difficult cases of disease. In most instances the plan displayed in the summary table of this chapter will suffice as powerful treatment and prevention. In terms of performance enhancement, the goal-specific programs of the next chapter can be added to the supplement foundation to deliver formidable results, as well. These specialized programs include ones for athletic power, muscle tone, and size improvement in addition to a stamina-enhancement component. You'll also find a tremendous natural libido-booster program, cognitive-performance support, and thermogenic facilitators that raise the potential of the foundation program if more aggressive weight-management strategies are required.

First and foremost, the nutraceutical-supplement element and the solid-ground dietary foundation of Ageless Performance must be applied to induce cellular correction, which facilitates the healing potential inherent in all of us. Correction of disease begins spontaneously once this balance is reinstated so that a condition-specific therapy, such as the boosters in the next chapter, may not even be required. In some cases, a booster may only be needed to initiate positive metabolic momentum for a short period. With this new biological efficiency the body's natural preventive chemistry is raised to maximum levels, acting as a shield against disease. This is the premise for prevention and anti-aging. Anti-aging is ultimately aggressive prevention.

If a condition-specific therapy is necessary, such as the administration of vanadyl sulfate (vs) and sodium metavanadate for diabetes, or s-adenosyl methionine (SAMe) for arthritis or depression, the results these specialized treatments induce will be helped by a metabolic system working toward balance and health—the corrected system. To continue with poor dietary and other lifestyle habits throughout therapy and afterward, whether the therapy is in the pharmaceutical or nutraceutical form, is to continue straining the body to the point where the diseased state will eventually be reestablished. A lifestyle that imposes metabolic inefficiency simply opposes therapy, causing the therapeutic strategy to be challenged by yet another hurdle. Insulin inefficiency, for instance, is a primary metabolic impairment that pushes against the positive chemistry of any proven therapy. Consequently therapy may be required continuously, or if disease is alleviated, the therapy will have to be applied again in the future. This progression is characterized by the typical alternation of remission and disease activity. By promoting metabolic correction, the *healed* state will more likely be maintained after therapy is terminated.

An ongoing requirement of a therapy such as the administration of acetylsalicylic acid (ASA or Aspirin) to reduce the danger of cardiovascular disease is a consequence of a dysfunctional metabolism. ASA therapy is needed to offset metabolic imbalance and is required indefinitely. The scientific facts previously outlined in detail convey this message conclusively. Dietary balance, however, will rectify cellular and metabolic imbalance, eliminating the necessity of unnatural hormone mediation via ASA.

You might be surprised at how similar many aspects of the therapeutic program are to the athlete's protocol. Protein intake, for example, is a vital fuel and building block for immune function and tissue renovation. Demand for dietary protein created by a body fighting disease might not be far off from that of a body recovering from the rigors of training. Adequate dietary protein, however, will be necessary for more than just tissue recovery. Properly supplied protein promotes balanced hormone response in the body, which includes anti-inflammatory potential. A healthy dietary protein component also helps put the brakes on the biological aging process. Ageless Performance isn't a Band-Aid for disease; it's a tuner of biological efficiency, and once that's accomplished the rate of biological aging slows down and the development of disease reverses itself. Simply put, the program outperforms any man-made drug by allowing the body to do what it does best on its own: heal, regenerate, and exist in a state of physical and mental well-being. Disease is merely a consequence of our blocking this natural course by unnatural interference.

If disease is chronic and competitive sport is a big part of the lifestyle, energy demands will be very high, and nutrient density of this energy must be equally elevated. Backing off from a competitive schedule for a short period might be a good idea to allow maximum recovery from disease. This tactic will heighten the intrinsic healing force as the nutrient-dense diet is directed full-force on the healing process instead of being spread thinly over two requirements—recovery from disease or rigorous training. That doesn't mean training has to be terminated altogether. One can persist with an active lifestyle that involves a maximum 30 to 45 minutes of training every second day for maintenance of the athletic condition. The lower oxidative stress experienced due to the decreased training schedule, in addition to the enhanced flow of nourishment to one biological focus, will accomplish recovery from disease more rapidly.

Of course, there will be less latitude to eat high-glycemic-index foods if the goal is recovery from illness regardless of whether exercise is regular or not. That's especially so if one's lifestyle doesn't include exercise. Regular activity in one form or another is important for the development and maintenance of physical and mental health even if disease challenges the body. A daily brisk walk might suffice as a start.

Some of the benefits of exercise have been previously discussed: the clearance of blood sugar, regulation of blood pressure, faster turnover of broken-down tissue, appetite control, energy expenditure, removal of debris through activation of the lymphatic system, and support of general physical and mental well-being. For those people struggling with diabetes or insulin resistance, a daily brisk walk is critical to recovery. Resistance training a few times a week will support lean tissue and better serum-glucose clearance, enhancing the body's ability to tolerate and overcome disease. This includes other diseases associated with insulin resistance such as biological aging. Remember, insulin resistance is bound to advance as we get older, so limiting its progression will slow the rate of biological aging and lower the risk of cardiovascular, cognitive, inflammatory, and respiratory diseases and, of course, diabetes.

Don't take obesity lightly; it's a disease just as diabetes is. In fact, the two go hand-in-hand. The prevalent goal of weight management must be a reduced risk of disease or disease management. The accumulation of body fat points to metabolic imbalance, especially if the gain is sudden. It isn't a result of chronological age. More likely, it's caused by *biological* aging—metabolic disarray.

If you're struggling with diabetes, insulin resistance, or weight management/obesity, you've aged biologically beyond your chronological years according to your internal chemistry. That means it's time to alter the pace before it's too late. The administration of vanadyl sulfate must be seriously considered. It's much easier to rectify diseases related to insulin inefficiency, including obesity, cardiovascular disease, and accelerated biological age, if insulin-activity enhancement is initiated at the beginning of therapy. This strategy allows more immediate metabolic assimilation of the corrective nutrients for a fast-paced recovery.

Administration of specialized supplements such as essential and fish-source omega-3 fats can contribute to disease amid the distressed insulin-inefficient metabolism unless precautionary measures are taken to increase the body's antioxidant support. Ageless Performance supplies a potent antioxidant arsenal and is designed to achieve recovery from insulin resistance even without the application of vs, which is optional and shouldn't be used as a substitute for dietary correction. Combining the corrective potential of the Ageless Performance diet and nutraceutical program with the specialized activity of vs is powerful therapy that shifts the recipient back in biological *time* quickly.

Extreme cases of insulin inefficiency or a diabetic state could make the degree of insulin resistance so severe that the corrective potential of Ageless Performance might not be as effective as it can be. In such instances the program might even fail to initiate correction without the assistance of vs. The benefit Ageless Performance can deliver to an individual with severely impaired insulin function (Type II diabetes) *without* concurrently administering vs is enhanced tolerance of the condition but not likely swift recovery.

That's where vs or pharmaceutical drugs such as metformin and glyburide can help spark the system toward a healthier state. The primary objective is to use these biochemical crutches temporarily and maintain the functional result with new dietary habits. However, some aggressive anti-aging strategies involve indefinite metformin administration to support insulin efficiency if insulin resistance is expected to be a problem based on familial history.

Metformin is often prescribed as a treatment for polycystic ovarian syndrome in women. Again, in this case, drugs are used to compensate for a condition that can be avoided. Nondrug, insulin-enhancing substances such as vs, alpha lipoic acid, and chromium likely reverse this syndrome as well as metformin does, but that hasn't been confirmed yet scientifically. However, a 2002 study has verified that n-acetyl cysteine (NAC), the powerful, natural, nontoxic antioxidant, can overturn this condition and improve insulin efficiency simultaneously. The study revealed that 1.8 g of oral NAC daily for five to six weeks will do the trick and without side effects (36). Nevertheless, the underlying message is still the obvious need for prevention in the first place—support of the primary hormonal gear of the body, insulin, before disease takes hold—and Ageless Performance helps achieve that.

The low-glycemic-index diet, in a sense, allows the body's systems to rest while correction occurs, much as a sprinter takes time off from running to heal a broken or sprained ankle. Rest frees the insulin/glucagon axis from the glycemic strain of the typical North American diet. Once more, vs can simply act as a priming agent to facilitate utilization and navigation of these vital nutrients from the inception of the program—vital nutrients that in turn are needed to correct the problem. Insulin health is crucial to nutrient assimilation—the very nutrients needed to create insulin health. Hence, the value of the vs primer. Ageless Performance's array of nutrients can then be used by an insulin-supported body to prompt that regenerative cycle, and the body can work its natural wonders to instill insulin self-sufficiency.

WORKING VS INTO THE CORRECTIVE PROGRAM

Vanadyl sulfate can be administered when initiating Ageless Performance. But first a physician must be consulted and then a legitimate health-inspection-certified version of vs has to be obtained. Approved vs, like all multi-vitamin and mineral formulations, has a drug identification number (DIN) assigned to it by a government health-inspection agency.

Start with 10 mg of vs taken with one meal of the day. vs is absorbed more efficiently when ingested on an empty stomach. However, it's tolerated better when taken with food. Since vs can induce gastrointestinal upset when consumed in larger doses in some individuals, it's advisable to begin administering it with meals for a few weeks before trying it on an empty stomach.

Increase the dosage to 10 mg with two separate meals for a daily total of 20 mg after a few days to one week. In the second week move to 30 mg per day—10 mg at a time taken with three separate meals. After another week or so, move the single dose up to 20 mg with each meal for a daily total of 60 mg. At any time vs can be taken on an empty stomach if the body will tolerate it. Refer to the administration table on page 408.

On week four of the therapy reach as high as 30 mg three times daily and persist for about a week with this 90 mg dose, then reduce the amount during the following week, staying on the regimen for 10 to 12 weeks. Practitioners have reported using as much as 150 mg of vs per day with tremendous success and only mild gastrointestinal distress as a side effect—a minor complaint compared to being afflicted by diabetes. This gastrointestinal distress isn't much different from the side effects the common diabetic drug, metformin, can cause.

Oddly vs is approved for over-the-counter sales in the United States just as other mineral supplements or multi-vitamin formulations are, but not in Canada. This is another example of Health Canada's sluggish response to essential nutraceuticals that can change the lives of millions with less than 50 cents per day and with only a two- or three-month therapy period as opposed to long-term dependence on expensive patented drugs. Almost three million people suffer from diagnosed diabetes in Canada, while in the United States the numbers are already in excess of 17 million. In both countries these statistics are climbing, and many more people struggle with the affliction but have never been diagnosed.

The supplementation of vs is an optional component of Ageless Performance and mustn't be substituted for medications such as metformin. It can, however, be administered in conjunction with metformin to enhance results. vs works through chemistry that's independent of metformin's facilitating cellular correction. Nevertheless, only when recovery is well under way can compensatory drugs like metformin be eliminated and only, again, with a health-care professional's approval and monitoring.

vs doesn't have to be used indefinitely. Its ability to stimulate transcription and membrane incorporation of glucose-transport sites in mice has been shown to correct the Type II diabetic state. These studies were referenced in previous chapters. After vs's use is terminated, the healed state persists in most cases. Human studies haven't revealed this retained activity scientifically yet—studies are still under way. But the anecdotal evidence suggests that the restoration of healthy insulin activity does continue similarly in humans. Scientific studies have demonstrated conclusively that vs does, however, improve insulin function and reverse diabetes while being administered and it does so safely. All of this documentation

VS Administration Strategy

Week	Mon.	Tues.	Wed.	Thurs.	Fri.	Sat.	Sun.
1 10 mg per day	10 mg with one meal	10 mg with one meal	10 mg with one meal	10 mg with one meal	10 mg, 2 times daily; 10 mg with two meals	10 mg, 2 times daily; 10 mg with two meals	10 mg, 2 times daily; 10 mg with two meals
2 30 mg per day	10 mg, 3 times daily; 10 mg with three meals	10 mg, 3 times daily; 10 mg with three meals	10 mg, 3 times daily; 10 mg with three meals	10 mg, 3 times daily; 10 mg with three meals	10 mg, 3 times daily; 10 mg with three meals	10 mg, 3 times daily; 10 mg with three meals	10 mg, 3 times daily; 10 mg with three meals
3 60 mg per day	20 mg, 3 times daily; 20 mg with three meals	20 mg, 3 times daily; 20 mg with three meals	20 mg, 3 times daily; 20 mg with three meals	20 mg, 3 times daily; 20 mg with three meals	20 mg, 3 times daily; 20 mg with three meals	20 mg, 3 times daily; 20 mg with three meals	20 mg, 3 times daily; 20 mg with three meals
4 90 mg per day	30 mg, 3 times daily; 30 mg with three meals	30 mg, 3 times daily; 30 mg with three meals	30 mg, 3 times daily; 30 mg with three meals	30 mg, 3 times daily; 30 mg with three meals	30 mg, 3 times daily; 30 mg with three meals	30 mg, 3 times daily; 30 mg with three meals	30 mg, 3 times daily; 30 mg with three meals
5 to 10 60 mg per day	20 mg, 3 times daily; 20 mg with three meals	20 mg, 3 times daily; 20 mg with three meals	20 mg, 3 times daily; 20 mg with three meals	20 mg, 3 times daily; 20 mg with three meals	20 mg, 3 times daily; 20 mg with three meals	20 mg, 3 times daily; 20 mg with three meals	20 mg, 3 times daily; 20 mg with three meals

is referenced thoroughly in previous chapters. In any event, vs can be employed as an occasional reset of insulin function.

The *short* restorative period of vs use helps to maintain insulin efficiency and is an active step toward the prevention of diabetes and other associated diseases. I use vs once every eight to 12 months for four to eight weeks at a time to ensure maximum insulin performance. Be cautioned, though: individuals who have experienced allergic reactions to sulfa-type antibacterial drugs have been known to experience reactivity to vs.

vs can help in the treatment of both Type I and II diabetes as can the Ageless Performance program as a whole. However, it's Type II (adult-onset) diabetes that can be completely reversed by this fabulous program. Of course, the specifications of the condition will dictate the level of recovery and the duration of the recovered state between cycles of vs. Additionally dietary habits will influence the integrity of the newly developed functional state. Poor habits result in rapid degradation and the necessity for vs or other drug intervention sooner rather than later between cycles and may promote the need for ongoing use of pharmaceutical or nutraceutical drugs. Type I diabetes, though, isn't likely to be reversed by Ageless Performance.

Rectifying a diabetic condition requires a lot of work. Label descriptions of foods and supplements have to be carefully scanned for ingredients that might have high glycemic indexes. Common high-glycemic-index carbohydrate additions to supplements that must be avoided if insulin resistance or diabetes is a problem are: glucose, dextrose, and maltodextrin; rice syrup solids; corn, potato, and rice starches; and extreme glycerine loads, maltose, and sucrose. Glycerine, a common sweetener and food additive, is a healthier factor than glucose if one must choose. Foods must be as close as possible to their whole and fresh states such as stone-ground rather than finely ground wheat. Bread made with whole, not finely ground, grains should be the first choice, and common additions to breads such as sugar, syrups, molasses, or unnecessary starches must be avoided.

Juicing of fruits and vegetables is also not a good idea while combating a progressive state of insulin resistance. Sugar from the natural fiber matrix of the food is released by juicing, allowing for faster delivery to circulating blood, which means a higher glycemic index for the same sugar that was once bound by natural fibers. Juicing is a great way to get a concentrated load of antioxidant and other nutrients, but it's better tolerated if insulin activity is supported in the body by a program such as Ageless Performance.

Sedentary folk on this anti-diabetic program require a protein intake of about 0.60 g per pound of body weight each day, which is measured as a sedentary therapeutic protein content (PC) or co-factor of 0.60 (0.60 g of protein x 170 pounds = 102 g of protein per day per pound of body weight).

THE VALUE OF PROTEIN QUALITY

An important factor to keep in mind is the quality of protein. Nutrition textbooks emphasize that the quality of dietary protein must be higher than average when disease is a challenge or the stage of development is such that growth is swift (37). The essential amino-acid portion of daily protein supplied to growing children, for example, should be more than 36% and at least 43% for infants. For sedentary adults, though, textbooks recommend only 19%. However, we rarely, if at all, see reference made to the increased demands for protein created by disease, trauma, injury, mental disturbances, and emotional and physical stress, even though the last two *boost* the demand for dietary protein. My recommendation is that we consume high-quality protein all the time in order to prevent disease. The suggestion to eat better quality protein to redirect the metabolism from a deficient state caused by less-than-optimal nourishment is absurd. Prevention is the best cure!

The quality of a protein source is determined by various factors such as the amino-acid profile. Contrary to misinformation from the marketing claims of some pharmaceutical and nutraceutical companies, amino-acid profile is *not* the dictating factor for biological value (BV) of a dietary protein. The delivery form of these amino acids is important, and the processing method strongly dictates its nature. People aren't going to calculate the proportion of essential amino acids in a protein source to determine the character of their daily intake. Nor are many of us about to think extensively about the quality of each and every protein source that enters our mouths.

We should, but we don't. That's why I recommend supplementing daily with at least one serving of a cold cross-flow, membrane-processed whey protein supplement—a whey protein isolate, not a whey concentrate. Each and every one of us, children and seniors, can ensure that quality building blocks reach biological construction sites by taking just a few minutes a day to stir a whey supplement into a glass of water.

Some experts tell us cooking heat can increase the digestibility of protein, but it can also contribute to amino-acid degradation and the binding of amino acids to each other to form insoluble complexes, rendering them unavailable for absorption. Processing of protein sources using excessive heat can make lysine unavailable for enzyme digestion, as cited in previous chapters. This reduces the entire bioavailability of a protein source. Even though the entire amino-acid profile of the protein source is displayed on the product label, including lysine, for instance, the amino acid isn't available to the gut absorptive process. The body depends grossly on such building blocks and can't replace them, leaving tissue and hormone regeneration incomplete when such sources are staples. Protein sources prepared for canning and dry preservation can be altered this way, too, something that's typical of kibble processing for dry dog and cat foods, as well.

Dietary protein sources can be subjected to alkali treatment, the opposite of acid treatment. Alkali treatment of protein can produce lysinoalanine complexes, a compound that isn't hydrolyzed by the gastrointestinal tract and is thought to cause severe growth retardation (38, 39). Acid hydrolysis to the point of peptide denaturation and extreme heat processing is another factor that reduces protein bioavailability (40, 41). Again, the preferred protein or amino-acid components might be contained in these extremely processed sources and listed on their product labels, but they're usually not available for absorption or not in the necessary proportions for tissue anabolism. The quality of a protein source is significant to how or whether or not the body can use it. You can't just determine how much protein you consumed in a day and leave that as your assessment for daily intake. Quality counts!

The storage of protein sources after they've been processed can facilitate reactivity—the Maillard reaction—which occurs if protein sources are mixed with sugar derivations. The resulting sugar/amino-acid complexes are nondigestible. Again, the amino acid might be detailed in the profile on a product label, but it won't be obtainable for absorption. In addition, newer findings have revealed that these indigestible complexes can also inhibit enzymes from digesting other viable protein (42, 43). I prefer sugar-free, pure whey protein sources as supplemental protein—no fructose, sucrose, maltodextrin, glucose, or dextrose.

The glutamine content displayed on the product label of a casein supplement, for example, is usually greater than in a typical whey protein isolate supplement, if listed at all. Casein naturally contains far more glutamine than whey. However, when blood glutamine levels are measured after the oral administration of casein versus whey protein isolate, serum glutamine is usually shown to be higher for the whey isolate group. Whey provides a higher peak for serum amino acid in the blood more quickly upon consumption, while casein is more slowly digested and only gradually absorbed. This higher profile for serum glutamine and essential amino acid promotes recovery of tissue more immediately. The rapid absorption is a function of various factors that contribute to the improved bioavailability for whey protein as opposed to casein. Obviously the whey protein isolate must be processed correctly to maintain its peptide integrity in order to deliver this extra beneficial nitrogen potential. Glutamine represents well over 50% of the amino-acid pool of human muscle. It's a major nitrogen-delivery system for the body. An influx of glutamine, as we've previously seen, is also important for cortisol down-regulation. That factor alone makes whey a better source of protein for anti-catabolic activity, muscle anabolism, brain preservation, and general recovery (44).

The controversy over whey- versus casein-based supplementation is extensive. Some experts claim that the slower release of amino acids into the bloodstream by casein is a better way to sustain a longer period of recovery. The problem is that if during this more gradual release essential amino acids take longer to make it into the blood for muscle or other tissue synthesis in the early phase of protein absorption by the gut, tissue synthesis will be limited. When these essential amino acids finally enter the bloodstream to meet the need, the other amino acids that were there previously might already have been metabolized by the liver.

The other difficulty is the need to supply an abundance of essential and other nitrogen-boosting amino acids during the window of opportunity—immediately after physical exertion. This issue pertains to those who are involved in regular athletic or job-labor physical activity, especially those individuals who are into intense physical sport. A limited absorption rate immediately after activity results in restricted recovery. Miss out on the window of opportunity and maximum recovery as well as optimal muscle and strength gains are compromised. As suggested before, the solution might be to consume two smaller whey isolate drinks right after the workout or other physical labor—one just after the session and another approximately 30 to 40 minutes later.

However, absorption isn't the ultimate factor determining the value of protein, either, or any other nutrient for that matter. The real test is retention of the nutrient in tissue. In other words, has the nutrient been incorporated into the tissues in need after digestion and absorption have taken place, or has the nutrient been discarded because of some unforeseen limitation? BV is a measure of this retention; that's why it's a great gauge of protein quality.

These factors have been carefully considered in the formulation of the entire Ageless Performance strategy, and not just for the protein component. The detailed description of protein bioavailability and retention potential simply serves as a model for every nutrient consumed. Contrary to the accepted adage, we're not what we eat. Instead we're what we're able to digest, absorb, and incorporate into our tissues. Ageless Performance is designed with this doctrine as a guide.

The proportion of essential amino acids in the dietary protein consumed by the health-conscious individual must be increased to compensate for any of the discussed impositions. A good-quality whey protein supplement can deliver an essential amino-acid portion in excess of 60% of its total protein content. If it's processed correctly through cold cross-flow extraction or ion-exchange isolation, then it's likely to deliver its high essential amino-acid component in a form that's easy to utilize. In my opinion the textbook-recommended 19% essential amino-acid share of daily protein for sedentary folk is much too little if potent disease prevention is a goal.

Insufficient quality of dietary protein contributes to the typical atrophy experienced by the elderly as much as insufficient protein quantity does.

414 • FRANCO CAVALERI

A long-term dietary shortfall leads to lean-body-mass degradation, immune impairment, disease, and poor recovery potential. The common gastric limitations experienced by the elderly amplify the problems that dietary shortages can induce.

The point is clear: quality protein is critical to prevention and recovery. Quality dietary protein delivers the building blocks and hormonal influence required to prevent disease. Again, just one serving of a whey protein isolate each day will raise the daily proportion of essential amino acids to healthier totals. This provides for better immune support, enhanced lean-mass recovery, increased antioxidant status, and improved preventive potential. It will even slow the pace of the biological clock.

Sedentary folk include those who work in offices whose jobs entail little physical activity. The level of stress such people are exposed to has to be accommodated for, which means a slightly higher protein intake might be required. Keep in mind that mental and emotional stresses increase demands for nourishment much as physical strain does. If you're fighting disease and maintaining an active lifestyle, you'll have to boost your daily protein intake to meet the higher compounded demand of multiple stressors.

Fast-pace walking is great exercise! If you're involved in a power-walking program that takes about one hour per session, you might find your dietary protein needs fall somewhere between Active and Sedentary, so choose a PC value between Active 1 and Sedentary 0.60. After you've determined your PC, calculate your protein requirements and from that value figure out your daily carbohydrate requirement. For example, if you run for 20 minutes three times a week and you don't want to commit to the full 1 g of protein per pound of body weight daily, you can decrease slightly to a PC of 0.8 g. The guidelines disclosed aren't rigid, since we're all biochemically, metabolically, actively, and genetically different. Use these suggested (tabulated or calculated) macronutrient quantities as starting points and make adjustments to fit your personal requirements, but don't deviate from the nutrient *quality* and proportions.

On the other hand, you might not have to change your protein intake from the recommendations, and a slight increase in the carbohydrate component might be enough to deliver the extra energy necessary for a more active lifestyle. However, if a diabetic state is the problem, raise the protein component marginally and maintain the suggested carbohydrate component as the low-glycemic-index, fiber-rich vegetable source exclusively. If your selection leaves you feeling run-down from the activity level by the end of the week and extraordinarily hungry at times, even after the minor carbohydrate adjustment, you might have to beef up your PC to 0.9 or to the recommended 1 and recalculate your needs altogether.

When activity includes regular resistance training more than two times a week in addition to walking or other cardiovascular pursuits, you'll have to default to the previously outlined Active program. In the Active program there are accommodations for weight management and guidance toward better insulin efficiency. Applying the vanadyl sulfate strategy to combat diabetes or simply as a preventive strategy while following the Active program is no different than the protocol with the Sedentary strategy. Merge Active and Sedentary (therapeutic) if you must for health reasons by using the Active dietary component with the nutraceutical supplementation program from the Sedentary therapeutic plan.

HEALTHY PARAMETERS

Keep in mind that we haven't compensated for obesity with the PC values in this category, as is the case for the previously discussed categories. It isn't appropriate to calculate a protein requirement for a body weight of 280 pounds if a large portion of the weight is attributable to fat mass. At 280 pounds the fat mass is likely to be a considerable percentage of body weight, even if the individual believes he or she is well muscled. If you're the king of muscle mass the way bodybuilder Paul Dillet is—at six feet two inches and close to 300 pounds, he's relatively fatless—you'll be calculating enormous daily protein needs. However, few people fall into this category. Fat mass doesn't need much protein for maintenance—in fact, relatively zero. If body-fat mass exceeds 20%, the PC-based formulas won't work. However, one thing few people appreciate is the fact that a big person carrying a large body-fat mass will typically also support a larger-than-average lean mass.

A big person works hard to bear that extra weight, and the adaptation process accommodates for the load by enhancing muscular strength and size. The proportions of this muscle mass, however, aren't like those produced by complete resistance-training strategies. Still, a big man or woman can pack a lot of muscle power. Maintaining this underlying muscle contributes to a healthier outcome when the fat weight is lost. But this lean-mass retention requires significant dietary protein to support it, and Ageless Performance is designed to maintain the healthy mass while the fat mass is melted away with little effort. Physical resistance training during body-fat reduction helps preserve the lean-muscle mass, as well.

TOP END OF THE PROTEIN SCALE FOR SEDENTARY FOLK

Daily protein intake for sedentary individuals with a high percentage of body fat should be set at a maximum of 110 g. The usual calculated protein requirement in the Sedentary category for a 220-pound person is 132 g for the day (0.60 x 220 = 132 g of protein), but if body-fat mass with this same weight is, say, 27%, then protein should be cut back to no more than 110 g daily. This quantity of protein is to be consumed over four or even five sittings (22 to 30 g per meal) where one or two of the meals are made up of a protein drink supplement, preferably a whey isolate beverage.

Ageless Performance is a good fit for children, as well; however, there must be an accommodation for the developmental stage and for growing adolescents to the end of their teens. The program to follow, whether the child is vigorous or not, is the active individual's guide outlined previously. Active children and adolescents might require a larger portion of dense carbohydrates to deliver the energy necessary for growth. Keep in mind, though, that this energy is a funtion of the primary need—nutrients. The daily carbohydrate intake of an active child might need to be increased slightly from the recommendations. Of course, the sources must be the low-glycemic-index carbohydrates as much as possible (under 70). Avoidance of refined foods can be difficult for children and teens since they've been programmed to adopt our new-age plastic foods and have developed addictions to them. Setting good examples at home is important!

BOTTOM END OF THE PROTEIN SCALE FOR SEDENTARY FOLK

Now that we have a top limit for daily protein intake, let's set the bottom end. Regardless of body weight, don't use a value lower than 75 g of total daily protein. Calculate carbohydrate requirements from this 75 g minimum and up to the maximum allowed. In a case where a sedentary adult weighs 105 pounds, for example, the usual protein calculation would amount to 63 g for the day (0.60 x 105 pounds). For sedentary individuals, though, automatically default up to a minimum 75 g of protein for the day and continue the calculation from there.

The carbohydrate portion for this category is calculated as in the previous programs. Use a carbohydrate co-factor (cc) of 2. Interestingly the cc for this category is higher rather than lower. This higher cc accommodation is due to a required higher nutrient-dense, fiber-rich food base. In addition, the fact that dietary protein levels are lower for this group necessitates an adjustment to a higher carbohydrate intake to spare protein for the recovery process. This strategy enhances *micro*nutrient density to help support recovery from disease and boost the preventive potential of the body.

The proportions between the dense carbohydrate and low-glycemic-index vegetable carbohydrates for each meal are left to each individual to pinpoint. These source proportions actually dictate how much digestible carbohydrate is consumed daily. The recommendation is to stay with low-glycemic-index vegetables and low-glycemic-index fruit as much as possible. Here's what the values should look like for a 170-pound sedentary individual battling disease: Sedentary cc = 2 (2 g of carbohydrates x 102 g of total daily protein = 204 g of dietary carbohydrates per day).

If you're in this category, make sure the high-glycemic-index carbohydrate intake doesn't exceed 30% of the carbohydrate total for the day. For a 105-pound person the dense source (higher glycemic index) supplies 60 g of the daily total and can come from potatoes, whole-wheat pasta, brown rice, kamut, or whole-grain rye bread. The low-glycemic-index, low-density carbohydrate sources (the vegetable medleys I've detailed previously) can comprise the rest of the daily carbohydrate intake. Make a note that a half cup of cooked brown rice or cooked whole-wheat pasta delivers about

25 g of carbohydrates. See Appendix A for guidance.

Fiber-rich vegetable carbohydrate sources slow the rate of glucose entry into the bloodstream and present a significant portion of their substance as nondigestible fiber. Preferably *all* of the carbohydrate choices by an individual fighting diseases, including obesity, will come from foods that are below a glycemic index of 60, ideally no higher than 55. Once again, refer to Appendix A for a list of carbohydrate sources.

THE ROLE OF EXERCISE IN THE BATTLE AGAINST DISEASE

Be aware that the high-glycemic-index foods (of the healthy category), such as brown rice and whole-wheat pasta, are best tolerated in a post-workout/walk meal. Plan the day so that the dinner meal is eaten immediately after an extensive walk or workout. These fine details play an immense role in the correction of health.

Keep in mind that dealing with a state of disease means less latitude regarding the consumption of dense, high-glycemic-index carbohydrate sources. However, exercise creates the opportunity for more latitude—the inclusion of high-glycemic-index foods in a post-exercise meal. A pre-workout whey protein drink will suffice for pre-exercise nourishment, with no other food for 60 minutes before the event. A local fitness center can provide guidance concerning a functional 30- to 40-minute light split routine, which might involve resistance training every second day. Sticking to a short, rigorous strategy for the program is an important feature as opposed to talking for 10 to 15 minutes between sets or exercises. This prevents hypoglycemia from setting in during the activity, preserving lean tissue in the body and ensuring better results from the training.

Plan the day so that dinner is eaten immediately after this short training session. No dietary carbohydrates after 7:30 p.m. can be consumed. Low-fat dietary protein is acceptable after this time. After a period of this aggressive correction, begin to include more high-density carbohydrates in the diet, but still abstain from carbohydrates after dinner. Some healthier sources of high-density carbohydrates are yams, sweet potatoes, oatmeal, and legumes such as beans.

The value of exercise is paramount if insulin resistance or diabetes is a problem. Exercise clears blood sugar, initiates the rebuilding of cellular glucose-transport systems, promotes a healthier dispersion of nutrients from the post-exercise meal, cultivates a positive mindset, pumps out healthy hormones and neurotransmitters, flushes the body of lymphatic toxins, and allows for the consumption of denser carbohydrate sources if desired. All of these claims are substantiated by previously mentioned scientific references. Limiting or omitting physical activity leads to restrictions in the diet and slows the rate of tissue turnover and debris removal from the body, decreasing the ability to recover from disease.

HEALTHY TIPS

The need to feed above the supply that Ageless Performance delivers might be caused by nibbling and snacking habits. If these desires are a problem, snack on low-glycemic-index fruit or vegetables such as apples, oranges, grapefruits, peaches, celery, cauliflower, broccoli, or a large mixed green salad. Snacking while fighting disease can also include low-fat or dry-curd cottage cheese or tuna (preferably fresh) topped with, if desired, my Heart Healthy Salad Dressing (see Chapter 9).

As nutrient and hormonal status improve, unnecessary snacking tendencies will disappear. Don't initiate the carbohydrate roller-coaster ride with high-glycemic-index snacks such as crackers, bread, cookies, juice, or dried fruit. These choices can easily derail positive metabolic momentum. Stick to snack foods that are nutrient-rich and alkalinizing. Appendix D displays such alkalinizing and acidifying foods.

Temptation can start the vicious circle of carbohydrate addiction. Don't take foods home from the grocery store that don't fit the new criteria. If unhealthy food is in the pantry, you're likely to snack on it. If the refrigerator and pantry are full of healthy, low-glycemic-index snacks, you won't have unhealthy alternatives to choose from. Most important, write out grocery lists before entering stores and stick to the plan.

What about a child's needs and desires? If you have a child, his or her needs aren't much different than your own. In fact, these strategies can offset much of the damage a child's typical junk-food diet can cause. At the very least take charge of the nourishment that goes into your child when he or she is at home. When you go out for dinner and eat outside of the healthy parameters, don't fret. However, don't take leftover pasta, cake, rice, white potatoes, and other foods that don't fit the healthy criteria home from the family get-together at a restaurant. To eat these foods on occasion is fine, but to keep them at home to binge on for days disrupts the healthy metabolic momentum that's been established, detouring the healthy course back to the addictive cycle.

If you're doing a labor-intensive job, you'll have to apply the Active program. If work involves construction, landscaping, mining, or other calorie- and nutrient-expensive labor, you'll have to increase intake to meet the demand. With the Active program the quality nourishment of the Ageless Performance dietary component will instill metabolic efficiency, and the desire to eat outside the right food choices will be easy to overcome. Again, the therapeutic nutraceutical plan can be incorporated into the Active dietary program as can the vanadyl sulfate strategy if required. The following table details the recommended starting points for the sedentary individual seeking therapeutic relief.

Review the different dietary suggestions for each weight class to get an idea of the choices that can be made to compose meals. Refer to the examples of quality protein sources on page 421 for an immediate reference for the type of protein required. An extended reference list indicating the quality and quantity of protein sources from which to choose is available in Appendix C.

MY FAVORITE—NUTRIENT-DENSE SOUPS

One of my favorite and convenient ways to get a calorie-restricted, nutrient-rich meal is through homemade soups or stews. Combine the nutrient bounty of low-glycemic-index vegetables such as green and red peppers, onions, squash, zucchini, garlic, celery, broccoli, cabbage, and cauliflower with the high-density carbohydrates of legumes such as a combination of beans (garbanzo, navy, soy, green, and blackeye). Add some diced yams or sweet potatoes. After the vegetable medley has had enough time to cook, it will turn into a rich vegetable stew. This mixture delivers complex low- and medium-glycemic-index carbohydrates and plenty of vitamins, minerals,

Dietary Recommendations for Recovery from Disease: Sedentary Individual

Body Weight in Pounds	Protein from High BV Sources	Total Daily Carbohydrates	Carbohydrates from Dense Sources: Brown Rice, Whole-Wheat Pasta	Carbohydrates from Low-Glycemic Vegetable Sources
240	110 g per day (men: 30 to 40 g per meal; women: 25 to 30 g per meal)	220 g	70 g total per day; example: 1/2 to 2/3 cup of cooked brown rice at one sitting (dinner or postwalk meal) plus 1 to 2 slices of whole-rye bread (breakfast)	100-plus g total per day; example: from vegetables as dinner medleys, raw vegetable snacks (i.e., 2 cups of mixed vegetables = approximately 20 g of carbohydrates; 1 cup of yams = 40 g of carbohydrates)
220	110 g per day (men: 30 to 40 g per meal; women: 25 to 30 g per meal)	Same as above	70 g total per day; example: 1/2 to 1 whole baked or steamed white potato (dinner or postwalk meal) plus 1 cup of oatmeal (breakfast)	100-plus g total per day; example: from vegetables as dinner medleys, raw snacks (i.e., 2 cups of mixed vegetables = 20 g carbohydrates); snack can include yams, sweet potatoes, or fruit
200	110 g per day (men: 30 to 40 g per meal; women: 25 to 30 g per meal)	Same as above	70 g total per day; example: 1 baked or steamed sweet potato or yam (dinner or postwalk meal) plus 1 cup of oatmeal (breakfast)	Don't include yams or sweet potatoes in the medley if the meal contains other dense carbohydrates such as pasta, rice, or white potatoes
180	108 g per day (men: 30 to 40 g per meal; women: 25 to 30 g per meal)	216 g per day	60 g total per day; example: 1/2 cup of cooked whole-wheat pasta at 1 sitting plus 1 to 1 1/2 cups of oatmeal (breakfast); never use instant oatmeal	Always compensate for the dense high-glycemic carbohydrates in the meal with the inclusion of a high-fiber vegetable medley
160	96 g per day (men: 30 to 35 g per meal; women: 25 to 30 g per meal)	192 g per day	45 g total per day; example: 1/2 cup of cooked whole-wheat pasta at 1 sitting plus 1 slice of whole-rye bread (breakfast)	100-plus g of vegetable medley throughout the day; low-glycemic-index fruits such as apples or oranges are allowed snacks between meals
140	84 g per day (men: 30 to 35 g per meal; women: 25 to 30 g per meal)	168 g per day	45 g total per day; example: 1/2 cup of cooked brown rice at 1 sitting plus 1 cup of oatmeal (breakfast)	100-plus g for the day of vegetable medley and fruit snacks; no dried fruit allowed
120	75 g per day (men: 30 to 35 g per meal; women: 25 to 30 g per meal)	150 g per day	45 g total per day; example: 1/2 cup of cooked brown rice at 1 sitting plus 1 cup of oatmeal (breakfast)	100-plus g for the day (i.e., 1 small orange = 15 to 20 g of carbohydrates; 1 small apple = 16 to 21 g of carbohydrates)
100	75 g per day (women: 25 to 30 g per meal)	150 g per day	45 g total per day; example: 1 cup of cooked yams at 1 sitting plus 1 slice of whole-rye bread (breakfast)	100-plus g for the day (i.e., 3 2-cup servings of low-glycemic vegetable medley plus 2 small fruits will meet the daily requirement for this category; this amounts to large food volume)

and phytoantioxidants. If these vegetables are prepared in large chunks, they're more likely to maintain their nutrient integrity. In other words, use whole mushrooms, whole small tomatoes, and larger pieces of broccoli and cauliflower, then add sprouts just before serving for additional unscathed, active nutrition.

To up the protein content of the stew, I add my common protein booster food, dry-curd cottage cheese, right into the soup while it's cooking. The addition of soy curd is also a great idea. Both types of curd deliver synergistic immune-supportive qualities. I make enough stew to last a few days and scoop my meal serving for reheating as needed. The vegetable protein sources in this soup are of reasonable quality but are still slightly limited. Soy protein, for example, is one of the better vegetable protein sources in terms of amino-acid profiles, but its biological value is quite a bit less than whey protein. Soy has a best BV of about 74, and whey can range between a low of 100 to a high of 159, depending on the processing method employed.

The added dry-curd cottage cheese (casein BV = 77) improves the BV score for the soy protein to increase the total for the soup meal. The BV for whole egg is 100; whole egg is the standard used to measure other sources comparatively. Since whole egg has a high BV (complete with highly bioavailable amino acids), it's a good idea to swirl a few eggs into the finished soup/stew to enhance the total protein quality. Better yet, swirl one whole egg into each large meal serving of the soup/stew to complement the quality and quantity of protein in the serving. This meal is thick with vegetables, sustenance, and satiety. You can also stir a few teaspoons of whey protein isolate right into your single serving of the stew. A good-quality whey isolate (plain version) will be relatively flavorless.

This convenient meal is quite easy to make. Just pour two liters of prepared liquid soup stock into a large stew pot. Buy the liquid concentrate in Tetra Paks at the grocery store. Avoid versions that have megaloads of MSG and unfamiliar preservatives. Add crushed and whole tomato as well as some vegetables and legumes. If more protein is needed in the soup, I sometimes bake or stir-fry some chicken or fish in a dab of olive oil and a few cloves of garlic, then add a pinch of seasoning. Eat the protein as a side dish to the soup, or add it into the serving bowl with the soup. An alternative is a whey protein drink to supplement the soup meal's protein total. If there are no vegetarians in your family, cook shredded chicken in the soup. Use a large bowl and don't be afraid to get your fill.

A good practice to get into is to stop eating halfway through a meal and take supplements. This mixes the supplements into the meal and also creates lag time to allow the stomach's stretch receptors to signal that the stomach is full. Sometimes we eat quickly and beyond our natural limits because this feedback signal doesn't make it to conscious awareness in time. Some of us get the stretch-receptor message quicker than others do. By the time the message registers, 10 more minutes of gorging takes place. Eat slowly and split the meal with a five- to 10-minute break to take supplements. *Feel* your fill.

EYEBALL ESTIMATION FOR THERAPY

Few of us have a nutritional almanac handy and few of us are prepared to weigh food for every meal. Who can blame us? Start meal planning by determining the protein requirement first. Use Appendix C as a convenient reference list of the more common protein sources. From these dietary protein volumes, determine carbohydrate requirements by volume estimation or employ macronutrient calculation. There's no excuse for procrastination; you might not have a nutritional almanac for reference, but you can work efficiently through the program with the reference appendices in this book.

Let's work through the dietary and lifestyle changes that must be put into practice for a sedentary 150-pound individual battling diabetes, someone who could lose a few pounds of fat to help reverse the condition. The midway point (between 140 and 160 pounds) for the protein requirement is 90 g daily. If we calculate the daily protein requirement using the PC value, the formulation looks like this: Sedentary therapeutic PC = 0.60 (0.60 g of protein x 150 pounds = 90 g of protein per day). Dividing the total daily protein value by five daily protein servings, we get 18 g of protein per meal. You might not have to sit and actually consume five meals in a day. Although this is the preferred protocol, it's difficult to commit to. Protein drinks can be taken between sitting meals to supplement the total daily protein intake—three meals and two drinks.

If we calculate the total carbohydrate requirement using the cc value, the formulation looks like this: Sedentary cc = 2 (2 g of carbohydrates x 90 g of total daily protein = 180 g of dietary carbohydrates per day). I've already mentioned that we all require different proportions of high-glycemic-index versus low-glycemic-index carbohydrates for the meal.

Employing the eyeball-estimation method, start out with the protein requirement to plan the meal. Twenty grams of protein (roughly 18 g per meal as calculated for the 150-pound sedentary individual) gives us the following list of choices: three to three and a half ounces (just under half a cup) of salmon; three ounces (one-quarter cup) of tuna; three ounces (one-quarter cup) of halibut; two whole eggs plus two egg whites; three ounces (one-quarter cup) of white meat chicken; and two-thirds of a cup of low-fat cottage cheese.

Precisely measure these quantities if you must for a week or so, but soon you won't need to reference volume for each meal because you'll develop an eye for your requirement. It isn't a tragedy to eat a little more than your protein requirement for a meal or two. The volume for each protein source listed above isn't a precise value, since the hydration and fat level can vary from time to time and type to type to affect the protein contribution. These volumes are estimations for convenience. As long as the protein sources suggested throughout this book are adhered to, the protein quality as well as the fat inherent in each source will support a healthy outcome.

The same plate size used for the active individual's program can be applied to this category. First divide the plate in half and then create quarter sections out of one of the halves for denser carbohydrate sources. For this category yams, sweet potatoes, oatmeal, and legumes are the best denser carbohydrate selections as opposed to pasta, rice, and white potatoes. The depth or height of each food category on the plate for the sedentary individual will be lower than that for the active person's meal if the same plate size is used. Logically less food—less nourishment—is needed for sedentary people.

Here's an example of a prepared meal plate for the sedentary individual seeking recovery from disease, including obesity. The same strategy will be applied if *mild* fat reduction is desired. The protein portion on the plate can include half of a chicken breast. The vegetable section might include one and a half cups of a low-glycemic-index vegetable mix, perhaps a variety of zucchini, cauliflower, broccoli, and mushrooms. This vegetable selection can be made up of one of the aforementioned vegetables also. An equal third portion of food will consist of the denser carbohydrate sources. The quantity of each third will be comparable in volume to the amount of protein on the plate, and the latter denser carbohydrate source will consist of beans and yams and/or sweet potatoes.

Food preparation is a significant factor because too many of us prepare our food to death and bury the goodness with unhealthy toppings. Making food as bland as possible delivers fewer calories. The vegetable medleys are best lightly stir-fried in a pan that's just been lightly wiped with a paper napkin moistened with olive oil. Short steaming periods are good, too. Add a little soy sauce or other seasoning. If you're not accustomed to eating this way, you'll eventually acquire a taste for it. The fatty, richer foods can be eaten once per week if desired.

Baking and broiling provide good-quality meals. Combining a protein source such as chicken with all of the colorful vegetables in a deep pot and cooking it in the oven with a cover allows the juices of the protein source to simmer the vegetables. Add a diluted mixture of lemon juice and a bit of soy sauce with herbal seasoning as well as some water occasionally to maintain the volume of natural gravy. This provides moistening and gravy without trans-fat saturation. Don't forget the Heart Healthy Salad Dressing and Spread (described in Chapter 9) as alternatives to butter and hydrogenated salad dressings. Don't cook with these specialty fat blends, since the flax component can't tolerate heat. If you must use commercial condiments, employ them sparingly and only occasionally, and when you do, dilute them with a touch of balsamic vinegar and olive and/or flax oil. There really isn't a time where less-than-healthy condiments are an absolute must. But a word of caution: don't cook with flax oil or other PUFA-concentrated oils. Olive oil is safe. Ghee is also a widely used safe cooking oil/fat. Essentially it's butter with all the milk solids removed; however, like butter, it's loaded with saturated fat and doesn't contain the antioxidants and other benefits associated with olive oil.

THE IMPORTANCE OF WATER

Water consumption hasn't been discussed in this book much, but it's more important than any one of the nutrients we've covered. You can *live* without any one of these nutrients for days, weeks, and even years, but you can't survive more than three or four days without water. Any level of hydration minutely below optimal results in suboptimal biological efficiency. The nutrient bounty of Ageless Performance is useless if the body is dehydrated. Maintain supple hydrated cells; in other words, drink all day. Don't allow yourself to be prompted by thirst, since this is a sign of dehydration, a state in which damage has already occurred.

The body is at least 90% water. Dehydration and the consequential thirst are often misinterpreted as hunger. Second, quenching thirst with cool fruit juices results in the overconsumption of high-glycemic-index sugars and unnecessary extra calories. Maintaining hydration with clean water maximizes nutrient delivery, appetite control, and biological efficiency. My common recommendation is to find a convenient water bottle that holds about 750 milliliters. Fill it in the morning with purified water or clean spring water and sip it all day. Make sure you consume two of these containers daily (1.5 liters or more) in addition to any other liquids you drink. If you consume coffee or tea, drink water before you indulge. Coffee and tea are natural diuretics, which means they promote water expulsion from the body. Compensate for this by increasing water intake. I prefer distilled water. The more common reverse-osmosis purified water is usually cheaper, but this filtration process, though quite advanced, still can't completely remove toxic trace metals like aluminum (45).

Interestingly a recent French study demonstrated that hydration level is directly related to protein synthesis and anabolic potential. The elderly are more vulnerable to dehydration, which leads to far more than just muscle reduction due to cell-volume loss. Muscle is mostly water; dehydrate the body and mass is lost. However, this study shows how anabolic potential declines significantly in the dehydrated state. Glycogenesis can't ensue, as I've described earlier, without sufficient water, and this also contributes to a considerable loss in muscle-mass volume and energy stores. In a sense, the French study illustrates that water can have an anabolic potential, but more accurately a deficit of water inhibits anabolism (muscle growth and maintenance) and energy storage in the young and old (46). What follows is a sample summary of the regimen for a sedentary individual fighting disease.

SAMPLE AGELESS PERFORMANCE REGIMEN FOR A SEDENTARY INDIVIDUAL REQUIRING THERAPY

7:45 a.m.—Breakfast

Whey protein beverage: 25 g serving of whey protein isolate; half teaspoon of psyllium husk stirred into three-quarters to one cup of purified water.

Substitute the above meal with a bowl of oatmeal—one cup of whole, unprocessed, non-instant oatmeal with a half cup of 1% cottage cheese on the side. Add a tablespoon of plain or vanilla-flavored whey protein isolate powder to the oatmeal if more protein is desired. Alternatively make an omelet with one whole egg, two egg whites, and three tablespoons of dry-curd cottage cheese stirred into the beaten eggs. Eat with a slice of whole-rye-kernel bread.

Supplements: multi-vitamin/mineral (multi-dose formulation to be taken more than once daily); vitamin C: 1,000 mg; curcumin: 600 to 700 mg (95% curcuminoids); bromelain: 200 to 300 mg (2,000 GDU); salmon oil: 3,000 mg; flax oil: 2,000 mg; vitamin E: 200 to 400 IU alpha tocopherol (in addition to the contribution by the ACES formula and the multi-vitamin formulation, this amount will suffice); alpha lipoic acid (R+): 100 to 200 mg; GTF chromium: 200 to 300 mcg; vanadyl sulfate: 10 mg (increase dose as detailed in the VS administration details on page 408).

One cup of coffee maximum (note: phytates from coffee antagonize mineral absorption).

Drink lots of purified water throughout the day.

10:00 a.m.—Snack 1

One apple.

11:00 a.m.—Snack 2

One whole egg plus one to two egg whites or one can of tuna or fresh lightly seared tuna topped with Heart Healthy Salad Dressing.

12:30 p.m.—Lunch

Component 1: sandwich choice—two slices of whole-rye bread or rye blend (ingredients profile might look like this: whole-kernel rye, purified water, whole-meal rye, whole-meal wheat, oat and barley flakes, linseed, non-iodized salt, sesame, yeast); half a can of tuna or chopped lightly seared fresh tuna (mustard and chives can be mixed into the tuna but no mayonnaise-type hydrogenated dressings); cucumber and tomato slices and lettuce. Alternatively use a meat filling for the sandwich such as unprocessed turkey breast or chicken breast from the previous night's dinner. A deviled egg sandwich also fills the need (with only a dab of mayonnaise, low-fat creamy cottage cheese, or a bit of low-fat sour cream).

Component 2: mixed green salad topped with sunflower and pumpkin seeds and the Heart Healthy Salad Dressing (olive and flax oil mixed with soy sauce, balsamic vinegar, and garlic); the salad can be large in serving size. Alternatively eat a leftover vegetable medley stir-fry planned the night before and made in abundance for the next lunch meal. By saving a portion of the chicken or fish protein consumed in the dinner meal of the previous day, this vegetable medley could be accompanied by a quality protein source for lunch to eliminate the need for a sandwich in this meal. Another possibility for this meal is a small portion of multi-vegetable soup to accompany the sandwich. In fact, a large enough bowl of this soup/stew with some extra protein, say, from chicken, egg, cottage cheese, and/or whey protein could serve as a complete, low-fat, healthy lunch itself, again eliminating the requirement for a sandwich.

Supplements: vitamin C: 1,000 mg; flax oil: 2,000 mg; salmon oil: 2,000 mg; curcumin: 600 to 700 mg (95% curcuminoids); bromelain: 200 to 300 mg (2,000 GDU); alpha lipoic acid (R+): 100 to 200 mg; GTF chromium: 200 to 300 mcg; vanadyl sulfate: 10 mg (increase dose as detailed in the VS administration details on page 408).

Antioxidant booster formula: one caplet might deliver 7,000 to 8,000 IU of beta-carotene; 150 to 200 mg vitamin C; 100 IU of vitamin E; and 50 to 75 mcg of selenium (ACES is a common fundamental antioxidant combination containing vitamins A, C, E, and selenium; this formula tops off the multi-vitamin/mineral).

2:00 p.m.—Snack 3

An apple, orange, or other low-glycemic-index fruit such as a pear, peach, or grapefruit.

Continue to drink a lot of purified water.

5:00 p.m.—Snack 4

Have a protein drink that can be prepared by placing the serving size of powder (20 g of powder, which usually equates to 14.5 to 16 g of protein) in a shaker cup that can be taken to work in a ready-to-mix dry form. Simply add water and shake. Don't forget to drink plenty of purified water on the way home from your workplace. Even if your job is indoors the bombardment from artificial light and air-conditioning will dehydrate and wear you down. The protein drink and hydration period will sustain you so that when you get home you can immediately head out for a brisk 40-minute walk before dinner. This is when fatigue might inhibit physical activity; however, if you push yourself into this walk, you'll likely return with more energy than before the exercise. Such exercise can easily become a habit if you persist during the first few weeks of this regimen. Work the walk up to a run by alternating short periods of walking with a few hundred yards of running, and soon you'll be jogging the whole way. If physical limitations impede the walk or run, get a good stationary cycle, perpetual rower, or stepper.

6:30 p.m.—Dinner

Start with a tossed salad topped with the Heart Healthy Salad Dressing. Wait five to 10 minutes, then proceed.

Half a chicken breast (steamed, broiled, baked, or lightly stir-fried strips); one to two cups of steamed or lightly stir-fried vegetable medley. Dinner could also include a denser carbohydrate source such as brown rice or whole-wheat pasta in a small quantity (half cup maximum; this amount can be increased as healthier insulin function is reestablished). The preferred dense carbohydrate sources are yams, sweet potatoes, or a half cup of legumes. Consume half of the above, take your supplements, wait five to 10 minutes, then finish the meal. Eat slowly to allow better food-volume control. *Feel* your fill to prevent overeating.

Supplements: vitamin C: 1,000 mg; flax oil: 2,000 mg; salmon oil: 3,000 mg; curcumin: 600 to 700 mg (95% curcuminoids); bromelain: 200 to 300 mg

(2,000 GDU); alpha lipoic acid (R+): 100 to 200 mg; GTF chromium: 200 to 300 mcg; vanadyl sulfate: 10 mg (increase dose as detailed in the VS administration details on page 408).

Antioxidant booster formula: one caplet might deliver 7,000 to 8,000 IU beta-carotene; 150 to 200 mg of vitamin C; 100 IU of vitamin E; 50 to 75 mcg of selenium.

8:30 p.m.—Late-Night Snack

The snack should consist of a protein source only. No carbohydrates are to be eaten past 7:30 p.m., since late in the evening they can interfere with the body's production of growth hormone during sleep. This snack can consist of a protein drink supplemented with 2 g (half a teaspoon) of glutamine and/or 2 g (half a teaspoon) of OKG to support growth-hormone secretions, lean-body-mass recovery, fat loss, gastrointestinal health, and immune function. The therapy-seeking individual would be served well with half a serving of whey protein isolate mixed in water as a late-night snack (15 to 20 g of whey protein isolate powder). If the daily protein intake is short, this drink can be topped off to a full serving to make up the total requirement. The snack can also consist of the previously described tuna or low-fat or dry-curd cottage cheese.

Supplements: vitamin C: 1,000 mg; curcumin (95% curcuminoids): 500 mg; bromelain: 500 mg; alpha lipoic acid (R+): 100 mg; GTF chromium: 200 mcg; grapeseed extract: 150 mg; calcium/magnesium: 250 mg/250 mg (one to two tablets supplying these elemental levels); salmon oil: 2,000 mg; flax oil: 2,000 mg.

Administration of melatonin a few minutes before bedtime will support the total antioxidant potential of the program and facilitate the cascade of a more youthful, restorative hormone profile. See the previous melatonin details for scientific rationale. Recommended melatonin supplementation: 1 mg for every decade past 25 years of age.

The above regimen provides the following macronutrient and caloric values for the day for a 150-pound, relatively sedentary person seeking recovery from disease.

Macro-Profile	Total Grams	Calories	% Calories
Protein	95	380	27%
Fat	50	450	32%
Carbohydrates	145	580	41%
Total	494	1,410	100%

With the addition of extra protein snacks, the above protein total can easily surpass 110 g for the day, but try not to exceed 110. This regimen is designed to deliver powerful therapeutic correction. If the exercise levels for such an individual progress to those previously outlined for the Active category (30 to 45 minutes of brisk walking or running five days a week), nutrient intake must reflect the requirement of the Active program. Such people should switch to the active individual's recommended dietary intake while maintaining the therapeutic nutraceutical supplement program.

HIGHER NUTRACEUTICAL INTENSITY FOR DIFFICULT CASES OF DISEASE

Daily doses of alpha lipoic acid (preferably R+) and curcumin deliver more powerful gene regulation of cyclo-oxygenase transcription amid free-radical density when they're combined. These nutraceuticals provide general antioxidant protection while down-regulating the production of inflammatory (PGE_2 prostaglandins from the omega-6, arachidonic acid) and cardiovascular-clotting (TXA—thromboxanes from the omega-6, arachidonic acid) hormones. They also contribute to insulin efficiency to work synergistically with GTF chromium.

Whey protein is an especially important inclusion to the supplement program when disease rages out of control, since it helps build protective glutathione levels and enhances insulin efficiency while the extra-dietary protein guides the correction of fat metabolism, lean-body-mass restoration, and immune-system activity. We've seen how this biochemistry unfolds in the body in previous chapters. In this antioxidant-rich and insulin-ameliorated environment, the essential and omega-3 fats (inherent in the food and supplement portions of the program) are able to find the right cellular metabolic path. Essential fatty-acid supplementation (linoleic and alpha linolenic acids from flaxseed, for instance) can be a futile attempt to correct health unless these metabolic accommodations are first addressed.

As you might have noticed, the fat intake in the program for sedentary people battling disease is actually slightly higher than that for active individuals. The incremental fat comes from the more aggressive polyunsaturated fatty-acid (PUFA) supplementation. The extra quantity of specialized fats is required to force cellular correction, which in the case of progressed disease has likely become severely imbalanced. It's crucial that molecular-distilled fish-fat supplements and organic, cold-pressed flaxseed oil are used as supplemental sources. These purification processes lower the risks associated with toxins that normally concentrate in the fat medium of animals and plants. This more aggressive therapeutic program can also be merged with the Active or Muscle-Building/Power Athlete strategies if so required.

Supplementation with these specialty nutrients in this therapeutic program amounts to the following aggressive daily totals: PUFA fat (flaxseed and salmon oils): 18 g; curcumin extract (95% curcuminoids): 2,600 mg; vitamin C: 4,000 mg; GTF chromium: 1,100 mcg; and alpha lipoic acid (R+): 700 mg. The rest of the supplements in the prioritized summary tables must accompany the aforementioned nutraceuticals in order to enhance results. However, the extreme doses listed above can be reduced to approximately half after recovery is achieved. Although recovery might take as much as a year for severely imbalanced cases, most people will experience positive metabolic changes within a week or so and more significant results within a few months.

COFFEE: YES OR NO?

The effects of coffee on health constitute a tremendous controversy. One expert advocates coffee consumption and another completely opposes it.

Confusion is understandable. Recent interviews of centenarians revealed that each one consumed coffee starting at a young age. Scientific data, on the other hand, has linked the overindulgence of coffee to endocrine disturbances, primarily those associated with impaired androgen activity in men. In these studies it was shown that avid coffee consumption could actually affect sperm count and testosterone secretion. More recent studies demonstrate, however, that sperm count isn't affected but sperm quality is. Motility of sperm might be enhanced by caffeine, but the sperm's ability to fertilize is reduced (47, 48).

Lower testosterone levels in men and higher estrogen potential in women are also somehow coffee-related (49). Increased sex-hormone-binding globulin (SHBG) levels and associated higher risks of breast cancer, endometriosis, and fibrocystic breast disease in female coffee drinkers have been identified in these studies. Higher SHBG levels, as we've seen, are connected to elevated estrogen activity in the body. Studies indicate increased cortisol production with coffee consumption, which might nominally reduce testosterone production (50). However, very little research points to significantly compromised testosterone levels due to coffee consumption. There might be an explanation for the hormone and sperm anomalies that has little to do with caffeine.

The University of Guelph in Ontario recently released new findings on coffee. This novel research identifies coffee as a contributor to the high rate of insulin resistance plaguing society. The study revealed that two cups of coffee consumed after a high-glycemic-index meal can induce insulin resistance to prolong the clearance of blood sugar (51). If these findings prove conclusive, the ill effects of coffee might include significant heightening of oxidative stress, promotion of insulin resistance, interference of hormone synthesis, and an increased risk of most of our epidemic diseases. But what explains the apparent resistance of those coffee-indulgent centenarians to these new coffee-related disorders? Once again, as we'll see, the explanation can be found in how we grow our food and how we treat our environment today in comparison to what these centenarians experienced when they were younger.

The cultivation of coffee and cocoa beans takes place primarily in countries where spraying with toxic pesticides is poorly, if at all, regulated.

The biological consequences of organochloride and organophosphate pesticides have been clear for decades, yet the agricultural bottom line still prevails over human health. Organophosphates are powerful neurotoxins. In fact, their original design was intended for chemical warfare as nerve gas.

In small doses organophosphates are effective killers of crop-destructive pests. Agricultural experts claim that this minuscule exposure doesn't damage the human biological system. But organophosphates aren't just in our food. They're sprayed in backyard flower and vegetable gardens, and in lumberyards to protect lumber from infestation.

Organophosphates are employed profusely in many countries that Canada and the United States import food from—coffee and cocoa bean producers included. Small but frequent neurotoxin exposure can accumulate to impose significant consequences. If you're a big coffee drinker, you're simply further concentrating your exposure to environmental- and food-borne toxicity. Ironically the Type II diabetic state impairs the natural enzyme system that protects us from incoming organophosphates (52). We can tolerate minute quantities of this neurotoxic compound, but not when our specialized enzyme systems are damaged. Adding this toxicity to a body that has difficulty detoxifying increases the danger of disease; however, if the metabolism were functional, this small exposure could be neutralized with ease.

Diabetes insipidus (a kidney/water-regulatory disorder that induces uncontrollable thirst) and hyperglycemia (high blood sugar *possibly* due to insulin resistance) can be attributed to organophosphates, as well. This toxicity is also associated with glucose in the urine. These symptoms point to kidney and pancreatic damage (53, 54). Organophosphate-induced hyperglycemia/insulin inefficiency *might* be the real cause for the findings at the University of Guelph. However, we don't know if the Guelph study used organically grown coffee that was confirmed to be organophosphate- or organochloride-free.

Organophosphates and organochlorides interrupt the endocrine system, impairing androgenic activity and facilitating estrogenic activity in the body. Organophosphate toxicity escalates cortisol levels, impairs thyroid output, and lowers follicle-stimulating hormone (FSH) secretions from the pituitary gland. The last-mentioned endocrine influence hampers sperm production and ovulation—in other words, fertility (55). Studies have revealed that some women today reach childbearing maturity earlier than ever before. That doesn't imply that the sole cause of this premature maturation is estrogenic toxicity from the environment. Today's better nutrition and advanced health care contribute to a more rapid development toward biological maturity to prepare women for childbearing sooner. However, other indicators demonstrate that environmental toxicity with these estrogenic compounds is a major factor in the development of associated diseases such as a high rate of breast and endometrial cancer and general endocrine imbalances in both men and women.

The cognitive implications of organophosphate and organochloride exposure are obvious. These chemicals stimulate neurons to death. The doses we're subject to today won't kill us immediately, but long-term exposure is significant. Cognitive disorders such as ADHD are likely consequences of many factors, including these pest poisons, as are other common neurological diseases such as Alzheimer's and Parkinson's. Elimination of just one of these contributing factors can give the body the break it needs to deal with the damage or at least cope longer.

Organophosphates damage neuron function in many ways to induce immediate cell death, and with low-level intoxication they initiate interference that can have long-lasting secondary consequences such as cognitive deficits (56, 57, 58, 59). In addition to displaying anti-cholinesterase activity (intense neuron firing), there is evidence that other neurological proteins are affected by these chemicals.

Studies of Mexican communities such as Tescopaco confirm that these facts are much more than probable. A study done by Elizabeth Gillette et al in 1994 confirmed the dangers of unregulated pesticide use. The rich soils of the Mexican Yaqui Valley seeded a successful farming community that proliferates today. Pesticide application here has become profuse and unregulated. In 1998 the results of the Gillette study were published in a peer-reviewed journal.

The valley's population experienced twice the birth defects and infant deaths of communities in the immediate outskirts. The valley girls' breast development was well under way at age seven—equivalent to young girls of age 12 in the outskirts. Breast development is estrogen-dependent (60). The same study revealed that the young men of the valley were physically immature for their age, with problems that included the late development of gonads.

The Gillette findings reveal that exposure to these toxins with the intensity that the Mexican locals experienced can have horrific consequences. North Americans might not be exposed to the degree that these Mexican communities are, but the small, frequent, multiple increments we receive from a variety of sources do reach considerable levels. For an infant or child this can lead to severe immediate consequences and repercussions that might appear later in life when compounded by other stresses.

The solution to the coffee problem, if you must indulge in the beverage, is to choose organic, freshly ground beans. Drink one cup before exercise to facilitate the burning of fat as an energy source during activity, sparing muscle glycogen and saving muscle from catabolism. A cup of coffee with a meal can improve dietary-induced thermogenesis (DIT), assisting the oxidation or "burning" of excess dietary fat (61). Caffeine also reduces the threshold for endorphin secretion, enhancing pain tolerance and performance potential (62). Moreover, the stimulant appears to increase lipolysis or fat breakdown independent of a meal (63). These coffee facts shed light on the value of eating organic as much as possible.

Other factors contribute to the effects of caffeine in the body today that might not have been issues in the past. Contraceptive pills can boost the half-life of caffeine, and estrogen-replacement therapy in postmenopausal women enhances caffeine's stimulatory influence to the point where in some individuals its consumption becomes intolerable (64). Cimetidine, a common drug employed to combat excess stomach-acid secretions, also interferes with the clearance of caffeine from blood (65). If you take these drugs, you might have noticed a newly developed sensitivity to coffee or caffeine-rich teas. Interestingly the amplified sensitivity and the likely increment of free fatty-acid mobilization that this factor might induce *could possibly* contribute to the risk of insulin resistance.

Now let's review the prioritized summary tables of the Ageless Performance program protocol, diet, and supplement regimen. The following table represents the basic program that can be applied for therapy or prevention. In the previous sample regimen the supplemental portion was intensified with an increased dose of selected nutraceuticals. Severe or difficult cases of diseases might require these small incremental adjustments, but recovery will still be facilitated for most cases with the smaller doses in the following table, though at a slower pace. If a more aggressive therapy is chosen, the program below is the one to fall back on once recovery is experienced.

PRIORITIZED SUMMARY TABLES FOR AGELESS PERFORMANCE

Priority #1: Instill and ensure insulin efficiency

	All Ages	Age 5 yrs+	Age 12 yrs+	Age 18 yrs+	Age 25 yrs+	Age 30 yrs+	Age 40 yrs+	Age 50 yrs+	Age 60 yrs+
Minimize consumption of processed food in the diet.	✓	✓	✓	✓	✓	✓	✓	✓	✓
Consume whole fresh foods as much as possible.	✓	✓	✓	✓	✓	✓	✓	✓	✓
Consume quality complete protein with every meal. (See Appendix C for the list of preferred protein sources.)	✓	✓	✓	✓	✓	✓	✓	✓	✓
Consume carbohydrate sources that rate below 55 on the glycemic-index scale. (See Appendix A for the glycemic-index table.) Higher glycemic-index meals/foods are allowed after activity/exercise only.	✓	✓	✓	✓	✓	✓	✓	✓	✓
Supplement every day with a quality multi-dosed multiple vitamin/mineral formulation to set a foundation for nutrient density of nourishment. (See Appendix B for guidelines for choosing a multiple.)	✓ children's formula	✓ children's formula	✓	✓	✓	✓	✓	✓	✓
Supplement with additional vitamin C to reach these maximums.			✓ Max per day 250 mg	✓ Max per day 750 mg	✓ Max per day 3,000 mg	✓ Max per day 4,000 mg	✓ Max per day 4,000 mg	✓ Max per day 4,000 mg	✓ Max per day 4,000 mg
Supplement with additional alpha lipoic acid (R+) to reach these maximums.					✓ Max per day 100 mg	✓ Max per day 150 mg	✓ Max per day 150 mg	✓ Max per day 250 mg	✓ Max per day 300 mg
Supplement with additional curcumin—turmeric (standardized to 95% curcuminoids).					✓ Max per day 350 mg	✓ Max per day 550 mg	✓ Max per day 1,000 mg	✓ Max per day 2,000 mg	✓ Max per day 2,000 mg
Supplement with additional GTF chromium.				✓ Max per day 100 mcg	✓ Max per day 200 mcg	✓ Max per day 500 mcg	✓ Max per day 500 mcg	✓ Max per day 600 mcg	✓ Max per day 600 mcg

The above doses are relatively aggressive *preventive* ones for most individuals. *Therapeutic* levels for recovery from disease might exceed those listed. Adjunctive doses for other condition-specific therapeutic applications are discussed in Chapter 16.

Priority #2: In addition to the previous primary priorities these secondary priorities will deliver additional value and bring the program closer to completion

	All Ages	Age 5 yrs +	Age 12 yrs +	Age 18 yrs +	Age 25 yrs +	Age 30 yrs +	Age 40 yrs +	Age 50 yrs +	Age 60 yrs +
Daily protein supplementation: high BV whey protein.		✓ Max per day two times 15g serving	✓ Max per day two times 15g serving	✓ Max per day two times 25 g serving	✓ Max per day four times 25 g serving	✓ Max per day four times 25 g serving	✓ Max per day four times 25 g serving	✓ Max per day three times 25 g serving	✓ Max per day two times 25 g serving
Additional antioxidant supplements; augment supplemental program to reach these maximums.					✓ Program for 25 years +	✓ Program for 30 to 49 years	✓ Program for 30 to 49 years	✓ Program for 50 years +	✓ Program for 50 years +

What follows are suggested antioxidant levels to enhance the protective strategy of conservative daily maximums; supplement multi-vitamin/mineral levels to reach these ultimate totals.

Program	Vitamin C	Vitamin E	Alpha Lipoic Acid (R+)	Selenium	Beta-Carotene	Vitamin A	Grapeseed Extract	Lycopene	CoQ10
25 years +	3,000 mg	800 IU	150 mg	200 mcg	15,000 IU	5,000 IU	200 mg	250 mg	30 mg
30 to 49 years	5,000 mg	1,000 IU	300 mg	300 mcg	35,000 IU	10,000 IU	300 mg	400 mg	50 mg
50 years +	8,000 mg	1,100 IU	450 mg	300 mcg	50,000 IU	10,000 IU	400 mg	500 mg	40 mg

The above general suggestions don't account for variable demands that individual lifestyles might create, i.e., more active lifestyles might require higher levels. Note: vitamin E levels are high in anticipation of the polyunsaturated-fat supplementation to come. My vitamin E levels reach as high as 1,500 IU on many days.

Priority #3: Addition of supplemental fats now that Priorities #1 and 2 have supplied the necessary micronutrient co-factors, antioxidants, and protein

	All Ages	Age 5 yrs +	Age 12 yrs +	Age 18 yrs +	Age 25 yrs +	Age 30 yrs +	Age 40 yrs +	Age 50 yrs +	Age 60 yrs +
Flaxseed oil: 1,000 mg gel capsule; additional flax oil in salads can support higher daily requirements.		✓ 2,000 mg per day	✓ 5,000 mg per day	✓ 6,000 mg per day	✓ 8,000 mg per day	✓ 8,000 mg per day	✓ 8,000 mg per day	✓ 8,000 mg per day	✓ 8,000 mg per day
Salmon oil: 1,000 mg gel capsule.		✓ 2,000 mg per day	✓ 5,000 mg per day	✓ 6,000 mg per day	✓ 10,000 mg per day	✓ 10,000 mg per day	✓ 10,000 mg per day	✓ 10,000 mg per day	✓ 10,000 mg per day

The above general suggestions don't account for variable demands that individual lifestyles might create, i.e., more active lifestyles might require higher levels and healthier diets might supply higher levels of active fats to warrant reduced supplemental doses. *Consult with a health-care professional before implementing this part of the program.*

Priority #4: Addition of specialized phytonutrients to facilitate eicosanoid-hormone balance and effective hormone communication

	All Ages	Age 5 yrs +	Age 12 yrs +	Age 18 yrs +	Age 25 yrs +	Age 30 yrs +	Age 40 yrs +	Age 50 yrs +	Age 60 yrs +
Grapeseed extract (75%+ proanthocyanidins).					✓ 100 mg per day	✓ 100 mg per day	✓ 250 mg per day	✓ 300 mg per day	✓ 350 mg per day
Bromelain (2000 GDU) facilitates curcumin absorption and delivers anti-inflammatory activity.					✓ 1,000 mg per day	✓ 1,000 mg per day	✓ 1,000 mg per day	✓ 1,000 mg per day	✓ 1,000 mg per day
ASA (optional).						✓ 20 mg per day	✓ 25 mg per day	✓ 40 mg per day	✓ 40 mg per day

Note that many of the above recommendations will change based on the state of health and type of disease. These values will have profound positive benefits. In Chapter 16 specific incremental values that may be necessary to induce recovery from progressed states of disease will be detailed. Curcumin and bromelain, for example, may be required temporarily in higher doses for cases involving severe inflammatory disease. These condition-specific programs will be outlined in the final summary in Chapter 16.

RECOMMENDATIONS

for Cardiovascular Disease, Asthma, Inflammation, Biological Aging, and Cognitive and Intestinal Disorders

Cardiovascular disease is closely linked to insulin resistance and obesity through the related chemistry. Treatment of cardiovascular disease calls for the same program detailed for previous conditions. The program designed for recovery from diabetes, insulin resistance, and obesity can be applied to treat unhealthy serum-lipid profiles (cholesterol, triglycerides), hypertension, and conditions affecting heart rhythm.

Balancing autocrine (hormones from polyunsaturated fats) chemistry leads to level hormone output and a self-sufficient biological system that begins to function normally at every stage, including regulated cardiovascular function and controlled broncho-reactivity to airborne irritants.

The program to apply for asthmatic conditions is the one outlined earlier in this chapter for the insulin-resistant/diabetic group. The additional component that helps correct the asthmatic condition is an aggressive dose of grapeseed extract. Grapeseed proanthocyanidins down-regulate leukotriene production by inhibiting the enzyme lipoxygenase (LOX), which is found in the fatty-acid pathway next to cyclo oxygenase (COX). Leukotrienes are produced from arachidonic acid to promote asthmatic symptoms. Use about 1,000 mg of a standardized (75% to 95% proanthocyanidins) version daily split over two to three doses (66, 67).

Ageless Performance supports a powerful anti-inflammatory hormone profile detailed in previous chapters. See the depictions of the fatty-acid metabolic pathways in Figure 12 in Chapter 10 and Figure 13 in Chapter 11. Correction of this biochemical pathway is crucial to recovery from diseases such as rheumatoid arthritis, osteoarthritis, and other chronic inflammatory conditions, as well as the aging process. Aging is a disease that can be accelerated by inefficient biochemical activity that pushes inflammatory prostaglandins to excessive levels and biological age to unnecessary extremes.

The aging process can be decelerated and even reversed with the alteration of this same biochemical activity. Anti-aging isn't mystical; accelerated aging is simply a result of poor metabolic function.

Various markers are used to assess biological age such as blood pressure and serum lipid levels (cholesterol and serum fat). These factors relate to cardiovascular health. Other markers of biological age include blood-sugar regulation or insulin efficiency and the measure of other hormone levels and activities. Visual and auditory functions are also markers of biological age. Antioxidant status of the body is yet another sign of biological age, as are bone density, muscle mass and muscle strength, immune-system efficiency, aerobic capacity, and body-fat-mass proportion.

Ageless Performance instills metabolic efficiency to maintain these markers at youthful status. Offsetting the typical pro-inflammatory hormone profile by down-regulating the production of inflammatory hormones and boosting the production of anti-inflammatory hormones allows cells to self-regulate without dependence on symptom-relieving drugs.

Disorders related to essential fatty-acid imbalance will retreat when the new functional biochemical balance takes over and reduces unwanted fat mass. The result is the institution of normal biochemical activity, the chemistry on which life depends, from which human life originally flourished. With this balance cells are better equipped to renovate themselves and reset biological pace. Positive youthful thinking and regular activity facilitate this achievement and maintain the new state.

Cognitive disorders can be ameliorated with the application of Ageless Performance, as well. Phosphatidyl choline and phosphatidyl serine can be added to the program in doses recommended in previous chapters and in Chapter 16. Other specialized nutraceuticals are also detailed for this category in Chapter 16. SAMe, too, improves neurological and inflammatory conditions, as do alpha lipoic acid and curcumin. The base program delivers tremendous support for cognitive function and for the battle against multiple sclerosis, ADHD, Parkinson's, Alzheimer's, and other forms of dementia.

Gastrointestinal-tract disorders such as inflammatory bowel diseases (IBDS), Crohn's, and colitis present unique challenges. The problem is to get the requisite nutrition into a body that can't absorb from a damaged gastrointestinal tract. IBDS tend to run in the family and are thought to have a strong genetic foundation, but here again we mustn't forget familial eating habits, lifestyle choices, and cultural influences that are common within the genetically linked group.

Diet must be altered to start the recovery process. The high-fiber diet that Ageless Performance provides, however, isn't the choice for recovery in this instance. An elemental diet, in most cases, must be employed, one that's predigested and in its elemental state so that the digestive process isn't heavily worked and absorption is effortless, allowing the intestines as much rest as possible.

Dairy products and beef must be eliminated. The best protein source, though it's dairy, is whey protein isolate (not concentrate) dissolved in purified water and cabbage juice with no added sweeteners or additives (30 g of whey per serving). Whey isn't as allergenic as casein can be. Furthermore, whey protein isolate has tremendous therapeutic value and contains relatively no lactose or arachidonic acid (omega-6 fat) in its isolated form. However, whey concentrates may contain some lactose and fat.

The common whey isolate supplementation isn't the best representation of elemental protein, since it isn't completely hydrolyzed. In order to eliminate allergenic potential of a protein source as much as possible, hydrolysis must be complete (68, 69, 70). In fact, this is the strategy used to create hypoallergenic protein sources whether from casein or whey—as close to 100% hydrolysis as possible. However, hydrolysis reduces the biological value of a protein source to extreme lows.

Again my recommendation is to use a cold cross-flow or ion-exchanged whey protein isolate that still contains intact di- and tripeptide units and results in a higher biological value. The product label description of the protein supplement must reveal these specifications. This undenatured supplement provides better assimilation and more tissue-retained protein. The Biologic Nutritional Research Inc. Web site (*www.biologicnr.com*) will lead you to sources that we approve.

If the gastrointestinal condition is such that this undenatured whey protein isolate can't be tolerated, the alternative must be the elemental, completely hydrolyzed, lactose- and fat-free whey. Use the tolerable protein source with the lowest degree of hydrolysis to save some biological value. Once again the first choice is the undenatured whey isolate. If this is tolerable, recovery will be faster. If it isn't tolerable, switch back to it when the condition is such that the more bioavailable protein can be digested without difficulty.

The cabbage juice base for this protein drink has to be freshly made each time. If desired, add some freshly juiced celery and a small piece of concurrently juiced apple for flavor. This beverage will be the daily elemental sustenance until gastrointestinal inflammation subsides, and it's the only time the juicing process is allowed as an exclusive nourishment alternative to fiber-rich food. On any other occasion juicing should be accompanied by natural fiber in the day.

Such a strategy allows nourishment to make its way to needy cells without irritating the intestines. When supplemental lactobacillus can be tolerated, its inclusion is important, since persistent diarrhea will abolish the friendly bacterial colony and reinoculation with supplemental probiotics as soon as possible will be required. To the life-support drink, add a few grams of glutamine and a couple of grams of ornithine alpha-ketoglutarate (OKG). These factors feed direct fuel to the mucosal lining for recovery and regeneration, which is important when food bulk is eliminated from the diet. The addition of fructo-oligosaccharide (FOS) is important, as well, since fiber elimination from the diet removes the fuel for friendly bacteria. FOS, a nondigestible fiber, feeds the friendly colony to support health in many ways, yet doesn't deliver irritating roughage to a vulnerable, inflamed intestine. The problem is that it can contribute to flatulence and must be used sparingly in the beginning. Use what you can tolerate, say, 200 mg at a time.

Transition of food in the gut stimulates mucosal cells to proliferate and regenerate. When solid food has been eliminated from the diet, dietary glutamine becomes imperative in supplemental form. It plays an important role in the conservation of structure and function of intestinal cells under normal and stressful conditions. Glutamine induces mucosal cell proliferation and robustness to maintain health and combat leaky gut syndrome (71). This supplement is also integral in the battle against rheumatoid arthritis and makes the gut less permeable to allergenic compounds that can seep into the systemic circulation (72).

Whey protein naturally contains an abundance of glutamine. Added glutamine is a good boost to this source. OKG is also a great addition to the elemental nutrient strategy, neutralizing ammonia production and contributing to the glutamine load of the drink. When OKG takes up ammonia, it becomes glutamine. OKG is also a potent supporter of growth hormone to enhance secretions and general recovery of the body from wear, tear, and disease. Drink this easy-to-digest-and-absorb drink three to five times daily to help alleviate the rigors of colitis, Crohn's, rheumatoid arthritis, and multiple sclerosis.

The high rate of absorption for this nutrient-dense liquid diet leaves behind little if any bulk and gives the intestines as much rest as possible. The aggressive levels of supplementation detailed for the therapeutic program must accompany this protein supplement beverage. If at all possible, a short period of an even more aggressive supplement program—essential fats and omega-3 fish fats, alpha lipoic acid (R+ type), and grapeseed extract—must be applied at levels even higher than previously outlined. Curcumin doses must be slightly raised, as well, simply because bromelain can't be administered orally when gastrointestinal inflammation is active. Bromelain is a proteolytic enzyme that digests vulnerable protein and irritates the inflamed gut. Since bromelain synergizes curcumin uptake, oral curcumin levels must be increased in its absence.

Don't use vanadyl sulfate during an inflammatory attack of the intestines and until several months after remission has been continuous. Alpha lipoic acid combats free-radical proliferation in the gut, counteracting that nasty inflammatory peroxynitrite free radical. When the body is challenged by any form of inflammation, alpha lipoic acid is an important supplement to use abundantly (300 mg plus daily). Again, the R+ form of alpha lipoic acid is the preferred isomer. Gut-initiated free radicals permeate the body in a flash. The site of inflammation is profuse with free radicals due to immune activity, perpetuating tissue damage and more immune activity. Oral glutathione must also be included in the supplemental regimen for gastrointestinal disease to help offset pesky gut free radicals that propagate exponentially within the intestinal lumen.

If diarrhea is persistent, an anti-diarrhea formula—even a little Imodium—will give the intestinal tract a chance to absorb the nutrient density. Polyunsaturated fats that can be flushed due to the combination of persistent diarrhea and fast-moving liquid nourishment must be supplemented diligently to help restore biochemical balance.

The only source of iron that can be safely tolerated with this condition is the Albion bisglycinate and lactoferrin. Any others will irritate sensitive intestines. In fact, recent studies show that in cases of experimental colitis, the wrong iron supplementation will increase intestinal inflammation and oxidative stress and even promote bleeding (73). Iron supplementation is crucial for ulcerated conditions, since bleeding can deplete the body of the precious metal quickly. Whey protein contains a significant dose of lactoferrin with each serving, and for that reason it's an important supplement to apply with this condition.

Supplementation with specialty nutrients for this therapeutic program amounts to the following aggressive daily totals: PUFA fat source: 22 g; curcumin extract (95% curcuminoids): 4,000 mg; vitamin C: 2,000 mg (ascorbyl palmitate only; 750 mg at a time maximum to prevent gastrointestinal disturbance); GTF chromium: 400 mcg; alpha lipoic acid (R+): 1,100 mg; grapeseed extract (95% proanthocyanidins): 400 to 500 mg; glutathione: 300 mg; bromelain: none; vanadyl sulfate: none.

Don't use this program as an alternative to drug therapy if pharmaceuticals like prednisone are required. Use this nutrient-dense elemental program without concern in conjunction with the therapy and include drugs such as Asacol (enteric-coated ASA) in high doses if necessary. The objective will always be to taper off prednisone slowly as a priority with, of course, a health-care professional's assistance.

Whenever prednisone is administered, make sure it's accompanied by adrenal support. Part of the reason for slowly reducing prednisone therapy as opposed to terminating it suddenly is the consequential expense to the adrenals of long-term use. The tapering allows the adrenals enough time to rebound in order to support the body with its own anti-inflammatory hormone cascade.

It's also important to administer concurrently the following adrenal support if prednisone or other corticosteroid-like drugs are being used or have been in use. In divided doses take: panax ginseng 4:1 main root extract (200 to 500 mg per day) for a 12-week period maximum; licorice root (1,000 mg per day); and vitamin C (extensive levels, more than 2,500 mg daily, which is already in the Ageless Performance program). This strategy protects the adrenal glands from severe atrophy, allowing faster reduction of corticosteroids so that the body can adjust more quickly to hormonal changes.

Once the inflammation goes into remission, slowly increase the fiber content of food. Start by employing the low-glycemic-index, whole-rye-kernel bread described in earlier chapters. This bread is easy on the intestines, supports healthy colon pH, and improves normal gastrointestinal function more quickly. As soon as the complete Ageless Performance dietary portion is achievable, stay with the high-level nutraceuticals displayed above for as long as possible. After several months, preferably a year, back off to the prioritized summary tables of dietary and supplementation protocols to maintain this new biological state.

Over the course of this book I've outlined in great detail what has to happen in order to live healthier. First and foremost, we have to free our minds from the self-imposed inhibitions that prevent us from identifying our potential. Meditation and visualization, as already pointed out, can help us find our paths. Most of us, including me, find it difficult to make the time to meditate and visualize. Ironically, when our lives are most hectic, meditation is most helpful. It slows us down to focus and helps us reset ourselves, allowing us to become much more productive. Second, using antioxidants, we have to neutralize the toxic interference that rises out of unhealthy emotional chemistry, negative thought, and external sources. Third, we have to nourish the conductive conduit from body to mind and mind to body so that our enormous atomic power can flourish.

As much as it's difficult for some people to fathom, disease can be accepted as a gift. Disease is the powerful message that guides us down our distinct paths. It's often a last attempt to force needed change in our lives. Listen to the message, heed the warning, and take the right road to recovery. If we can muster the strength to dive deep enough within us, we'll discover the essential roots of our pain, the root of our disease. Doing so, together with proper nutrition and lifestyle, will help us leave disease behind forever and allow us to achieve our individual universal purpose.

16

CONDITION-SPECIFIC THERAPIES

Ageless Performance is the foundation of biochemical health, hormonal balance, and cellular correction. It's the core from which therapeutic chemistry can be generated. The miracles of healing and enormous physical feats are built into us—healing and performance that are limited by our restricted thinking and incomplete nourishment.

This potential can be tapped when mental inhibitions are removed. An adult elephant is held captive by a mere peg in the ground that restrains it as successfully as if it were a baby. As an adult, the elephant could easily rip the peg out of the ground, but brainwashing as a juvenile prevents it from doing so. In a similar fashion our parents, peers, and experiences inform our limitations in life.

Imagine journeying through life not knowing about limitations. When would you stop striving for your goals if you couldn't conceive of restrictions? I look back at the progression I experienced from the inception of my first business to the point when I sold it. I started out literally knocking on unfamiliar doors and with no business experience whatsoever. The workload I imposed on myself was unbelievable to most people. At the time I didn't know this was a difficult task. I didn't fathom the government-regulatory implications and difficulties that would eventually throw up roadblocks. I couldn't imagine I'd be managing 23 people on a national campaign within a few years. The evolution and turnover of programs were so complex that if I'd known what I was about to embark on perhaps I would have chosen an easier goal.

However, because I had confidence in myself I knew I could work my way through any of the upcoming challenges. Without knowing what lay ahead, I had no conception of limitation. I knew that anything was possible, but the possibility depended on me and nothing else. Step by step, as challenges presented themselves, I worked through them. It's when you reflect on the totality of the challenges that difficulty begins to appear.

Now I understand that the unfathomable is possible, and my business model is ready for reapplication. One could look back and conclude that the workload was too great and that to undergo it again isn't acceptable. On the other hand, one could reason that the second time around should be easier since the model is already set and the trials and errors have already been endured. It all depends on how historical experiences are interpreted and then applied to current situations. This is the essence of positive mindset or paradigm control—you *really* are in charge. And even if your life seems to be out of control, you can manage that state. In fact, failures, as many of us perceive them, are merely hidden victories. They reveal the methods we want to avoid, directing us down a more reasonable path. This is the sort of paradigm shift in thinking that sets the foundation for success in business, health, athletics, career objectives, and personal relationships. Not recognizing failure for the guidance that it is only creates the potential for one to repeat the dead-end experience.

The same situation prevails when embarking on recovery from disease. If we think the task will be long and arduous and the positive result out of reach, it won't be attainable. If we believe positive results are within us, we'll extract them by overcoming each challenge that comes our way, each hurdle between us and the healthy outcome. However, if we look back at where we started and measure the distance we've come and how far we have to go, we might conclude that the task is too difficult and not within our capabilities. In fact, disease itself is sometimes a final attempt by that inner guiding beacon to force us into making positive changes. It's a formidable fire alarm. Heed it and act on it. Better yet, if we pay attention to the more subtle intuitive warnings that always precede disease, we might avoid illness.

The fact remains that all of us have always had the potential to prevail, but somewhere along the line some of us were taught that we couldn't. Any individual who thinks this way merely has to reprogram himself or herself to believe. It's really that simple: reprogram the outcome we wish for ourselves. See it every day. Talk ourselves into this state of mind each day. Know that it's achievable. I was taught that life holds limitations. I was told that certain things weren't possible. However, I knew instinctively that this was untrue and I stuck to my navigational gut feeling early on.

I was stubborn. I reprogrammed. I set my goals. I knew I could achieve. I knew I could recover from disease. The thought that must prevail at all times in order for true success to be accomplished is that achievement, recovery, and personal growth *don't* come at the expense of other people. This concept is also applicable to business and health. If we attempt to hoard business opportunities and personal health to the exclusion of other people, true success will never be attained. Some believe this is outlandish thinking, but if we realize that active projection of harm toward other people must first pass our own inner litmus tests, then we can understand that our hearts always feel the essence of our intentions, propelling an inner chemistry much like that of stress chemistry—in other words, our harmful actions injure us before they harm others. If something doesn't feel right, it usually isn't. If we persist with behavior that doesn't feel true, the chemistry of that feeling will eventually affect our cellular chemistries. This transformed chemistry manifests altered cell activity and physiology. Ultimately, if this condition persists long enough, it will lead to disease.

Remember, though, we can also evoke recovery in much the same way: we're all composed of power-packed atoms that can initiate recovery, healing, and performance. This potency harbors far more than just the atomic configuration of ATP or creatine-phosphate. Every gram of our beings is an atomic embodiment with a core that relies on the elemental configuration of vitamins, minerals, phytonutrients, and other essential nutrients. Therapy *is* an attempt to bring this miracle to the surface. Therapy *isn't* the application of an external medication that imitates bodily tissue and replaces biochemical activity. Therapy *is* the priming of our intrinsic healing capacity, the deployment of that deep-seeded miracle. An ongoing need for drugs is usually a coping mechanism required because we've somehow incapacitated our own inner potential. Accelerated aging is caused by the same inhibition.

The key to powerful prevention and anti-aging is immediate deployment of immune activity when it's required to stop any degree of microbe proliferation, ensuring that free-radical propagation can't gain momentum and cause damage to our bodies. This process requires that the tissues and biological systems and the cells and cellular chemistry of our bodies must function at optimal capacity with all the biochemical feedback systems in ready and alert mode. Ageless Performance supports this level of vitality, transforming the body into a complete bioenergetic system.

Today we fear biological and chemical warfare more than ever. Our best defense against these scourges is to be immune and antioxidant-alert. Fully saturated glutathione stores protect the brain, the liver, and the entire biological network from chemicals such as nerve gases as well as from microbes as pervasive as the severe acute respiratory syndrome (SARS) coronavirus. I've demonstrated how powerful this strategy is with irrefutable references. Ageless Performance also provides this protection, but the strategy requires proactivity. Prevention is the most powerful antidote in these cases. Nutraceuticals protect against mutated microbes simply by sanctioning the most powerful antidote here, as well—empowerment of our own immunity.

Many of us have left health to chance, hoping to combat the rigors of contemporary life without the application of an active strategy, allowing our bodies and minds to limp along in a substandard state, and relegating ourselves to a biological age beyond chronological time. But there comes a point in the advancement of degeneration where even aggressive programs such as Ageless Performance can't reverse the damage on its own. This state requires specialized building blocks and system-specific nutraceuticals to jump-start the biological systems and mediate the penetration of Ageless Performance.

The main program and the slight variations we've discussed in past chapters erect a therapeutic foundation that prompts the body to resurrect its inherent potential, promoting healing and prevention of many diseases that have reached epidemic proportions. In most cases Ageless Performance will be enough to reverse biological age and instigate a completely new level of life.

We've touched upon how Ageless Performance combats and halts severe inflammatory conditions such as Crohn's, ulcerative colitis, and osteo and rheumatoid arthritis. We've seen how the program provides insulin health and how it can reverse insulin resistance and diabetes. We've seen how cardiovascular disease can be reversed with what seems to be a spontaneous adjustment. We've seen how Ageless Performance can generate eicosanoid-hormone balance to advance respiratory and cognitive health and efficient energy metabolism. And when it comes to diabetes or severe insulin resistance, we've seen how the application of vanadyl sulfate in short bursts can act as a priming agent for recovery. Severe diabetes and states of insulin resistance won't need much more assistance than the previously discussed plans.

Ageless Performance isn't about symptomatic relief, nor is it about using special herbal extracts or nutrients to fight disease, though we'll touch on a few specialized nutraceuticals as important treatments for specific diseases in a moment. Ageless Performance is about creating self-sufficiency to prevent the onset of disease and allowing the body to prevail when disease has successfully penetrated. With this efficiency glands don't need to oversecrete hormones (like insulin) and the body can function with greater effectiveness. Ageless Performance delivers this priming for better cell response in the body.

In this primed state everything works quickly and completely when specialized therapies are implemented. The application of Tribulus terrestris and methoxyisoflavone for testosterone, libido, and lean-muscle enhancement depends on this primed foundation for optimal results; pigeum and saw-palmetto extracts for prostate protection work their wonders more thoroughly when the Ageless Performance foundation is in place; and the administration of creatine, glutamine, and HMB for athletic performance is most effective when backed by Ageless Performance, as are thermogenic strategies for fat loss. You might have used these specialized nutraceuticals in the past with nominal results, but try them after you've primed yourself with Ageless Performance for three weeks to a month and the results will be a lot different. The following target-specific and condition-specific therapies will work far better once this efficiency is in place, if they're required at all.

In some cases of disease the wear and tear of time have taken their toll and the specialized building blocks and cell resuscitators of the following protocols will be essential requirements for recovery. The degree of *essentiality* for the condition-specific therapies that follow is classed as either Essential or Optional. The highlighted italic suggestions are ones I include in my program on a regular basis to boost the Ageless Performance base program for greater protection and a more aggressive approach to anti-aging.

MATTERS OF THE HEART

Ageless Performance provides the most thorough heart-health program available. If the strategy is applied in its entirety, no other requirement is needed. Remember: longevity is highly dependent on the undisturbed operation of the cardiovascular system, and Ageless Performance is already designed with this consideration as a priority.

Optional

- *Acetyl l-carnitine: 1,000 mg two to three times daily.* Carnitine forms part of the transport system for fats into the mitochondria for oxidation as energy. That doesn't mean it can be employed as a fat-loss facilitator. It only increases fat oxidation when demands are extreme, i.e., exceptional activity intensity (1). Carnitine supplementation can enhance endurance performance potential for athletes, especially when combined with caffeine (2, 3). The inclusion of caffeine for endurance enhancement boosts mobilization of fats for carnitine transport and subsequent oxidation. Carnitine inhibits the collection of fat in the heart muscle (4, 5). Supplementation with carnitine can improve angina and lower LDL cholesterol (6, 7). Use l-, not d- or dl-carnitine.
- Hawthorne berry.
- Garlic extract.
- Cayenne.
- *Folic acid: 2 to 5 mg daily.* Folic acid has recently been shown to improve nitric-oxide production and to control free-radical activity more effectively in endothelial cells (8).
- *Panax ginseng 4:1 main root extract: 100 mg two to three times daily.*

- Soy protein. Soy protein can lower LDL, raise HDL, ameliorate arterial health, and reduce the risk of atherosclerosis and arteriosclerosis.

ARTHRITIS

The Ageless Performance diet is anti-inflammatory in nature. The diet activates production of anti-inflammatory hormones and slows the manufacturing of inflammatory hormones while the antioxidant nutraceuticals mediate the same activity. Curcumin and alpha lipoic acid (R+ isomer preferred) inhibit inflammatory PGE_2, and grapeseed extract, as previously referenced, is critical to the recovery and protection of joint connective tissue, as well, through nitric-oxide regulation and cox inhibition.

Grapeseed's considerable potential for prevention and recovery in this category is commonly overlooked simply because few people experience positive results with this herb. The reason is that the doses necessary for significant results frequently aren't applied. Capsule strategies often only deliver 75 or 100 mg of a low-grade extract. In order to get the required power punch for therapy, 10 to 15 of these capsules are needed daily, something that isn't likely to happen. Grapeseed is included in the Ageless Performance foundation in reasonable doses of 150 to 450 mg daily. In combination with the synergistic activity of the rest of the program, this daily dose is highly effective.

When disease is active, however, such as in the case of arthritis, a daily dose of 800 to 1,200 mg of a standardized extract (75% to 95% proanthocyanidins) is called for to provide the bounty of catechin, cyanidin, delphinidin, and other anthocyanins of the grape. Extracts from other parts of the grape have proven to be of tremendous therapeutic and protective value, as well, such as the grapeskin. Extreme body weights will require doses that exceed 1 g daily for recovery and pain relief. Such amounts must be split into two doses.

ASA is a cheaper alternative to grapeseed extract and has been shown to relieve pain but, as we've seen, chronic, high-dose ASA administration can lead to problems. As previously referenced, ASA interferes with joint-tissue construction while masking pain, and it presents a risk of severe intestinal aggravation when used for prolonged periods. Apply Ageless Performance to reverse the condition. Use 20 to 40 mg of ASA only in conjunction with the complete program, which includes grapeseed extract. Glucosamine supplementation is a good alternative to ASA, delivering anti-inflammatory activity and reducing the pain associated with arthritis. SAMe and chondroitin are good, too. Try them with the Ageless Performance base in place.

Rheumatoid arthritis is thought to originate from a leaky gut releasing undigested food particles into the bloodstream. These particles, possibly along with microbes, eventually deposit in tissues to elicit an immune response. The allergic reaction eventually causes a massive autoimmune attack of joint tissues. Hence, we can see a link between gastrointestinal diseases such as Crohn's and colitis and joint afflictions such as arthritis. Intestinal health is critical to general biological well-being. One of the prevalent features of the Ageless Performance design is the support of intestinal health.

Osteoarthritis is a very different disease from rheumatoid arthritis, since the latter is autoimmune in nature. Ageless Performance sets a perfect foundation for recovery and relief from rheumatoid arthritis. Flaxseed oil, omega-3 fish oils, alpha lipoic acid, curcumin, and grapeseed extract play major parts in the correction of this condition. Use the doses detailed in the aggressive therapeutic program of Chapter 15 for a month or two and back down to the doses detailed in the prioritized summary tables (also in Chapter 15). The aggressive doses can be cycled for four weeks on every 10 to 12 weeks, or as required.

The rest of the supplements in the prioritized summary tables must accompany these highlighted nutraceuticals in order to enhance the result. Bromelain must be used as a curcumin enhancer and as an anti-inflammatory agent in the doses described in the prioritized summary tables. SAMe is required in similar doses for rheumatoid arthritis as for osteoarthritis to deliver recovery support from the damage the former causes. As seen in previously detailed, research-supported data, SAMe repairs the damage to synovial cells caused by this autoimmune condition.

Although all of the above factors could be added to the program to deliver phenomenal results, chondroitin sulfate, SAMe, and glucosamine are the priority additions (and in that order). Chondroitin sulfate, like SAMe, stimulates the reconstruction of cartilage tissue. Glucosamine sulfate is the more appropriate inclusion over glucosamine HCl. SAMe is just as important but is often cost-prohibitive. If the expense of the therapy isn't a factor, SAMe is an essential inclusion. These additional ingredients can be cycled eight weeks on and four weeks off with the Ageless Performance base as a constant.

Essential for Osteoarthritis

- Glucosamine sulfate: 1,000 mg two times daily. Sulfur is a critical component of protein tertiary and quaternary structure, contributing to the gel-like property of cartilage. Since glucosamine facilitates sulfur's incorporation into the matrix, and sulfur availability is required to complete the function of ordinary glucosamine, glucosamine sulfate is the logical preference over glucosamine HCl. Glucosamine HCl, the hydrochloride version of glucosamine, is missing the sulfur component and requires the concurrent administration of MSM for optimal results.
- Chondroitin: 1,000 mg two times daily. Chondroitin stimulates chondrocyte synthesis of proteoglycans and cartilage. Glucosamine synthesis tends to decline with age, in part due to the nitric-oxide factor previously discussed. This contributes to the age-related development of osteoarthritis. Ageless Performance maintains healthier cell function throughout the body to lower the risk of cell dysfunction of this kind. The inclusion of these specialty ingredients over the Ageless Performance foundation will deliver miraculous results. The additional ingredients might only be needed temporarily as long as the base program is continued indefinitely.
- *SAMe: 200 to 400 mg two to three times daily.* SAMe resuscitates chondrocyte activity and is a powerful pain reliever; it's a logical addition to glucosamine administration, since it facilitates the assimilation and incorporation of glucosamine.
- *MSM: 3 g two to three times daily.* If food in the diet is whole and not overcooked, MSM supplementation won't be required every day. A full day's dose a few times weekly mixed in a protein drink will suffice.

ASTHMA

Individuals suffering from asthma will receive tremendous relief from Ageless Performance.

Optional

- Quercetin: 750 mg two to three times daily. Quercetin delivers powerful anti-inflammatory and antihistamine activity and helps to control skin and other allergies (9, 10).
- Licorice root.
- Green-tea extract.
- *Grapeseed extract (90%+ proanthocyanidins): 150 to 250 mg two to three times daily* (already in the Ageless Performance program).
- Ephedra extract equivalent to 11 mg ephedrine two to four times daily. Ephedra is to be used with caution and must be monitored by a health-care professional.

BONE DENSITY/OSTEOPOROSIS

Ageless Performance is designed to enhance and maintain optimal bone health. Exercise is an important factor for bone health.

Essential

- Calcium/magnesium mineral supplementation (over and above the multi-vitamin/mineral's content).
- Zinc supplementation. Usually already added to the calcium/magnesium formula (over and above the multi-vitamin/mineral's content).
- Vitamin D: 200 IU. Usually already added to the calcium/magnesium formula (over and above the multi-vitamin/mineral's content).
- Ipriflavone: 200 to 300 mg two to three times daily. Ipriflavone (7-iso-propoxy-isoflavone) facilitates bone mineralization, bone-building, and maintenance of bone health regardless of age and stage of development.

Studies show that ipriflavone's activity is on the osteoclast, inhibiting this cell's bone resorption activity. Osteoblasts are another group of specialized cells involved in the composition of bone matrix; ipriflavone promotes activity by these cells (11, 12, 13). Ipriflavone can be employed if osteoporosis requires treatment. It's not suggested as a preventive nutraceutical. Still, in order for ipriflavone to be fully effective the raw materials for bone mineralization must be made available without limitation. Use isoflavone supplementation in the form of water-processed soy protein supplementation as a preventive nutraceutical.

- Isoflavones support bone density with a similar activity to ipriflavones and can be used as a preventive strategy (14, 15).

DEPRESSION

Exercise, meditation, and visualization are important facets of Ageless Performance and are critical to the relief of the depressed state. The Ageless Performance nutraceutical foundation is exceptional support for recovery from depression.

Optional

- SAMe: *200 mg two to three times daily.* SAMe supplementation maintains health and longevity in many ways. Supplementation with SAMe provides healthier dopamine and serotonin secretions (16, 17).
- Gingko biloba. Recently shown to deliver MAO activity, gingko is now rated as an important protective and anti-proliferation factor for dementia such as Alzheimer's, especially in conjunction with vitamins A, C, and E. This particular report indicates that research has conclusively demonstrated that antioxidants will play a huge role in the battle against dementia (18, 19).
- St. John's wort. Improves serotonin activity safely to be effective against mild depression (20). Note that all proper studies done with St. John's wort indicate it's a successful application in the treatment of mild depression. However, it's not as effective as some pharmaceuticals are

when dealing with deeper cases of depression. The same goes for hydroxy citric acid (HCA), which is now recognized as a serotonin re-uptake inhibitor, assisting in the amelioration of mild depression without the common side effects associated with most pharmaceutical antidepressants.
- Phosphotidylserine.

COGNITION/MENTAL FUNCTION/DISORDERS OF CNS ORIGIN

The Ageless Performance foundation supplies a bounty of nutrients to support cognitive health. Protection and maintenance of the brain is critical to the anti-aging potential of the program. Life extension or anti-aging initiatives are normally centered around brain health, so much so that common pharmaceutical drugs such as deprenyl (selegiline hydrochloride) have become crucial to the anti-aging strategy. Deprenyl is a monoamine-oxidase inhibitor that blocks the enzyme acetylcholinesterase, which is responsible for chewing up acetylcholine (a critical neurotransmitter) in the synapses of the neurons. Blocking the destruction of this neurotransmitter prolongs the transmission of its message. The activity of this drug promotes the bioavailability of brain dopamine, as well. The dopamine level in the brain tends to decline with age, and this shortfall has now been identified as a major element in the biological aging process.

Such drugs deliver antidepressant capabilities, cognitive-enhancing capacity, general brain and mentation preservation, and even aphrodisiac activity. Typically deprenyl, or selegiline, is an approved pharmaceutical prescription treatment for Parkinson's and Alzheimer's patients but has become more accepted as a significant preventive factor that adds tremendous synergy to the nutraceutical anti-aging strategy. As an anti-aging or dementia-preventive agent, deprenyl is applied in 1 to 5 mg quantities weekly from age 30 to 40 years and often raised to 1 mg daily after age 40—of course, always with monitoring by a professional experienced in this field. The dose is often increased to as high as 10 mg daily for those as old or older than 80. As a therapeutic agent for the previously mentioned diseases, it's often used with other drugs in doses as high as 20 mg daily.

Research now indicates that nutraceuticals can deliver some of the positive brain-preservation activity that deprenyl provides. Huperzine A, also known as Chinese club moss or Huperzia serrata, imparts activity similar to a monoamine-oxidase inhibitor. In addition, studies performed on humans and animals with this substance demonstrate that the nutraceutical protects neurons against environmental toxins such as organophosphate pesticides, which are terrible nerve toxins and have already been described a few times in different contexts. Huperzine A acts as an important neuro-protective against overstimulation by other common factors, including stress hormones, malnourishment, and biological aging. The aging process is now seen as a factor in the decline of acetylcholine output by neurons, and when this neurotransmitter becomes short in supply, memory, mood, and general cognition are also reduced. As these brain functions weaken, the body follows suit quickly. Preserving brain function is vital to longevity, and the avoidance of mental deterioration is critical in the prevention of Parkinson's and Alzheimer's, which can develop at an exponential rate once neuron damage has been sustained.

Optional

- SAME: *200 mg two to three times daily.*
- Phosphotidylserine: 200 to 500 mg two to three times daily.
- *Acetyl l-carnitine: 500 mg two to three times daily.* Acetyl l-carnitine protects neurons from neuronal death and supports acetylcholine production and cognition. It even improves learning capacity in aged test animals (21).
- Thiamine: 100 mg two to three times daily (over and above the multivitamin dose).
- Gingko biloba.
- Huperzine A.
- Selegiline hydrochloride: 5 mg weekly (1 mg per day maximum).
- Additional powerful neuronal mitochondria-protecting antioxidants that have recently become accepted tools for cognition preservation in the brain are phenyl-N-butyl nitrone and N-t-butyl hydroxylamine (22). Keep an eye out for these antioxidant power punches; they're known to protect the mitochondria of cells.

PROSTATE HEALTH

With Ageless Performance as the potent foundation, the following combination will deliver a tremendous therapeutic outcome in the pursuit of prostate health.

Essential

- Zinc: 20 mg two times daily (over and above the multi-vitamin/mineral levels).
- *Pygeum africanum extract (90% sterols): 100 mg two to three times daily.*
- *Saw-palmetto extract (85% to 95% sterols): 100 mg two to three times daily.*
- Stinging-nettle extract: 150 mg two to three times daily.
- Isoflavones. Soy isoflavones have been shown to deliver powerful prostate protection as previously detailed and referenced.
- Reminder: The italicized neutraceuticals of the prostate-health and other categories above are recommended additions as a preventive measure for men over the age of 30. They're the nutraceuticals I add to my Ageless Performance foundation.

BREAST/ENDOMETRIAL HEALTH

Ageless Performance is significant protection against diseases such as cancers of the breast and endometrial tissue. The following tissue-specific factors can be added to the fundamental program.

Essential

- Flaxseed meal: grind three to four tablespoons and eat them *immediately* upon grinding two to three times daily. Flaxseed meal is rich in lignans. Clinical research reveals that lignans (their metabolites in the body, enterodiol and enterolactone) are very potent antioxidants effective in the prevention and therapy of breast cancer, cardiovascular disease, and osteoporosis (23, 24).

- Soy protein isolate. The water-extracted isolation process maintains the protective isoflavone activity of this supplement.
- Isoflavone (extracted). Isoflavones provide protection from breast and endometrial cancers. Isoflavones have extremely mild estrogenic activity, docking on estrogen-receptor sites to prevent the full power of the hormone from delivering its action to the occupied sites.

MENOPAUSAL SYMPTOMS

Again, the Ageless Performance base is exceptional support through menopause, with exercise playing a critical role in the maintenance of health during and after this transition. Keep in mind that estrogen helps maintain insulin health; upon reaching menopause, insulin resistance is more likely to advance, increasing the risk of the secondary diseases previously discussed. Studies show that insulin resistance is more likely to develop with low estrogen levels, but it's also more probable with extremely high levels (25). The contraceptive pill and excessive estrogen replacement therapy can both induce insulin resistance, according to these reports.

Optional

- Isoflavones from soy protein or pure isoflavone extraction. The mild estrogenic activity of isoflavones helps alleviate some of the symptoms associated with menopause and also protects against the now higher risk for osteoporosis and heart disease. Important: seek professional health care for progesterone and *mild* estrogen-replacement therapy that might be required.
- Black cohosh.
- Chasteberry extract (Vitex).
- Don Quai.

EXTRA SUPPORT TO COUNTER OBESITY

Ageless Performance sets the stage for efficient metabolic activity, which includes thermogenic activation. The program will certainly melt away unwanted pounds, but in some cases a little boost might be required to prime the brown adipose fat cells' thermogenic potential. Ephedra, caffeine, and ASA are common applications that can have side effects. If used over long periods and without professional assistance, such drugs can pose serious risks. In some cases they can have immediate health consequences without warning if cardiovascular or cerebrovascular problems previously exist. Ephedra has also been known to increase the danger of prostate aggravation. The better alternative is Ageless Performance, which stimulates and maintains thermogenic activity safely. To enhance the thermogenic potential of the Ageless Performance foundation, the herb Citrus aurantium (CA) can be employed safely instead of ephedra. However, caffeine is still required to support the adrenergic activity of CA.

Optional

* *Citrus aurantium (standardized to 6% to 11%): 400 to 450 mg three to four times daily.* CA has been used as an Eastern remedy for millennia to treat gastrointestinal disturbances. Today it's recognized more for its powerful adrenergic activity and stimulation of thermogenesis. CA has become widely accepted as an alternative to ephedra, since its activity isn't as likely to cross the blood-brain barrier and stimulate the central nervous system the way ephedra can. Like ephedra (ephedrine is the main active alkaloid), CA must be used with methylxanthine (caffeine) sources such as kola nut, guarana seed, and/or coffee. The interactive biochemical activity of these combinations is thoroughly discussed in previous chapters of this book. Once prostaglandin health is established, there is no requirement (or mild 20 mg doses only) for ASA to block excess PGE_2. Omega-3 fish oils, combined with sufficient levels of grapeseed extract, curcumin extract, and alpha lipoic acid, will get the job done in place of ASA megadoses. Many of these herbs are part of the Ageless Performance strategy already.

- Guarana-seed extract (standardized to 22% methylxanthines): 500 mg two to three times daily. Guarana (a natural caffeine source) is a safe and powerful thermogenic application.
- White-willow-bark extract and 20 mg of ASA.

GOUT

Ageless Performance is a perfect solution to gout. Applying the low-fat, fiber-rich, low-glycemic-index diet will facilitate recovery and maintain relief. Alpha lipoic acid, curcumin, and grapeseed extract, which are part of Ageless Performance's strategy, protect tissues from damage and provide balanced eicosanoid-hormone production. Ageless Performance also promotes the establishment of healthy body-fat mass, an important factor in the regulation of gout. Don't allow body-fat levels to decline rapidly if weight reduction is employed—no more than a loss of two to three pounds per week.

Essential

- Quercetin: 300 mg two to three times daily. Quercetin's activity is comparable to that of the drug allopurinol. It inhibits uric-acid production and delivers anti-inflammatory and antihistamine relief. Studies show that kaempferol also impedes xanthine-oxidase activity and uric-acid production (26).
- Ginkgo biloba: 200 mg two times daily. Ginkgo biloba contains both quercetin and kaempferol (27).
- Sources of anthocyanidins and proanthocyanidins protect tissues from damage, i.e., grapeseed extract, blueberries, cherries.
- Folic acid: 15 to 40 mg daily (orthomolecular doses). Folic acid, as research indicates, delivers more powerful xanthine-oxidase and uric-acid inhibition than allopurinol (28).
- A low-purine diet must be adhered to. The Ageless Performance protocol can function as a great foundation as long as high-purine foods are avoided. Steer clear of organ meats, red meat, shellfish, yeast, mackerel,

sardines, herring, anchovies, dried beans, peas, mushrooms, and spinach.
- Chicken, turkey, and fish not listed above can be consumed in extremely small quantities. Protein supplementation such as a whey isolate is suggested once daily if other protein sources have been eliminated.
- Abundant water consumption to dilute uric-acid concentrations.
- No alcohol or caffeine.

PEPTIC ULCERS

The clean, immune-supportive, pH-buffering activity of Ageless Performance can prevent peptic ulcers. However, an immune system that's faltering due to strain from physical and mental stress and environmental- and food-borne toxicity will allow infiltration by Helicobacter pylori bacteria. Increased gut acidity can break down gut membranes and promote the formation of an ulcer. The acidity can be attributed to the diet, including the direct effects of coffee, ASA, tobacco, processed foods, and alcohol (29, 30). However, more often than not, the acid accumulation and inability to tolerate acidity is a result of other factors such as ASA-induced damage to the mucosal membranes. Helicobacter pylori bacteria are thought to contribute to the stress on the mucosal membranes and the development of duodenal and gastric ulcers.

Essential

- Eliminate or change the mental dynamic of stress. Meditation and visualization techniques for stress management and healing are crucial, especially if the condition is chronic.
- Glutamine and OKG. Glutamine, as referenced previously, is an important immune and gastrointestinal fuel that promotes mucosal cell proliferation and regeneration. OKG is an ammonia scavenger that produces glutamine and ornithine when it takes on free ammonia and is metabolized. It also supports growth-hormone secretions and therefore general recovery from disease.
- Freshly juiced cabbage and broccoli in the amount of one liter per day

for the blend. Add a half teaspoon of glutamine, a half teaspoon of OKG, and one tablespoon of whey isolate to each 250 mL serving of cabbage juice. Drink four servings daily. Cabbage and broccoli promote protective mucosal secretions and have antibacterial properties (31, 32).

- Licorice root: 500 to 750 mg before each meal. This is a powerful remedy for peptic ulcers. However, the licorice root must be chewed to form a paste in order for it to induce a corrective result. Chewable tablets are available. Significant recovery will take a few weeks to appear. Licorice root also provides mild anti–Helicobacter pylori activity (33). Chew the licorice root 10 to 15 minutes before each meal and persist with this application for several weeks after recovery is established. Make sure the Ageless Performance foundation is maintained.

LIBIDO

A nutrient-rich diet and regular exercise promote physical and mental wellness and also support a healthy libido. Ageless Performance helps maintain effective insulin function, which is critical for a healthy libido (34). Sex drive varies among individuals and is motivated and impaired by a multitude of factors that range from physical to psychological. Although some nutraceuticals can enhance libido, they usually only work if the biological and psychological fundamentals are in operative condition.

Prostate protective protocols such as those previously detailed must be used when Tribulus terrestris is administered; this precaution is needed to reduce the risk of dehydrotestosterone (DHT) imposition on the prostate. Pygeum extract blocks DHT influence on the prostate (35). Saw-palmetto-berry extract is also shown to reduce COX activity in the prostate gland (36).

In addition to DHT protection, anti-aromatase activity must be administered when testosterone action is enhanced to reduce the incidence of estrogen production from the extra testosterone. The body will try to maintain its preferred testosterone-to-estrogen ratio. If testosterone rises drastically, estrogen levels can increase due to aromatase activity—the conversion of testosterone to estrogen by enzymes. This problem is significant among people who use exogenous testosterone therapy (steroids), especially if administration is poorly monitored.

There are other factors that regulate testosterone in the body to prevent elevated activity for prolonged periods. For those people who want to raise testosterone levels beyond normal output, good luck, unless exogenous testosterone sources are used. It's quite difficult to boost lean muscle and strength above normal solely through naturally secreted testosterone. The body is quite meticulous at regulating this hormone. Some tricks will be discussed in upcoming pages. Applying them can work quite well, but don't expect the immediate anabolic potential of testosterone analogues such as the common steroid drugs. The long-term results, however, are very impressive and quite comparable to synthetic steroid use when the post-administration downward spin the steroid will produce is accounted for.

Essential for Men

- *Tribulus terrestris: 350 mg two to three times daily.* Studies show that Tribulus can increase sexual desire by raising testosterone, by penile nitric-oxide enhancement, or by both methods (37, 38). Use applications that deliver a furostenol content of 40% or more. The same herb can differ drastically. Tribulus grown in one part of the world might not have the same activity as that cultivated in another. Climate and soil conditions play a large role in the pharmacology profile of herbs. By using standardized versions of herbs as suggested, the desired pharmacological activity is more likely to be achieved.

- *Panax ginseng 4:1 main root extract: 200 mg two times daily (for 30 days on and 30 days off).* Studies indicate that a good ginseng extract such as the one described here can enhance sperm motility and endurance, likely increasing the chances for conception (39). Ginseng has been known as a sexual enhancer for millennia, but exciting new studies completed in 2002 have revealed that it modulates penile nitric oxide to improve erections in ways similar to Viagra's effect, though Viagra has a power-punch application. The general biological adaptogenic benefits of ginseng are also partly attributed to its nitric-oxide influence in endothelial (blood vessels) and neurological tissues (40). Ginseng's merits are apparent after extended use. The difference between ginseng and drugs such as Viagra is that the latter works relatively immediately, while the former is subtle and provides a maintenance program rather than an aggressive stimulatory regimen. Tribulus is much faster-acting than ginseng.

- *Arginine: 600 to 1,000 mg orally three times daily concurrently with the above recommended doses of Tribulus terrestris (use the HCl or alpha ketoglutarate forms of arginine).* The key to results from Tribulus is concurrent administration of arginine. As we've previously seen, arginine is a precurser to nitric oxide, and while Tribulus stimulates nitric-oxide production in the penis, it requires an abundance of arginine in order to deliver maximum results. After a three- to four-day priming period, arginine doses can be dropped to two per day.
- *Yohimbe-bark extract: 300 to 500 mg per dose.* The inclusion of yohimbe-bark extract (yohimbine) is also an extremely powerful cumulative boost. Use standardized versions delivering at least 2% yohimbine alkaloids. Remember to consult a physician before applying these powerful strategies.
- Methoxyisoflavone: 500 mg two times daily.
- DHEA (after age 35): 25 mg daily.
- Muira puama.
- SAMe.

Essential for Women

- SAMe.
- DHEA: 25 to 100 mg daily as a slight boost for female testosterone production.
- Tribulus terrestris (works for some women, but reports of menstrual-cycle disturbances are common).
- Epimedium grandiflorum.
- Epimedium brevicorm.

CANDIDIASIS

The yeast, Candida albicans, is a common problem that contributes to symptoms that might be misdiagnosed. Poor immune function and/or gastrointestinal damage can allow this yeast to proliferate beyond controllable levels and enter the body systemically. The symptoms of this occurrence are general malaise, mental and emotional disturbances, irritability, digestive disorders, abdominal cramps, gas, bladder infections, frequent vaginal infection, and further immune-system impairment (41, 42).

It's easy to see how these symptoms can lead to the misdiagnosis of depression, chronic fatigue syndrome, or gastrointestinal diseases of various kinds, followed by the application of unnecessary drugs. If treated symptomatically, each of these conditions simply comes and goes and the root of the problem is rarely addressed.

A common cause of this yeast infiltration is prolonged antibiotic use that isn't followed by the restorative inoculation of friendly probiotic bacteria (acidophilus, bifidus). Antibiotics reduce the proficiency of friendly bacteria in the intestinal tract, allowing Candida to proliferate uncontrollably. High-glycemic-index, processed diets support Candida by feeding it carbohydrate nourishment. At the same time the processed diet fails to deliver the special fibers required by friendly bacteria, further impairing the bacteria's potential to keep the yeast at bay. The nutrient-scant North American diet is unable to support immune function in the body, causing it to falter in its attempt to protect itself from invasion—again, allowing the opportunistic yeast a window of opportunity.

The North American way, accompanied by prolific antibiotic use, supports candidiasis and explains the growing frequency of its diagnosis. Steroid hormones such as corticosteroid-type prednisone also increase the risk of candidiasis, likely due to the steroid's immuno-suppressive effects (43). A 2002 Swiss study shows that estradiol facilitates Candida resistance to anti-fungal agents (44). For women on prednisone and estrogen replacement or the contraceptive pill simultaneously, Candida is sure to infest with ease.

Essential

- Oil of oregano is one of the more effective therapies in the treatment of candidiasis. Make my effective slurry consisting of diluted oil of oregano in distilled water with the addition of psyllium husk. Drink this slurry two or three times daily. This is my unique way of creating a nutraceutical suspension of the treatment so that the oil of oregano in the slurry can slowly and carefully caress the entire length of the intestine as it makes its way down and out. Add extracted garlic oil to this suspension to further enhance the potential. Administration of probiotics *must immediately* follow the use of the oil-of-oregano suspension treatment. Use the suspension for three to four days and start the probiotics with the last administration dose of the slurry, persisting with the probiotics for several weeks.

- Caprylic acid.
- Garlic extract in abundance.
- Probiotic administration two times daily for three weeks as described above (lactobacillus acidophilus and bactobacillus bifidum).
- Fructo-oligosaccharide (FOS): 3 g twice daily for three weeks.
- Note: Before accepting a diagnosis and/or drugs for chronic fatigue or inflammatory bowel disease, make sure candidiasis has been eliminated from the list of possible causes.

COMMON HORMONAL MANIPULATION

With the application of Ageless Performance each and every cell of the body functions with a higher efficiency to respond better to hormone stimulation. Still, many of us might want to consider a more powerful therapy to maintain youthful profiles of endocrine hormones. However, exogenous sources of hormones aren't alternatives to a healthy lifestyle. Maintaining hormonal balance with Ageless Performance puts off the need for hormone therapy so that when and if you do apply the treatment it can be done with much lower doses.

Estrogen-blocking flavones have made a groundbreaking entrance into the preventive, therapeutic, and sports-nutrition fields. However, the innovation isn't that new. These anti-aromatase (preservation of testosterone and suppression of estrogen production in the body) or estrogen-blocking flavones have been known for a couple of decades. Methoxyisoflavone (5-methyl-7-methoxyisoflavone) hit the bodybuilding magazines with claims that it and other similar flavones would deliver "more muscle than ever." The buzz created quite a sensation for methoxyisoflavone-fortified protein drinks. Administration of methoxyisoflavone to livestock resulted in phenomenal lean-muscle gains, increasing feed efficiency and setting in motion the unfounded frenzy for human bodybuilding applications.

Subsequent studies of human-administered methoxyisoflavone showed suppression of corticosteroid-induced catabolism to enhance nitrogen retention. Although some manufacturers display this molecule as a mystical muscle builder, its method of activity isn't that mysterious. However, by keeping the pharmacology under wraps, manufacturers can lull consumers with the mystique and ensure they won't look around for similar anti-aromatase compounds that demonstrate better results.

Methoxyisoflavone actually refers to a great variety of different estrogenlike flavones. These methoxyisoflavones can block an enzyme that converts testosterone into estrogen, *possibly* leading to higher-than-normal testosterone levels in the body. The chemical variations of these aromatase-inhibiting flavones are 5-methyl-7-methoxyisoflavone; 5,7-dihydroxy-4-methoxyisoflavone; 5,6,7-trihydroxyflavone; and 5, 7-dihydroxyflavone, or chrysin (45). Methoxy, as it's often termed, blocks aromatization. If testosterone levels rise quickly (whether by oral or injected exogenous testosterone or testosterone analogues, i.e., steroids), the body attempts to convert the extra testosterone into estrogen to maintain functional natural proportions. This can lead to the estrogenic or female-like characteristics (gynecomastia—breast development in men) that androgenic substances ("anabolic steroids," as they're often loosely called) can induce when abused. By blocking this conversion of testosterone to estrogen, not only is testosterone activity protected but the negative effects associated with high estrogen levels can be eliminated or at least reduced.

In 1993 I found and began using a product called chrysin (5, 7-dihydroxy-flavone), an extremely expensive natural flavone. Studies performed at the University of Minnesota in 1993 compared chrysin, methoxyisoflavone, and a pharmaceutical aromatase inhibitor, aminoglutethimide, to show that chrysin was a much more powerful estrogen blocker than methoxyisoflavone. It was also discovered to be far more effective than a pharmaceutical drug (aminoglutethimide) used to combat estrogen-dependent carcinoma (46).

Additional studies conclude that the hydroxyflavone-type complex of chrysin is a significantly more potent blocker than the isoflavone-type complex of methoxyisoflavone (47).

In another more recent 1997 study at Tulane University Medical Center in New Orleans, these flavones were shown to have similar activity to tamoxifen, another pharmaceutical estrogen blocker used in anti-cancer therapies (48). That meant these flavones could also compete for estrogen-binding sites, preventing estrogen from inducing its powerful activity in the body. This estrogen-site competition is different from anti-aromatase activity.

In the bodybuilding world, tamoxifen is usually known by the brand name Nolvadex, which is commonly used in conjunction with testosterone or testosterone-analogue administration. Nolvadex is then employed by athletes to block estrogen accumulation from the unnaturally elevated testosterone levels. Isoflavones extracted from soy, for example, have anti-aromatase activity, as does hesperetin, but they're not nearly as effective as specialized flavone compounds such as methoxyisoflavone and chrysin. These estrogen-blocking, anti-aromatase flavones are important adjunctive supplements when testosterone levels are elevated by herbal remedies such as Tribulus terrestris or other pharmaceutical applications. I utilized this research with a meticulous scientific craft in my bodybuilding heyday to compete successfully. Furthermore, these substances serve as powerful anti-cancer agents for women.

The controversy over whether or not these flavones cause cancer or are anti-carcinogenic should be put to rest based on the above findings. Obviously their extremely weak estrogenic influence and their estrogen-competitive characteristics make them valuable protective agents for women. For the fetus and the developing infant, however, the mild estrogenic effect might cause some developmental problems.

TESTOSTERONE AND MUSCLE MASS

Although Tribulus terrestris and other testosterone-enhancing herbs are often used with the intention of building muscle, the attempt isn't usually successful. Enhancement of muscle size and strength in relation to serum-testosterone alteration is a lot more complex than just raising testosterone levels. Libido enhancement is a lot easier to achieve, and Tribulus will certainly lift the spirits if the right extract is employed. Again, safe sexual enhancement means using an estrogen blocker and prostate protection while applying Tribulus.

As we've seen, zinc and magnesium supplements deliver muscle-mass-enhancing potential. These minerals are important factors if optimal testosterone activity is desired for libido improvement, sport, or general health. Another regulatory agent the body uses to down-regulate serum-testosterone activity is sex-hormone-binding globulin (SHBG). This hormone binds to circulating testosterone to inhibit or prevent it from docking on testosterone receptors. Such inhibition prevents testosterone from delivering its masculine message. In fact, more than 90% of the circulating testosterone is tied up by this hormone, which means that when more testosterone is pumped into the body, more SHBG is produced to down-regulate the activity.

The key to gaining testosterone activity for anabolism as well as libido enhancement is the freeing of testosterone from SHBG. Age plays a role in this dynamic, and studies have shown that the aging male tends to produce more SHBG, leaving less testosterone free for action (49, 50). Research also indicates that body-fat mass likely contributes to excess SHBG and therefore lowers free testosterone (51). Lean physiques produce more efficient testosterone activity!

If testosterone could be freed from SHBG, levels of the former wouldn't have to be elevated significantly to enhance libido and gain muscle. The common formulation of zinc monomethionine aspartate and magnesium aspartate is said to do just that, but the activity might not be extremely potent. More research will have to confirm that this action is what it's claimed to be. I'm not convinced yet that this is how the minerals work. I believe they simply provide for normal receptor-site activity for these hormones as I've detailed and referenced in previous chapters.

Nevertheless, estrogen blockers such as chrysin and methoxyisoflavone can prevent estrogen levels from rising to support testosterone and to create compounding results. Green tea can be added to the list of estrogen blockers and testosterone enhancers, as well. A 2002 study demonstrated that megadoses of green-tea extract increase circulating luteinizing hormone and testosterone in rats. More than likely it would do the same in humans if the dose were high enough. Aromatase activity is identified as a primary factor (52).

Studies show that the amount of SHBG is related to serum-estrogen levels; higher serum estrogen can significantly boost SHBG production and interfere with testosterone (53). As men age, the quantity of testosterone in proportion to estrogen tends to decrease. In other words, relative estrogen levels increase. Continuing youthful athletic, sexual, and mental performance depends on the maintenance of youthful hormone proportions more than it depends on individual hormone quantity. Apply these estrogen-blocking, SHBG-regulating and testosterone-enhancing strategies at the same time with the complete prostate-protective herbs and a more youthful biological age and performance will be preserved.

This strategy is obviously logical: when estrogen is prevented from rising after serum testosterone is boosted, SHBG levels might not escalate as dramatically, allowing for a higher degree of free testosterone. The process involves far more than just muscle mass, strength, and sex drive. It also promotes mental well-being, fat incineration, cardiovascular fitness, and bone health, since testosterone vigor is now linked to these structures and functions, as well (54, 55).

Androstene supplementation requires the same precautionary measures as Tribulus terrestris does—estrogen blockers and prostate protection. Androstenedione is available in different variations, with 19-norandrostene-diol serving as one of the safer and more effective forms. Essentially androstenediol is a testosterone (steroid hormone) precursor that can cause systemic testosterone levels to increase when consumed orally (56, 57). However, even with the application of androstenedione (or "andro," as it's called in the gym), improving serum-testosterone levels isn't that simple. Age, for example, can impair luteinizing hormone secretions in the male, which might affect testosterone status in the body. Luteinizing hormone from the pituitary gland directs testicular testosterone production. Studies reveal that impaired feedback mechanisms in the aging brain might be the endocrine problem, and taking precursors like androstene orally can't combat such hormonal arrhythmia (58). Maintaining optimal brain health is critical to hormone balance throughout the body, as well.

There are many factors that influence how androstenedione is used in the biochemical pathway of steroid synthesis. In fact, it can just as easily produce estrogen as much as testosterone (59). One theoretical (anecdotally and not scientifically proven) way to push androstenedione production toward testosterone is to supplement concurrently with Tribulus terrestris (60). Although studies differ regarding luteinizing hormone elevation by Tribulus, the herb does have some sort of aphrodisiac effect. The above research shows incremental serum-testosterone levels when Tribulus is taken with androstenedione, as well, while other independent studies demonstrate that the effect of Tribulus on libido is likely due to penile nitric-oxide induction and not luteinizing hormone induction (61).

Both testosterone enhancement and nitric oxide will have cumulative erectile effects. But my interpretation of the available research indicates that the penile nitric-oxide elevation of Tribulus is irrefutable science, though its luteinizing hormone enhancement is still questionable. That's why I keep highlighting my theoretical standpoint for the testosterone-elevating capacity of Tribulus. Take Tribulus (800 mg plus per day), small amounts of androstenedione (200 mg per day), arginine (1,000-plus mg per day), and ginseng (400 mg per day) for synergistic up-regulation of libido.

However, when and *if* circulating testosterone levels are successfully boosted through this strategy, there is a consequence: the natural production of the hormone is shut down. The body carefully monitors these hormones through complex feedback mechanisms. Part of the brain, the hypothalamus, acts like a thermostat to regulate many hormones in the endocrine system. The hypothalamus instructs the pituitary gland to secrete luteinizing hormone, which in turn flows to the testicles to stimulate testosterone manufacturing. If circulating testosterone levels reach the body's set point or limit, the hypothalamus halts pituitary secretions of luteinizing hormone. Subsequently the production of testosterone can cease.

Androstenedione supplementation is extremely controversial, since for proper use it's considered a drug that requires monitoring by a professional. Some experts don't think andro is worthwhile or that it even works. The research is highly conflicting, with some positive results and lots of research that indicates andro isn't effective at all. However, the same can be said of creatine. A good deal of research shows that creatine isn't helpful from an ergogenic standpoint. But creatine does work quite well when used properly as a muscle and power enhancer.

Andro might very well be in the same boat, although the side effects of its extreme use are likely problematic, since the endocrine system is being manipulated. Andro became popular a few years ago among bodybuilders as a testosterone booster, but lack of results by those applying it incorrectly and the fact that it was raised to drug status in some countries have caused its status to diminish.

Some experts claim that even if testosterone levels are raised, the enhancement delivered by these strategies doesn't support an increase in muscle mass. I can say from personal experience that it does, but only if the entire anabolic scheme is applied and the functional biochemical foundation of Ageless Performance is in place.

Based on my investigative research, in order to build and maintain muscle, serum-testosterone levels have to be raised and then maintained at this higher level without extreme decline. This means that nutraceutical products such as androstene, Tribulus, arginine, stinging nettle, and saw palmetto must be used frequently each day—three to four evenly spread doses. By using the frequent daily-dose system, testosterone levels can be kept high without fluctuation. Although each facet of the strategy I've outlined is supported by scientific data, the muscle gains attributed to this complete daily multiple-dose, multiple-factor scheme haven't been scientifically proven. Anecdotal results, however, are quite impressive. This multiple-nutraceutical-sustaining strategy will be put to the clinical test shortly.

Once testosterone is boosted even minutely, its potential conversion to estrogen by blocking aromatase activity must be accounted for. In addition, any elevated testosterone must be freed from the inhibitory SHBG. Lastly testosterone receptor sites must be functional. The described multi-dose, multi-ingredient strategy does just that.

Tribulus terrestris might support the testosterone gain. In order for Tribulus to work at all for strength and muscle gains, I found that I had to consume large quantities, say, 400 to 600 mg of the 40% to 45% furostenol (saponins) herb at least four to five times daily—up to 3,000 mg per day. In other words, keep priming testicular production with multiple doses throughout the day (one dose every three hours or so) to keep levels high consistently.

Remember, the science supporting whether or not Tribulus actually increases testosterone significantly is controversial, but I do know that something does occur regarding endocrine and nitric-oxide activity. And if Tribulus is applied as I've done, it seems to work. Again, this isn't scientifically founded. As soon as testosterone levels drop (theoretically), however, the extra muscle support and mass (minuscule for the day) declines, as well. One megadose of the herbal strategy in the morning only causes levels to peak and fall drastically before the end of the day, and it doesn't account for testosterone release from the inactivating binding protein.

For muscle and strength, take the Tribulus supplement in multiple daily doses with 20 to 30 mg of zinc daily and, if possible, use the zinc monomethionine aspartate/magnesium aspartate blend as a source to possibly assist with the freeing of testosterone. Additionally employ methoxyisoflavone or chrysin with the mix (10 mg per pound of body weight per day of either or a combination of the two). This is a much heavier dose of the isoflavone than is typically advocated, and it's necessary in order to promote the best results.

The bodybuilding testosterone program looks like this: Tribulus terrestris, androstenedione (in small doses), methoxyisoflavone, chrysin, pygeum extract, and saw-palmetto extract. Ageless Performance will deliver enough protein and other muscle-building co-factors to facilitate protein synthesis; muscle health, size, and power; libido improvement; and cardiovascular and mental health. But don't forget the prostate protection detailed earlier.

DHEA (dehydroepiandrosterone) is another drug that arrived in the marketplace with a big bang. Not only has DHEA become a popular anti-aging supplement, but athletes are gobbling up the claims made for its purported ability to enhance endurance and muscle mass. Don't confuse DHEA with DHA (docosahexaenoic acid), the omega-3 polyunsaturated fatty acid produced from linolenic acid. DHEA is a precursor hormone used by the body to produce steroid hormones, and its blood levels have been shown to decline significantly with age (62).

However, DHEA supplementation mustn't be applied until serum DHEA, or more specifically DHEA-sulfate levels, are tested and blood levels are monitored on occasion thereafter. Excessive blood DHEA-sulfate levels can cause hormone proportions to fly out of control, actually facilitating biological aging and increasing the risk of disease. DHEA activity is more complex than we care to admit, and supplementation is a delicate endeavor. Despite this, multiple studies reveal the considerable benefits of DHEA supplementation.

DHEA supplementation enhances cognitive function. Levels in the brain drop significantly with age and have also been shown to be low in cases of brain disease. DHEA supplementation improves learning and memory in cognitive aging. Studies have prompted researchers to investigate the potential benefits of DHEA in dementia like Alzheimer's (63).

Low DHEA levels in both men and women are linked to the development of insulin resistance and therefore diabetes. Supplementation with DHEA improves insulin efficiency in these cases (64). Although DHEA levels seem to decrease fairly consistently in men with age, the decline is consistent in women until menopause, at which point it drops more rapidly (65).

This decrease in DHEA is responsible for the reduction in peripheral androgen and estrogen production. These substances are manufactured in the peripheral cells of the body for use within those very cells. DHEA supplementation can improve and maintain post-menopausal bone and vaginal health. Recent research indicates that in men supplementation can even prevent prostate disease (combined with androgen blockade) and is able to prolong significantly the life of those with advanced prostate cancer.

DHEA supplementation in men must be accompanied by large doses of pygeum and saw-palmetto extracts and estrogen blockers like chrysin and/or methoxyisoflavone. For women reports show that DHEA supplementation can reduce the growth of breast cancer as well as prevent breast and uterine cancers but must be taken in conjunction with abundant lignan, soy isoflavones, and chrysin (66). Interestingly the skin is one of the major organs of DHEA conversion to androstenedione and then testosterone for women. Healthy skin is therefore important for much more than just looks. It's an active endocrine organ. In fact, the skin is now considered the largest organ of the body (67). DHEA is generated in the adrenal cortex, and studies show that it can attenuate the damage in the brain caused by stress (68). This means DHEA can combat stress-induced learning impairment, memory deficit, mood disorders, and possibly even catabolism, but stress itself, if mismanaged, may impair its availability, too.

Supplementation with DHEA also increases IGF-1 (insulinlike growth factor) to normal levels in the brain to support healthier hypothalamus (neuroendocrine) function, but IGF-1 levels in the available research weren't seen to rise in the blood. This indicates that DHEA levels and IGF-1 in the brain might play a role in general endocrine regulation and that small supplemental doses of DHEA might combat the detrimental decline of brain DHEA that occurs with age (69).

However, as I've cautioned already, don't jump to uncontrolled mega-DHEA supplementation. Consult with a qualified physician before administering conservative doses, starting with 25 mg once daily (in the morning with polyunsaturated-fat supplements) and not exceeding 100 mg per day. In conjunction with the testosterone/anti-aromatase protocols discussed above, mild DHEA supplementation might be a good application for those over the age of 35. But don't forget—use DHEA with methoxyisoflavone and/or chrysin and abundant lignan consumption. Men must use pygeum and saw-palmetto extracts in addition to these estro-protective agents. Ageless Performance serves as a great foundation for correct DHEA supplementation to work from, as well.

AFTERWORD

We've entered an era where self-help and self-education have taken on prevalent roles in our lives. Our minds and bodies interact continuously through signs. The key to optimal health and maximum performance is to open the communication conduits to these messages. They're subtle, but using them can transform our lives profoundly.

The realization that we have tremendous potential within us to prevent disease, induce healing, and perform feats of athletic magnificence has inspired a proactive society that doesn't necessarily accept the habits and theories of previous generations. Just knowing that this potential resides within us is the first step toward healing and maximum life potential. The next step is to understand how we can remove the hindrances and facilitate full activation of this potential. Dealing with some elements such as undertaking active lifestyles and adopting wholesome diets will improve health, but identifying and rectifying more factors such as mental state and vitamin and mineral supplementation will boost vitality further.

As technology advances, the world around us changes, and so do environmental influences on humanity. These include the social impositions caused by denser populations, new and foreign technological byproducts, less-active lifestyles, and lower nutrient density of foods. As a result, our outlooks on health, disease, and fitness must be modified, as well, and to default to conventional medicines and nutritional recommendations that were designed decades ago without first recognizing the true causes of our new-age diseases is foolhardy. Many of our essential nutrients, the definition of essential status, and the nutritional recommendations first advocated emerged almost 90 years ago. Of course, these concepts and suggestions have evolved but haven't kept up with the rate of alterations to our environment, social states, and foods. The types of toxicity we face today—commercial pollution, household chemicals, food-borne pesticides, and adulterated food—have created a demand for protective antioxidants, a need that Ageless Performance fulfills, providing a beacon that sheds light on what would otherwise be a dark, dire situation.

If you haven't read all of *Potential Within* but have jumped into the program, you'll experience results. However, I urge you to read the entire book to gain greater insights into how this remarkable program functions and especially how the mind can ignite the complete process. The struggle to achieve more energy, better health, lower body fat, and enhanced athletic performance doesn't have to be difficult, not if you embrace the life-changing strategies of Ageless Performance and allow your potential within to truly blossom.

APPENDICES

APPENDIX A: GLYCEMIC INDEX

Use the Glycemic Index (GI) Table below to guide you to healthy carbohydrate sources. Eat low-index carbohydrate sources throughout the day (an index less than 60) and only eat higher glycemic levels after an intense workout. If disease, including obesity, plagues you, eat foods that have an index less than 55 until the illness is under control.

The standard in the glycemic index is pure glucose, which rates 100. The italicized entries in the table highlight the foods that must be adhered to for each category when disease, including obesity, is active or an aggressive prevention strategy (anti-aging) is applied. Water, by the way, has a glycemic index of *zero*, so drink it abundantly.

Food	GI	Food	GI
Breakfast Cereals			
Puffed wheat	120	Oatmeal (instant)	85
Rice Krispies	120	Cheerios	74
Cornflakes	112	Raisin Bran	73
Weetabix	109	*Oatmeal*	*49–54*
Shredded wheat	97		
Breads/Grains/Pasta			
Millet	100+	Couscous	64–66
White bread	90–100	*Brown rice*	*55–65*
Whole-meal barley bread	93	*Bulgur*	*50–65*
Whole-meal rye bread	85–90	*Wild rice*	*50–55*
Whole-wheat bread	85–95	*Whole-wheat pasta*	*37–60*
White rice	80–88	*Whole oatmeal*	*49–54*
Corn	65–80	*Whole-rye kernel*	*47*
Buckwheat	65–70	*Whole-grain rye bread*	*42*
Wheat kernel	65–70	*(no additives)*	
White-flour pasta	60–67	*Barley*	*25–36*
Fruit			
Date	100–105	*Grape*	*45–50*
Apricot (extra ripe)	90–95	*Apricot*	*35–50*
Raisin	80–95	*(less than ripe)*	

Banana (ripe)	85–90	*Pear*	*34–40*
Papaya (ripe)	75–81	*Peach*	*29–40*
Mango (ripe)	75–81	*Plum*	*35–36*
Pineapple	55–66	*Grapefruit*	*25–30*
Banana (green)	*55–60*	*Cherry*	*22–25*
Cantaloupe	*55–60*	*Blueberry*	*18–20*
Orange	*40–55*	*Raspberry*	*18–20*
Apple	*40–50*	*Strawberry*	*18–20*
Watermelon	*40–50*		
(medium ripeness)			

Vegetables

Potato (instant mix)	100+		
Potato (baked)	93–100	**Legumes**	
Parsnip	90–95	Canned baked bean	60–70
Carrot	85–95	*Fresh baked bean*	*48–55*
French fry	75–80	*Pinto bean*	*39–60*
Corn	60–80	*Green bean*	*45–50*
Beet	60–70	*Navy bean*	*38–40*
Yam (baked)	*50–62*	*Tofu*	*35*
Sweet potato (baked)	*50–56*	*Garbanzo Bean*	*30–55*
Green pea	*44–50*	*Lentil*	*30–40*
Asparagus	*22*	*Kidney bean*	*30–40*
Squash	*15–20*	*Black bean*	*30–35*
Tomato sauce	*15*	Lima bean	*30–35*
Kale	*15*	*Soybean*	*17–30*
Celery	*15*	*Almond*	*25*
Peppers	*15*	*Walnut*	*15–20*
Lettuce	*15*	*Peanut*	*14–20*

Dairy Products

Tofu ice cream	100+	Whole milk	30–39
Dairy ice cream	70–80	*Plain nonfat yogurt*	*15–32*
Plain yogurt	33–40	*Dry-curd cottage cheese*	*15–18*
Nonfat milk	32–39		

Seeds

Pumpkinseed	*20*	Sesame seed	*20*
Sunflower seed	*20*		

Protein Drinks in Water

Soy protein isolate	15	Casein protein supplement	15
Whey protein isolate/ concentrate	15		

Common Snacks

Rice cake	110+	Oatmeal cookie	75–80
Shortbread	88–90	Soda cracker	75
Jellybean	80–85	*Dark chocolate*	*60–70*
Pretzel	80–83	*Custard*	*60*
Soda pop	75–90	*Popcorn*	*55*
Bagel	75–85		

Sweeteners

Maltodextrin, maltose	110+	Unprocessed molasses	55–60
Glucose	100	Fructose	23
Corn syrup (solid)	85	*Licorice-root extract*	*5–10*
Processed honey	80	*Fructo-oligosaccharide*	*0*
Sucrose (table sugar)	70	*Stevia*	*0*
Unprocessed brown sugar	60–65	*Neohesperidine DC*	*0*
Unprocessed honey	58		

APPENDIX B: MULTIPLE-VITAMIN/ MINERAL GUIDELINES

In order to select the right multiple-vitamin/mineral, you must consider your activity level, age, and health status. I've divided the requirements into two activity levels: preventive/active/stress and extremely active/high stress. Keep in mind that mental stress is just as taxing on the body as physical stress, both of which raise nutrient demands significantly. Disease, as well, is classified as a body stress. Regardless of whether you're active or not, you'll fall into one of these two categories.

Even the best multiple-vitamin formulations don't deliver requisite levels of vitamins E, D, and C, and if they include alpha lipoic acid, grapeseed extract, curcumin, and bromelain, the levels won't be high enough. That means additional supplementation with these factors will be needed to make up the requirement for maximum prevention, therapy, recovery, and athletic performance. Make a note of the suggested forms and quantities of vitamins E, D, and C and crosscheck with the totals in the Ageless Performance prioritized summary tables in Chapter 15 to determine which nutrients you may need to supplement over and above what you find in the following table.

A one-pill dose (multi-vitamin/mineral) three times daily will suffice for most individuals with higher stressed, more active, and disease-infiltrated lifestyles. Typically to get the required nutrient intake from these multi-vitamins, it's necessary to take two pills per dose three times daily. The multi-vitamin should give you this sort of instruction on the label. If your commitment is less than wholehearted, the two daily doses (two multi-vitamin/mineral pills at breakfast and two at dinner) will be the most convenient strategy.

Multi-Vitamin/ Mineral Recommendations

Vitamin/Mineral/Antioxidant	Per Pill	Per Two-Pill Dose	Per Day (One Pill, Three Times Per Day), Lower Stress/Activity	Per Day (Two Pills, Three Times Per Day) High Stress/Activity
Vitamins				
Beta-Carotene (Provitamin A)	10,000 IU	20,000 IU	30,000 IU	60,000 IU
Vitamin A	800 IU	1,600 IU	2,400 IU	4,800 IU
Vitamin D$_3$ (Cholecalciferol)	80 IU	160 IU	240 IU	480 IU
Vitamin E (D-Alpha Tocopherol)	100 IU	200 IU	300 IU	600 IU
Vitamin C (Magnesium Ascorbate, Ascorbic Acid, Ascorbyl Palmitate)	100 mg	200 mg	300 mg	600 mg
Vitamin B$_1$ (Thiamine)	20 mg	40 mg	60 mg	120 mg
Vitamin B$_2$ (Riboflavin)	20 mg	40 mg	60 mg	120 mg
Niacinamide	20 mg	40 mg	60 mg	120 mg
Vitamin B$_6$ (Pyridoxine)	25 mg	50 mg	75 mg	150 mg
Pantothenic Acid	20 mg	40 mg	60 mg	120 mg
Vitamin B$_{12}$ (Hydroxycobalamin)	25 mcg	50 mcg	75 mcg	150 mcg
Folic Acid	750 mcg	1,500 mcg	2,250 mcg	4,500 mcg
Biotin	500 mcg	1,000 mcg	1,500 mcg	3,000 mcg
Minerals				
Calcium (Bisglycinate, Citrate)	70 mg	140 mg	210 mg	420 mg
Magnesium (Bisglycinate, Citrate)	60 mg	120 mg	180 mg	360 mg
Potassium (Citrate, Malate)	10 mg	20 mg	30 mg	60 mg
Zinc (Histidinate, Citrate)	5 mg	10 mg	15 mg	30 mg
Manganese (Citrate, Malate)	1 mg	2 mg	3 mg	6 mg
Iron (Bisglycinate, Lactoferrin)	0.5 mg	1 mg	1.5 mg	3 mg
Copper (Bisglycinate, Citrate)	0.33 mg	0.66 mg	1 mg	2 mg
Chromium (GTF, Nicotinate, Citrate)	100 mcg	200 mcg	300 mcg	600 mcg
Selenium	50 mcg	100 mcg	150 mcg	300 mcg
Molybdenum	15 mcg	30 mcg	45 mcg	60 mcg
Citrus Bioflavonoids	50 mg	100 mg	150 mg	300 mg
Other Important Inclusions*				
Alpha Lipoic Acid				
N-Acetyl Cysteine				
Grapeseed Extract				
Bromelain				
coQ10				
Other Enzymes and Other Flavonoids				

* These antioxidant and enzyme inclusions are common in multi-vitamin formulations. However, because little tablet room is left over in these formulas, these additional ingredients rarely make it into the formulation in efficacious levels; they're simply *window dressing* for the label claims. As we've seen, though, they're important to the Ageless Performance strategy and must be supplemented with additional sources. Again, determine what your needs are by referring to the appropriate prioritized summary table in Chapter 15 and make the necessary additions to your daily multiple strategy.

APPENDIX C: PROTEIN SOURCES

Choose protein sources that are high in biological value (BV) for as many meals of the day as possible. The lower BV protein sources such as soy (74 or lower) can be combined with the higher BV proteins such as casein or chicken (77 or higher) to create high-quality combinations. Preferred protein choices are italicized. The criteria for these selections results in a supply of protein that's either low in fat and high in protein quality or rich in omega-3 fats and high in protein quality (BV). The portions displayed in the following tables are designed to deliver *approximately* 20 g of protein per serving. Eighty-four grams is the common serving size for each source. These values represent the typical minimum-protein requirement per meal.

The volume of the protein source making up the minimum 20 g of protein is an *averaged* volume that can be used to *estimate* your serving size. The volume of a protein source delivering 20 g can change significantly based on the fat content, hydration level, and method of preparation. Keep in mind that the excess arachidonic acid will be delivered with beef fat. All sources are displayed as cooked (baked or broiled) unless otherwise stated and from the leaner cuts unless specified.

After the upcoming table of quality protein sources, you'll find a second table displaying the nutrient values of various fast foods that you must avoid. This second table reveals how much fat and calories are delivered by fast foods when they're used to reach daily protein requisites.

Recommended Protein Sources

Protein Source	Biological Value (BV)	Serving Portion	Serving Portion by Volume	Calories	Protein in Grams	Carbohydrates in Grams	Total Fat in Grams	Saturated Fat in Grams	Polyunsaturated Fat in Grams	
									Omega-3	Omega-6
Salmon (Atlantic)	80-83	84 g	0.5-0.6 cups	155	22		7	1.1	2.6	0.6
Herring (Atlantic)	80-83	84 g	0.5-0.6 cups	172	20		10	2.2	2.2	0.2
Trout	80-83	84 g	0.5-0.6 cups	162	23		7	1.3		0.2
Tuna (can, light, wtr)	80-83	84 g (drained)	0.5-0.6 cups	99	22		1	0.2	0.3	
Tuna (bluefin, fresh)	80-83	84 g	0.5-0.6 cups	150	25		1	1.4	1.0	0.1
Flounder	80-83	84 g	0.5-0.6 cups	100	21		1	0.3	0.6	0.1
Halibut (Atlantic)	80-83	84 g	0.5-0.6 cups	166	20		7	2.2	2.2	0.2
Shrimp	80-83	84 g	0.5-0.6 cups	84	18		1			
Red Snapper	80-83	84 g	0.5-0.6 cups	90	20		1.1	0.2		0.1
Lingcod	80-83	84 g	0.5-0.6 cups	84	18		1.2	0.2		0.1
Chicken (breast, no skin)	79-80	84 g (small broiler)	half breast	142	27		3	0.9	0.1	0.7
Chicken (dark, no skin)	79-80	84 g (small broiler)	2 drumsticks	164	24		6	0.7	0.1	1.2
Turkey (light meat, no skin)	79-80	84 g	0.6 cups chopped meat	137	26		3			0.5
Beef Tenderloin (lean)	80-81	84 g	0.6-0.7 cups chopped meat	179	24		10	3.2	0.3	
Beef Shank (regular)	80-81	84 g	0.6-0.7 cups chopped meat	224	26		15	4.8	0.1	
Bison	80-81	84 g	0.6-0.7 cups chopped meat	122	24		4	0.8		0.4
Pork Chops (lean)	79-81	84 g	0.6-0.7 cups chopped meat	196	26		10	3		0.2
Ham (cured, lean)	79	84 g	0.6-0.7 cups chopped meat	227	19		19	6.8	0.2	0.6
Bacon (lean)	79	3 slices	3 slices	110	5.8		11	3.3	0.8	1.6
Egg (whole, large)	100	2 eggs	2 eggs	155	13		12	2.5	0.1	5
Egg (white)	88	2 whites	2 whites	31	7.5					1.3
Yogurt (plain, low fat)	75-77	500 g	2 cups	250	20	36	4	2.3		
Cottage Cheese (low fat)	77	150 g	0.6 cups	112	16	6	2.5	1.7		
Cottage Cheese (dry curd)	77	120 g	0.5 cups	97	21	2	0.6	0.2		
Whey Protein Isolate (powder supplement)	100-159	30 g (powder)	1 serving	117	26	1	1			
Whey Protein (concentrate powder supplement)	90-110	30 g (powder)	1 serving	123	22	3	2.5			
Soy Protein Isolate (powder supplement)	74	30 g (powder)	1 serving	113	25	1	1			
Casein Protein Isolate (powder supplement)	77	30 g (powder)	1 serving	117	26	1	1			

Fast-Food Blood-Vessel Chokers

Fast-Food Protein Source	25 g Serving of Protein	Fat	Calories	40 g Serving of Protein	Fat	Calories
Church's Chicken	breast (fillet)	34 g	608	2 large thighs	41 g	580
Del Taco	combo/deluxe	25 g	530	2 servings chicken fajita	22 g	870
Kentucky Fried Chicken	2 drumsticks (original recipe)	18 g	280	breast (extra crisp)	29 g	505
Kentucky Fried Chicken	6 wings (spicy)	33 g	471	5 chicken strips	26 g	570
McDonald's	ham, egg, cheese on a bagel	23 g	550	2 Quarter Pounders	42 g	860
McDonald's	Big Mac	32 g	570	3 Filet-o-Fishes	78 g	1410
Skipper's	fish fillet (2 servings)	20 g	350	baked salmon	11 g	270
Harvey's	1 chicken sandwich	16 g	419	2 cheeseburgers	36 g	830
Jack in the Box	1 Jumbo Jack hamburger	37 g	590	7 chicken breasts	24 g	504
Godfather's Pizza	half a small, thin-crust, cheese-only pizza	18 g	540	half a small, stuffed, cheese-only pizza	33 g	930
Burger King	bacon cheeseburger	22 g	400	1 Big King Burger	42 g	640
Subway	6-inch chicken breast sandwich	6 g	342	2 parmesan chicken wraps	10 g	666

APPENDIX D:
ALKALINIZING AND ACID-FORMING FOODS

As we've seen, foods can have a tremendous influence on the body regarding hormonal and acid/alkaline balance. Maintaining acid/alkaline balance (pH balance) is critical to optimal biological function. The body functions within a very narrow range of pH and, if even slightly altered, biochemical havoc sets in to impair system efficiency.

Since the byproducts of metabolism tend to induce acidosis, we must, as much as possible, feed our bodies with buffering foods. Buffering foods promote alkaline/acid balance and must be relatively alkaline in nature to oppose the acidosis our bodies create under even normal operating conditions. This is especially important for athletes and people exposed to highly stressful lifestyles. Larger volumes of dietary protein and fat, as well as strained metabolic activity from exercise, require greater buffering or pH-balancing potential from our diets.

With greater levels of physical activity, more protein is required in the diet and, again, more of the alkaline foods are required to neutralize the potential acidosis created by the extra physical and metabolic activity. Have a look at the following chart to get an idea of the types of foods you must consume in abundance. You'll notice that the recommendations are pretty much those made throughout this book—low-glycemic-index, fresh vegetables and fruits.

Lower Acid-Forming Alkaline Foods (Consume Abundantly)	Higher Acid-Forming Foods (Consume Moderately or Eliminate)
Kale	Alcoholic Beverages
Garlic	Beef
Onion	Chicken
Broccoli	Lobster
Cauliflower	Pork
Squash	White/Red Potato
String Bean	Soybean
Sweet Potato	Pea
Yam	White Rice

Lower Acid-Forming Alkaline Foods (Consume Abundantly)	Higher Acid-Forming Foods (Consume Moderately or Eliminate)
Lentil	Puffed Rice
Navy Bean	Corn
Fava Bean	White Pasta
Carrot	Puffed Wheat
Grapefruit	White Bread
Blueberry	Rye
Apple	Orange
Fig	Coffee
Pear	Soda Pop
Strawberry	Chocolate
Apricot	Most Processed Food
Guava	
Turkey	
Saltwater Fish	
Water	
Green Beverage Supplement	

GLOSSARY

Acetyl coenzyme A (acetyl COA): Condensation product of coenzyme A and acetic acid; found in animals, bacteria, and plants; plays a huge role in intermediate metabolism for energy production, growth, et cetera.

Acetyl l-carnitine: A chemical, an acetic ester of carnitine that facilitates movement of acetyl COA into mammalian mitochondria during the oxidation of fatty acids; supplementation known to preserve and restore cognitive health.

Acetylsalicylic acid (ASA): Odorless, white bitter drug used to reduce pain, fever, and inflammation; sometimes employed to prevent blood-clotting; also known as Aspirin.

Adenosine triphosphate (ATP): Nucleotide present in all living cells; serves as an energy source for many metabolic processes.

Adipocyte: Fat-storage cell; animal connective-tissue cell specialized for the synthesis and storage of fat.

Advanced glycosylated endproduct (AGE): Accumulates over time on plasma lipoproteins and vascular wall components and plays an important role in the development of diabetes and age-related cardiovascular and other diseases.

Alanine: Nonessential amino acid that can be manufactured by the body from other sources as needed; involved in the energy-producing breakdown of glucose; found particularly concentrated in meats.

Alpha ketoglutaric acid (AKG): Family of compounds containing an oxo group with the general structure of 1,5-pentanedioic acid; keto acid or skeleton of glutamine; displays ammonia-scavenging (clearing) activity.

Alpha linolenic acid: Omega-3 fatty acid; 18-carbon chain containing three double bonds; found in plants and animal tissues and involved in formation of prostaglandins; one of the two essential fats for humans that must be supplied by diet; in short supply in the North American diet; more vulnerable to processing than linoleic acid (omega-6).

Alpha lipoic acid: Coenzyme in the oxoglutarate-dehydrogenase complex of the citric-acid cycle; powerful antioxidant in both lipid (fat) and aqueous mediums; recycles other antioxidants such as vitamin E to active state; supports insulin activity; abundant in red meat.

Alpha tocopherol: Yellow, viscous, odorless, oily liquid chemical that deteriorates on exposure to light, health, and oxygen; most often obtained from wheat germ oil or by synthesis; biologically exhibits the most vitamin E activity of the tocopherols and is an antioxidant that retards rancidity by interfering with the autoxidation of fats.

Amine: Any of a group of organic compounds derived from ammonia by replacing one or more hydrogen atoms with a hydrocarbon radical.

Amino acid: A class of organic molecule that contains an amino (NH) group and can combine linear arrays to form proteins in living organisms; building block for tissues, hormones, and other biochemicals; can now be produced by biotechnology in bulk using fermentation and biotransformation.

Amyloid precursor protein (APP): Alzheimer's disease patients are characterized by extensive accumulation of amyloid in the brain, and it's thought that this protein may contribute to neuron degeneration; also appears in the brains of older Down's syndrome patients.

Antioxidant: Synthetic or natural substances that protect the body from free-radical damage, degradation, disease; added to products to prevent or delay deterioration by action of oxygen in the air; rubber, paints, vegetable oils, and prepared foods commonly contain antioxidants.

Arachidonic acid: Omega-6 fatty acid; 20-carbon chain polyunsaturated fatty acid with four double bonds; nonessential dietary component for humans; precursor for biosynthesis of prostaglandins and thromboxanes (eicosanoid hormones); building block for cell membranes; made from linoleic acid in the body.

Arginine: A nonessential amino acid and a major component of protein that becomes essential when the body is under stress or is injured; lack of dietary arginine can result in depressed growth; supplementation has been shown to ameliorate blood pressure and libido.

Attention-deficit hyperactivity disorder (ADHD): Diagnosis applied to people who consistently display certain characteristic behaviors over a period of time; most common behaviors are inattention, hyperactivity, and impulsivity.

Autocrine hormone: Eicosanoid hormones; secretion of a substance, such as a growth factor, that stimulates the secretory cell itself and those in close proximity; made from cellular polyunsaturated fats.

Beta-carotene: Also known as provitamin A; an antioxidant that protects cells against oxidative damage that can lead to cancer and other diseases; found commonly in carrots, sweet potatoes, spinach, and tomatoes.

Biological value (BV): Rating system used to measure the nutritional value of a protein, usually calculated in comparison to the nutritional value of egg protein (BV = 100); measurement based on the body's retention of protein; one of the more accurate, more appropriate methods to date; protein sources are assigned values that reflect their biological value to the human body; example of a high number—150 for whey protein isolate; example of a low number—49 for most beans (soybean = 74).

Branched-chain amino acid (BCAA): There are three types of BCAA: L-Isoleucine, L-Leucine, and L-Valine, which must be present in muscle cells to promote efficient protein synthesis in nature; BCAAs help increase bioavailability of complex carbohydrate intake and are absorbed by muscle cells for anabolic muscle-building and anti-catabolic activity.

Butyric acid: Acid with an unpleasant odor that occurs in butter, cod liver oil, sweat, and other substances; short-chain (four-carbon), relatively stable fat.

Carnitine: Compound that transports long-chain fatty acids across inner mitochondrial membranes; also called vitamin Bt or vitamin B$_7$.

Carotenoid: Accessory lipophilic photosynthetic pigment in plants and bacteria; possesses powerful antioxidant activity; protects body against free radicals.

Casein: Protein isolated from milk; amphipathic polypeptides of around 200 amino acids; biological value 77.

Catabolism: Any destructive metabolic process by which organisms convert substances into excreted compounds or fuel sources.

Catalase: Enzyme that breaks down hydrogen peroxide into a less toxic compound.

Chatecholamine: Any of a group of chemicals that include epinephrine and norepinephrine produced in the medulla of the adrenal gland; usually manufactured when body is under stress.

Chelate: (Noun) compound that has a ring structure that usually contains a metal ion held by coordinate bonds; (verb) to combine with (a metal) to form a chelate ring; to react so as to form a chelate ring.

Cholesterol: White crystalline substance in animal tissues and various foods normally synthesized by the liver; a constituent of cell membranes and precursor to steroid hormones.

Choline: Base that occurs as a component of phospholipids, especially in animals, and is essential to liver function.

Cholinesterase: Enzyme that hydrolyzes choline esters and that's found especially in blood plasma.

Chondrocyte: Differentiated cell responsible for production and secretion of extracellular matrix of cartilage of joints.

Chrysin: Also known as Flavone X; inhibits aromatase, which is a naturally occurring enzyme in the body that converts testosterone and even androstenedione into estrogen; accelerated aromatase activity is undesirable for men because it leads to decreased testosterone levels, sabotaging the efforts of the serious bodybuilder; displays anti-cancer activity.

cis fat: Most desirable type of fat; found in most unmodified dietary sources such as olive and flaxseed oils.

Citrus aurantium (CA): Fruit commonly known as bitter orange; used to treat digestive and circulatory problems; also displays powerful thermogenic activity through its noradrenergic influence; used in place of ephedra for safe fat loss.

Coenzyme Q10 (coQ10): Powerful antioxidant that assists in oxidation of nutrients within cells to create energy; sometimes prescribed as a complementary therapy to combat AIDS-related conditions and as an adjunct to statin drug prescription.

Co-factor: Nonprotein substance that enzymes require to function; also called coenzymes or metal ions.

Coleus forskohlii: Member of the mint family; recognized as the only plant source with the diterpene compound known as forskolin; possesses ability to stimulate synthesis of Cyclic AMP, which facilitates a response inside the cell from the signal a hormone may induce on the cell surface (cell membrane).

Conjugated linoleic acid (CLA): Modified version of an essential fatty acid; displays antioxidant activity and anti-cancer potential and facilitates thermogenesis or fat loss.

Corticoid: See *corticosteroid*.

Corticosteroid: Any of the steroid hormones produced by the adrenal cortex or their synthetic equivalents such as cortisol and aldesterone.

Creatine: Compound made by the body; used to store energy in the form of creatine phosphate; in supplemental form used to enhance muscle size and strength; recently recognized as an anti-inflammatory and cognition enhancer.

Curcumin: Active component of turmeric; studies have proven this antioxidant inhibits HIV replication by blocking the long-terminal repeat region on HIV's genes; promotes powerful antioxidant activity and has anti-inflammatory properties.

Curcuminoid: Natural anti-inflammatory plant extract; used for centuries for effective pain relief without side effects; extracted from turmeric; see *curcumin*.

Cyclic AMP (cAMP): Messenger chemical within cell that relays signal internally received by a hormone on the cell's surface.

Cyclo oxygenase (cox): Enzyme protein complex present in most tissues that catalyzes two steps in prostaglandin biosynthesis and produces prostaglandins and thromboxanes from arachidonic acid; acceleration of this enzyme leads to common cardiovascular and inflammatory diseases; ASA or Aspirin works its wonders by inhibiting cox.

Cysteine: Amino acid that contains a thiol (SH) group; in intracellular enzymes the unique reactivity of this group is frequently exploited at the catalytic site; promotes antioxidant activity.

Cytokine: Any of a class of immunoregulatory substances such as lymphokines that are secreted by cells of the immune system.

Dehydroepiandrosterone (DHEA): Precursor of androgens and estrogen and the most abundant steroid in the body's circulation; declines with age.

Dehydrotestosterone (DHT): Byproduct of testosterone metabolism known to deliver detrimental activity to the prostate if elevated; implicated in hair loss.

Deprenyl: Prescription drug used as an anti-parkinsonian agent; also used as a cognition preserver in anti-aging programs.

Desaturase enzyme: Catalyzes desaturation of polyunsaturated fatty acids; deficiency results in unbalanced and poor hormone regulation; involved in prostaglandin and other eicosanoid-hormone production in cells.

Dietary-induced thermogenesis (DIT): Increase in energy expenditure following ingestion of food; also known as specific dynamic action, thermic effect of food.

Dihomo gamma linolenic acid (DGLA): Omega fatty acid found in mother's milk and organ meats such as spleens, kidneys, and adrenals; made from linoleic acid (omega-6).

Dimethylsulfoxide (DMSO): Highly polar organic liquid chemical solvent that can penetrate plant and animal tissues and preserve living cells during freezing; used as a topical anti-inflammatory in veterinary applications.

Disaccharide: Sugar made up of two monosaccharides (single sugars); sucrose and lactose are examples of disaccharides; sucrose is made of one glucose molecule and one fructose molecule.

Docosahexaenoic acid (DHA): Polyunsaturated fatty acid found predominantly in cold-water fish oils that supports insulin function and heart and brain health when supplemented.

Dopamine: Drug used to treat hypertension and stimulate cardiac and urine output; secreted by brain as a neurotransmitter.

Eicosanoid hormone: Unsaturated fatty acid containing 20 carbon atoms; able to induce profound physiological effects at extremely low concentrations such as production of pain and fever and regulation of blood pressure; effects are often intracellularly mediated by cAMP but isn't transported in the bloodstream; acts in same environment in which it is synthesized; different from endocrine hormone; see *autocrine hormone*.

Eicosapentaenoic acid (EPA): Omega-3 polyunsaturated fatty acid found in fish oils; supplementation supports healthy omega-3 to omega-6 balance, eicosanoid-hormone balance, anti-inflammatory activity, and heart health.

Elaidic acid: Unsaturated monobasic transisomer of oleic acid; trans fat derived from essential fat when hydrogenated.

Endocrine hormone: Hormone produced by endocrine system; manufactured by a gland to affect tissues and/or systems distantly located.

Endogenous: Developing or originating within an organism or arising from causes within the organism.

Epinephrine: Cardiac drug used for cardiac arrest; also known as adrenaline; secreted under stress by body; "fight or flight" hormone.

Exogenous: Developing or originating outside the organism, as in an exogenous disease.

Folic acid: Abundant in liver and green plants; growth factor for some bacteria and an essential nutrient for hormone health.

Follicle-stimulating hormone (FSH): Hormone secreted by pituitary gland; in women it stimulates ovarian follicle (egg) development and the release of estrogens; in men it stimulates the production of sperm.

Forskolin: Chemical from plant coleus forskohlii that possesses anti-hypertensive abilities, inhibits platelet aggregation, and contains smooth-muscle relaxant properties; also promotes release of hormones from pituitary gland and heightens cAMP activity of cells.

Free radical: Chemically active atom or group of atoms with charge that seeks to gain or release electrons to achieve more stable configuration, damaging large molecules in cells; has unpaired electrons that must be paired for biochemical stability to exist; can promote oxidation.

Fructo-oligosaccharide (FOS): Nondigestible, soluble-fiber carbohydrate that supports growth of beneficial gut bacteria; passes through small intestine into the large intestine.

Fructose: Six-carbon sugar found in plants; a monosaccharide with a low-glycemic-index rating of 23.

Gamma linolenic acid (GLA): Omega-6 fatty acid produced in the body; abundant in primrose and borage oils.

Gingko biloba: Extracted from gingko biloba tree and believed to have regulating effect on entire vascular system; most commonly used for its apparent ability to regulate blood flow to the brain, legs, and other extremities; may also promote metabolism of cerebral and neuro-sensorial cells.

Glucagon: Hormone secreted in response to a fall in blood-sugar levels; can induce hyperglycemia.

Glucocorticoid: Any of a group of corticoids, such as cortisone, that produce many effects of stress response; level of circulating glucocorticoids is most commonly employed physiological measure of stress; anti-inflammatory and antioxidant activity in low doses but catabolic at higher levels.

Glucosamine: Amino sugar used as a building block for various body tissues, including joint tissues; displays anti-inflammatory activity.

Glucose-tolerance factor (GTF): Organic complex of chromium with dinicotino-glutathione; dietary compound linked with maintenance of glucose tolerance; increased dietary GTF in normal individuals augments action of insulin; shown to reduce insulin requirements in some diabetics.

Glucose-transport site (GLUT-4): Insulin stimulates glucose transport in fat and muscle cells by triggering transport by these sites; damage to these transporters of blood sugar results in insulin resistance and Type II diabetes.

Glutamine: One of 20 amino acids commonly found in proteins; supplementation supports positive nitrogen balance, immune function, and gastrointestinal health; supplementation of glutamine is valuable when body and mind are stressed.

Glutathione peroxidase: Detoxifying enzyme that eliminates hydrogen peroxide and organic peroxides.

Glyburide: Oral hyperglycemic agent; a diabetic drug.

Glycemic index (GI): Classification of foods based on their blood-glucose-raising potential; higher GI indicates that a food raises blood sugar faster and higher.

Glycerine: Oily, viscous liquid existing in natural fat and oil; used as an ointment, as a solvent, as a vehicle for medicines, and as an adulterant in wine and beer; has carbohydrate-like activity in the body.

Glycosaminoglycan (GAG): Macromolecule found on surface of eukaryotic cells; thought to play a role in a cell's recognition of other cells; building material for connective tissue.

HDL cholesterol: High-density lipoprotein cholesterol (the "good" cholesterol).

Heparin: Drug that interferes with blood-clotting.

Homocysteine: Amino acid that irritates blood vessels, causing blockages in arteries; impairs cognitive health and induces inflammation and can be overproduced by a body that lacks vitamins or is overfed with animal meats.

Hydrocortisone: Chemical used as injection or topically in treatment of inflammation, allergies, asthma, and shock.

Hydroxy citric acid (HCA): Ingredient found in weight-loss supplements; derived from the Garcinia cambogia plant and believed to inhibit enzyme that allows carbohydrates to be stored as fat; modified form of citric acid; involved in the metabolism of carbohydrates and displays mild MAO-inhibitor activity.

Hydroxymethylbutyrate (HMB): Metabolite of amino acid leucine; regarded as natural anti-catabolic, muscle-building/fat-loss aid; also displays anti-inflammatory activity.

Hypercholesterolemia: High level of cholesterol in the blood.

Hyperglycemia: High level of glucose in blood that may indicate diabetes is out of control.

Hyperinsulinemia: High blood insulin level.

Hyperlipidemia: Elevated concentrations of any or all of the lipids (i.e., cholesterol) in plasma.

Hypoglycemia: Low blood sugar.

I-kappa-b: Family of inhibitory proteins that bind to transcription factors and modulate their activity; affects gene activity.

Insulinlike growth factor (IGF-1): Polypeptide with considerable sequence similarity to insulin; capable of eliciting comparable biological responses and is involved in protein synthesis and general metabolic health.

Ipriflavone: Synthetic flavonoid derived from the soy compound daidzein; promotes the incorporation of calcium into bone and inhibits bone breakdown.

Isoflavone: Isomeric form of flavone in which the benzene group is attached to the 3 position of the benzopyran ring instead of the 2 position; therapeutic and preventive value within the cardiovascular and cerebrovascular systems; protects prostate and breast tissues against cancer; found in soy, red clover tops, and kudzu root.

Ketogenesis: Metabolic production of ketones or ketone bodies.

Ketone: Any of a class of organic compounds having a carbonyl group linked to a carbon atom in each of two hydrocarbon radicals.

Ketone body: Ketone-containing substance produced by fatty acid, protein, and carbohydrate metabolism in the liver; used as fuel by muscle and brain tissues.

Ketone stick: Urine-testing strip that contains a special chemical that changes color if ketones are detected in urine.

Ketosis: Metabolic production of abnormal amounts of ketones.

Krill oil: Oil from the krill, a crustacean that thrives in waters off Antarctica; supplies EPA, DHA, and antioxidant activity.

Lactoferrin: Iron-binding protein.

LDL cholesterol: Low-density lipoprotein cholesterol (the "bad" cholesterol, if elevated).

Leucine: Most abundant amino acid found in proteins; a branched-chain amino acid.

Leukocyte: White corpuscle in blood; spherical, colorless, nucleated immune cell involved with host defenses.

Leukotriene: Any of a group of hormones originating from arachidonic acid that are thought to mediate allergic responses, causing lung constriction and muscle contraction in asthma.

Ligand: Group, ion, or molecule coordinated to a central atom or molecule in a complex.

Linoleic acid: Omega-6 fatty acid found in plants and animal tissues and involved in formation of prostaglandins; one of the two essential fats for humans that must be supplied by diet; occurs abundantly in typical North American diet and tends to survive processing better than linolenic acid (omega-3).

Lipid: Any of a group of organic compounds, including oils, fats, waxes, sterols (i.e., cholesterol), and glycerides, that are insoluble in water but soluble in organic solvents.

Lutein: Yellow substance extracted from egg yolks; powerful antioxidant that helps to protect eyes.

Lycopene: Linear, unsaturated hydrocarbon carotenoid; major red pigment in tomatoes and other fruit; powerful antioxidant with affinity for prostate and cardiovascular protection.

Lymphocyte: White blood cell derived from stem cells of lymphoid series.

Lipoxygenase (LOX): Enzyme that catalyzes reactions between linoleate and other fatty acids (i.e., omega-6, arachidonic acid) and oxygen to form hydroperoxy fatty-acid derivatives (leukotrienes) involved in asthmatic activity.

Lysine: Amino acid that's the only carrier of a side-chain primary amino group in proteins; has important structural and chemical roles in proteins.

Lysinoalanine complex: Unnatural amino-acid derivative during processing of foods that can cause impairment of metabolism, including kidney dysfunction and retarded growth.

Medium-chain triglyceride (MCT): Fat with an unusual chemical structure that allows the body to digest it easily; absorbed intact and taken to the liver where it's used directly for energy, similarly to carbohydrates; different enough from other fats in that it can be used as a fat substitute by people (especially those with AIDS) who need calories but are unable to absorb or metabolize normal fats; popular among athletes as a performance enhancer, but there's still no consistent evidence that MCT is effective in this role.

Melatonin: Hormone secreted by pineal gland; powerful antioxidant and insulin supporter.

Metformin: Hypoglycemic agent used in treatment of noninsulin-dependent diabetes mellitus that doesn't respond to dietary modification; typical Type II diabetic drug; recently used as weight-management aid.

Methionine: Neutral amino acid essential in human nutrition.

Methoxyisoflavone: Nonhormonal supplement expected to decrease cortisol levels dramatically, increase protein synthesis and nitrogen retention, and block aromatase activity to preserve testosterone.

Methylsulfonylmethane (MSM): Administered to individuals experiencing stress-response symptoms, including gastrointestinal upset, inflammation, skin maladies, and joint damage; natural sulfur source.

Mitochondria: Intracellular organelle responsible for energy production and cell respiration; powerhouse of the cell, producing ATP.

Monoamine: Amine compound containing one amino group, especially a compound that functions as a neurotransmitter.

Monoamine oxidase (MAO): Enzyme in cells of most tissues that catalyzes the oxidation of monoamines such as norepinephrine and serotonin; desaturates these neurotransmitters.

Monosaccharide: Simple sugar unable to be hydrolyzed to smaller units (i.e., glucose and fructose).

N-acetyl cysteine (NAC): Acetylated version of cysteine; an antioxidant that helps to maintain glutathione status in the entire body; supports healthy lung function and protects against development of lung ailments; bolsters liver and cognitive health.

Neuropeptide: Peptide with direct synaptic effect or indirect modulatory action on nervous system.

Neurotransmitter: Molecule utilized for signaling between nerve cells (synapse) or neurons.

Nitric oxide: Soluble, highly reactive gas formed by natural chemical and physical reactions in atmosphere; produced in cells from arginine, an amino acid; passes through cell membranes and is often used as biological signal; in the brain it plays a role in development and neuron-to-neuron signaling and probably contributes to the formation of memories; involved in regulation of various bodily systems.

Nitric-oxide synthase: Enzyme that catalyzes the formation of nitric oxide from oxygen and arginine.

Nonsteroidal anti-inflammatory drug (NSAID): Anti-inflammatory agent (i.e., ibuprofen, ASA) that inhibits the production of prostaglandins.

Noradrenalin/norepinephrine: Hormone that's a neurotransmitter for most of the sympathetic nervous system.

Nuclear-factor-kappa-B (NF-kappa-B): Regulates expression of genes, most of which encode proteins that play important role in immunity and inflammation; involved in brain function, particularly following injury and in neurodegenerative conditions such as Alzheimer's disease.

Nutraceutical: Any food or food ingredient considered to provide medicinal or health benefits, including the prevention and treatment of disease.

Nutrient-deficiency craving (NDC): State induced by deficiency of a nutrient.

Oleic acid: Monosaturated fatty acid found in olive oil; displays cardio-protective activity; good/stable cooking oil.

Omega-3 fat: Unsaturated fatty acids in which the first double bond (point of unsaturation) is found at the third carbon from the methyl end; often limited in the diet; alpha linolenic acid (essential fat) is an omega-3 fatty acid derived from animal and seed oils; DHA and EPA are omega-3 fatty acids.

Omega-6 fat: Unsaturated fatty acid in which the first double bond (point of unsaturation) is found at the sixth carbon from the methyl end; often abundant in the diet; linoleic acid (essential fat) is an omega-6 fat.

Omega-9 fat: Unsaturated fatty acid in which the first double bond (point of unsaturation) is found at the ninth carbon from the methyl end; sometimes mistaken for an essential fatty acid; humans produce a limited amount; found abundantly in olive oil (oleic acid is omega-9); supplementation or abundant consumption is associated with arterial health, cholesterol balance, improved general cardiovascular system, insulin efficiency, and improved glucose maintenance, as well as enhanced immune-system function.

Organochloride: Chlorinated hydrocarbon used as a pesticide; toxic to body in many ways, including neurotoxicity.

Organophosphate: Phosphorus-containing organic compound that inhibits cholinesterase; used in insecticides and war gases; extremely toxic to endocrine function and neurological system.

Ornithine alpha-ketogluterate (OKG): Combination of amino acids ornithine and glutamine; ammonia scavenger; supplementation improves protein retention, wound repair, and immune function by increasing levels of anabolic (growth-promoting) hormones such as insulin and growth hormone.

Oxalate: Salt of oxalic acid found in kidney stones in people with primary hyperoxaluria or oxalosis.

Oxidant: Molecule or atom that accepts electrons in an oxidation-reduction reaction and can cause cell/tissue damage.

Peptide: Compound of two or more amino acids in which alpha-carboxyl group of one is bound to the alpha-amino group of the other.

Peroxynitrite free radical: Toxic chemical produced when nitric oxide reacts with free radicals; often at center of inflammatory conditions.

Phaseolamine: Derived from extract of northern white kidney bean and has ability to inhibit action of alpha-amylase, the enzyme needed to convert starch to glucose; can reduce glycemic index of meals.

Phosphodiesterase: Group of catalytic enzymes that play a wide role in cellular processes.

Phospholipid: Major structural lipid of most cellular membranes.

Phytase: Enzyme that hydrolyzes phytate, the primary storage form of phosphorus in plant seeds and pollen; phytates can interfere with mineral absorption.

Phytate: Component of seeds and grains; anti-nutrient that can bind to iron and other minerals and disrupt the body's ability to absorb them.

Proanthocyanidin: Flavonoid complex derived from bark of French maritime pine tree; quashes the three specific types of dangerous free radicals—superoxide, hydroxyl, and nitric oxide; also derived from grape-seed extract.

Prostacyclin: Unstable prostaglandin released by mast cells and endothelium; potent inhibitor of platelet aggregation; an eicosanoid hormone.

Prostaglandin: Any of a group of components derived from unsaturated 20-carbon fatty acids via cyclo-oxygenase pathway that are extremely potent mediators of a diverse group of physiologic processes; autocrine hormone derived from omega-6 fatty acid.

Proteoglycan: High-molecular-weight complex of protein and polysaccharide, characteristic of structural tissues of vertebrates, such as bone and cartilage; also present on cell surfaces and partakes in cell-to-cell communication.

Quercetin: Mutagenic flavonol pigment found in plants; possesses antioxidant and antihistamine activity.

Reactive oxygen species (ROS): Radicals and nonradicals constantly formed in body that kill bacteria and inactivate proteins; implicated in various diseases when left uncontrolled or in absence of antioxidant activity.

Resistin: Adipocyte-derived cytokine implicated in insulin resistance and glucose intolerance.

Resveratrol: Ingredient of red wine, red grapeskin and seeds, and purple grape juice; natural antioxidant known to protect against illnesses and diseases, including neurodegenerative afflictions such as Parkinson's or other dementias, cancer, and intestinal and heart disorders.

Retinal: Aldehyde derivative of vitamin A that combines with opsins in retina to form visual pigments.

Retinol: Vitamin A, a fat-soluble vitamin that can't be synthesized by mammals and some vertebrates and must be supplied by diet; intermediary in vision cycle and plays role in growth and differentiation.

Ribose: Five-carbon sugar used by the body to make adenosine and the basis for making ATP; often supplemented to improve heart health and performance.

S-adenosyl-methionine (SAMe): Amino acid manufactured in brain and other tissues from another amino acid, methionine; donates methyl groups to other chemical compounds in the body, including neurotransmitters, changing them into alternate compounds; SAMe is "recycled" through an ongoing re-methylation process; production is impaired in depressed people; supplementation displays antidepressant activity; also promotes anti-inflammatory activity and is a powerful antioxidant.

Selenocysteine: Amino-acid derivative; the natural sulfur of cysteine is replaced by selenium.

Selenomethionine: Essential trace mineral in the human body; important part of antioxidant enzymes that protect cells against free radicals produced during normal oxygen metabolism; amino-acid derivative.

Serotonin: Organic compound found in the brain, blood serum, and gastric mucous membranes; active in vasoconstriction and transmission of nerve impulses.

Sex-hormone-binding globulin (SHBG): Glycoprotein synthesized by the liver; circulating androgen and estrogen concentrations influence SHBG synthesis; binds testosterone to inactivate it.

Sodium metavanadate: Oral vanadium-based hypoglycemic agent.

Squalene: Found in nature; sources include olives, palm oil, and wheat germ oil; largest concentration is from deep-sea shark liver oil; used to strengthen and support immune system; serves as an antioxidant and as an improver of skin complexion.

Statin drug: Slows endogenous production of cholesterol to reduce serum (blood) cholesterol.

Sucrose: Common table sugar made up of fructose and glucose; disaccharide.

Superoxide dismutase (SOD): Any of a range of metallo-enzymes that catalyzes formation of hydrogen peroxide and oxygen from superoxide, protecting cells against superoxide-induced damage.

Superoxide free radical: Formed when oxygen is reduced by transfer of a single electron to its outer shells; main significance is that it's a chief source for generation of hydrogen peroxide.

Syndrome X: Insulin resistance and its associated secondary diseases.

Taurine: One of most abundant amino acids in body; found in central nervous system, skeletal muscle, brain, and heart; not found in vegetable protein; inhibits and modulates neurotransmitters in brain; supplementation known to support insulin activity, cognition, and heart health.

Thermogenesis: Physiologic production of heat in body.

Thiol: Molecular group containing sulfur; involved in antioxidant and catalyst activity.

Thromboxane: Group of eicosanoids produced from arachidonic acid by action of cyclo oxygenase; together with prostaglandins make up prostanoid subgroup of eicosanoids; induces platelet aggregation and clotting.

Thyroxine: Thyroid hormone.

Tocotrienol: Vitamin E fraction; an antioxidant and anticoagulant that possesses some alpha tocopherol activity.

Trans fat: Formed when liquid vegetable oil turns into a solid; found most commonly in margarine or shortening; food companies use trans fat instead of oil because it can reduce costs, extend a product's storage life, and improve flavor and texture; contributes to development of disease; formed during hydrogenation.

Tribulus terrestris: Herb derived from Tribulus plant that helps improve impotence, libido, male infertility; clinically proven to enhance energy and vitality; may help build muscle and strength; also known to induce ovulation.

Tumor necrosis factor (TNF): Cytokine found in synovial cells and macrophages; occurs in inflammatory diseases and also as a response to endotoxins from bacteria.

Type I diabetes: Chronic condition in which pancreas makes little or no insulin because beta cells have been damaged and body is unable to use glucose for energy; insulin must be injected daily, and a diet plan, exercise, and blood testing for glucose must be employed regularly.

Type II diabetes: Milder form of diabetes with more gradual onset; usually develops in obese individuals over age 35; responds well to dietary regulation and/or oral hypoglycemic agents and can be reversed.

Uncoupling protein (UCP3): Specialized mitochondrial protein that causes fat-derived energy to be dispensed as heat in thermogenic process instead of forming ATP from food energy; this activity results in calorie expenditure by the body independent of exercise/fat loss without physical work.

Uric acid: Minor endproduct of nitrogen metabolism in body that's found in small amounts in urine; gout in humans is associated with abnormal levels of uric acid in the system; saturation of uric acid in bloodstream may result in kidney stones when acid crystalizes in the kidney.

Vanadium: Soft, silvery white metallic element used in steel alloys that occurs in several complex minerals, including carnotite and vanadinite; possesses anti-diabetic activity.

Vanadyl sulfate (vs): Unusual compound derived from trace-mineral vanadium that has insulinlike effects and insulin-potentiating properties.

Xanthine oxidase: Enzyme normally found in liver and not free in the blood; metabolic pathway for uric-acid formation.

NOTES

Chapter 3: History Doesn't Have to Be Repeated

1. C. W. Hunt et al., "Effect of Cattle Diet on Escherichia Coli o157:H7 Acid Resistance," *Applied and Environmental Microbiology* 65.7 (1999): 3233–35.

2. H. R. Feiz and S. Mobarhan, "Does Vitamin C Intake Slow the Progression of Gastric Cancer in Helicobacter Pylori–Infected Populations?" *Nutrition Reviews* (Washington, D.C.) 60.1 (2002): 34–36.

3. Pierre Pannunzio, "Thiamine Deficiency Results in Metabolic Acidosis and Energy Failure in Cerebellar Granule Cells: An In Vitro Model for the Study of Cell-Death Mechanisms in Wernicke's Encephalopathy," *Journal of Neuroscience Research* 62.2 (2000): 286–92.

4. S. C. Hung et al., "Thiamine Deficiency Can Cause Neural Impairment: Thiamine Deficiency and Unexplained Encephalopathy in Hemodialysis and Peritoneal Dialysis Patients," *American Journal of Kidney Disease* 38.5 (2001): 941–47.

5. E. Wenzel et al., "Effect of Heat-Treated Proteins on Selected Parameters of the Biotransformation System in the Rat," *Annals of Nutrition and Metabolism* 46.1 (2000): 9–16.

6. M. Friedman, "Chemistry, Biochemistry, Nutrition, and Microbiology of Lysinoalanine, Lanthionine, and Histidinoalanine in Food and Other Proteins," *Journal of Agricultural and Food Chemistry* 47.4 (1999): 1295–1319.

7. L. W. Kroh and A. Schulz, "News on the Maillard Reaction of Oligomeric Carbohydrates: A Survey," *Nahrung* 45.3 (2001): 160–63.

8. Robert S. Goodhart and Maurice E. Shils, eds., *Modern Nutrition in Health and Disease*, 5th ed. (Philadelphia: Lea and Febiger, 1973) 95.

9. Marie V. Krause and L. Kathleen Mahan, *Food, Nutrition, and Diet Therapy: A Textbook of Nutritional Care*, 7th ed. (Philadelphia: Saunders, 1984) 119.

10. Corinne H. Robinson et al., *Normal and Therapeutic Nutrition*, 17th ed. (New York: Macmillan, 1986) 178.

11. Krause and Mahan, *Food, Nutrition, and Diet Therapy*, 119.

12. U. Nageli and J. C. Somogyi, "Anti-Thiamine Effect of Coffee," *International Journal for Vitamin and Nutrition Research* 46.2 (1976): 149–53.

13. S. Pattanavibag and P. Ruenwongsa, "Effect of Tea Consumption on the Levels of Alpha-Ketoglutarate and Pyruvate Dehydrogenase in Rat Brain," *Experientia* 38.7 (1982): 787–88.

14. Elizabeth Hall and Marion Perlmutter, *Adult Development and Aging* (New York: John Wiley, 1985) 101.

15. I. Elmadfa et al., "The Thiamine Status of Adult Humans Depends on Carbohydrate Intake," *Experimental and Clinical Endocrinology and Diabetes* 109.6 (2001): 330–36.

16. T. Kamihara and I. Nakamura, "Regulation of Respiration and Its Related Metabolism by Vitamin B_1 and Vitamin B_6 in Saccharomyces Yeasts," *Advances in Biochemical Engineering/Biotechnology* 29 (1984): 35–82.

17. K. J. Meador et al., "Evidence for a Central Cholinergic Effect of High-Dose Thiamine," *Annals of Neurology* 34.5 (1993): 724–26.

18. R. G. Mair et al., "Impairment of Olfactory, Auditory, and Spatial Serial Reversal Learning in Rats Recovered from Pyrithiamine-Induced Thiamine Deficiency," *Behavioral Neurscience* 105.3 (1991): 360–74.

19. M. K. Gaitonde et al., "Decreased Metabolism In Vivo of Glucose into Amino Acids of the Brain of Thiamine-Deficient Rats After Treatment with Pyrithiamine," *Journal of Neurochemistry* 24.6 (1975): 1215–23.

Chapter 4: A Radical Generation

1. P. S. Wong et al., "Inactivation of Glutathione S-Transferases by Nitric-Oxide-Derived Oxidants: Exploring a Role for Tyrosine Nitration," *Archives of Biochemistry and Biophysics* 394.2 (2001): 216–28.

2. Ricardo Gredilla et al., "Effect of Short-Term Caloric Restriction on H_2O_2 Production and Oxidative DNA Damage in Rat-Liver Mitochondria and Location of the Free-Radical Source," *Journal of Bioenergetics and Biomembranes* 33.4 (2001): 279–87.

3. W. J. Durham and M. B. Reid, "Generation of Reactive Oxygen and Nitrogen Species in Contracting Skeletal Muscle: Potential Impact on Aging," *Annals of the New York Academy of Sciences* 959 (2002): 108–116.

4. J. S. Noh et al., "Neurotoxic and Neuroprotective Actions of Catecholamines in Cortical Neurons," *Experimental Neurology* 159.1 (1999): 217–24.

5. T. G. Hastings and M. J. LaVoie, "Dopamine Quinone Formation and Protein Modification Associated with the Striatal Neurotoxicity of Methamphetamine: Evidence Against a Role for Extracellular Dopamine," *Journal of Neuroscience* 19.4 (1999): 1484–91.

6. P. Dandona et al., "Effect of Hydrocortisone on Oxygen Free-Radical Generation by Mononuclear Cells," *Metabolism: Clinical and Experimental* 47.7 (1998): 788–91.

7. J. Gasic-Milenkovic et al., "Protein 'AGEing'—Cytotoxicity of a Glycated Protein Increases with Its Degree of AGE Modification," *Zeitschrift für Gerontologie und Geriatrie* 34.6 (2001): 457–60.

8. S. Gupta et al., "Hyperglycemia Increases Endothelial Superoxide That Impairs Smooth Muscle Cell Na+-K+-ATPase Activity," *American Journal of Physiology: Cell Physiology* 282.3 (2002): C560–66.

9. T. Inoguchi et al., "High Glucose Level and Free Fatty Acid Stimulate Reactive Oxygen Species Production Through Protein-Kinase-c-Dependent Activation of NAD(P)H Oxidase in Cultured Vascular Cells," *Diabetes* 49.11 (2000): 1939–45.

10. Priya Mohanty et al., "Glucose Challenge Stimulates Reactive Oxygen Species (ROS) Generation by Leucocytes," *Journal of Clinical Endocrinology and Metabolism* 85.8 (2000): 2970–73.

11. P. Riederer et al., "Advanced Glycation Endproducts Change Glutathione Redox Status in SH-SY5Y Human Neuroblastoma Cells by a Hydrogen-Peroxide-Dependent Mechanism," *Neuroscience Letters* 312.1 (2001): 29–32.

12. M. H. Helmy et al., "Effect of Selenium Supplementation on the Activities of Glutathione-Metabolizing Enzymes in Human Hepatoma Hep G2 Cell Line," *Toxicology* (Amsterdam, Netherlands) 144.1–3 (2000): 57–61.

13. T. Chepda et al., "Synergy Between Ascorbate and Alpha Tocopherol on Fibroblasts in Culture," *Life Sciences* 69.14 (2001): 1587–96.

14. S. Khanna et al., "Alpha Lipoic Acid Supplementation: Tissue Glutathione Homeostasis at Rest and After Exercise," *Journal of Applied Physiology* 86.4 (1999): 1191–96.

15. Mujgan Cengiz and Salih Cengiz, "The Effect of Vitamin C Administration on Erythrocyte Glutathione and HbA1c Levels of Type II Diabetic Patients," *Cerrahpasa Tp Dergisi* 31.4 (2000): 211–15.

Chapter 5: Nature Holds the Keys

1. D. Thompson et al., "Prolonged Vitamin C Supplementation and Recovery from Demanding Exercise," *International Journal of Sport Nutrition and Exercise Metabolism* 11.4 (2001): 466–81.

2. M. Otsuka et al., "Ascorbate Indirectly Stimulates Fatty-Acid Utilization in Primary Cultured Guinea Pig Hepatocytes by Enhancing Carnitine Synthesis," *Journal of Nutrition* 124.5 (1994): 732–37.

3. "Ascorbic Acid Increases the Density of the Acetylcholine Receptor on Muscle Cells," *Nutrition Reviews* (Washington, D.C.) 47.12 (1989): 378–79.

4. A. G. Clark et al., "The Effects of Ascorbic Acid on Cartilage Metabolism in Guinea Pig Articular Cartilage Explants," *Matrix Biology* 21.2 (2002): 175–84.

5. J. M. May, "How Does Ascorbic Acid Prevent Endothelial Dysfunction?" *Free Radicals in Biology and Medicine* 28.9 (2000): 1421–29.

6. M. McCann et al., "The Nitric Oxide Hypothesis of Aging," *Experimental Gerontology* 33.7–8 (1998): 813–26.

7. Brian Bandy et al., "Bioflavonoid Rescue of Ascorbate at a Membrane Interface," *Journal of Bioenergetics and Biomembranes* 33.4 (2001): 269–77.

8. S. Taddei et al., "Vitamin C Improves Endothelium-Dependent Vasodilation by Restoring Nitric-Oxide Activity in Essential Hypertension," *Circulation* 97.22 (1998): 2222–29.

9. Max Hansen et al., "The Effect of Grapeskin Extract on Oxidative Status," *British Journal of Nutrition* 84.4 (2000): 505–13.

10. Lester Packer et al., "Enzyme Inhibition and Protein-Binding Action of the Procyanidin-Rich French Maritime Pine-Bark Extract, Pycnogenol: Effect on Xanthine Oxidase," *Journal of Agricultural and Food Chemistry* 48.11 (2000): 5630-39.

11. E. Maneiro et al., "The Effect of Sulphate Chondroitin on the Production of Nitric Oxide by Human Arthrosic Chondrocytes," *Revista Española de Reumatología* 28.1 (2001): 12–17.

12. M. F. McCarty et al., "Sulfated Glycosaminoglycans and Glucosamine May Synergize in Promoting Synovial Hyaluronic Acid Synthesis," *Medical Hypotheses* 54.5 (2000): 798–802.

13. U. Çakatay et al., "Effect of an Alpha Lipoic Acid Supplementation on Oxidative Protein Damage in the Streptozotocin-Diabetic Rat," *Research in Experimental Medicine* 199.4 (1999): 243–51.

14. V. E. Kagan et al., "Dihydrolipoic Acid, a Universal Antioxidant Both in the Membrane and in the Aqueous Phase: Reduction of Peroxyl, Ascorbyl, and Chromanoxyl Radicals," *Biochemical Pharmacology* 44.8 (1992): 1637–49.

15. G. K. Zoloev et al., "The Function of Endogenous Protective Systems in Patients with Insulin-Dependent Diabetes Mellitus and Polyneuropathy: Effect of Antioxidant Therapy," *Bulletin of Experimental Biology and Medicine* 130.10 (2000): 437–41.

16. M. W. Roomi et al., "Cytotoxicity of Lipoic Acid and Dihydrolipoic Acid Against Malignant Murine Leukemia Cells: A Comparison with Ascorbic Acid and Dehydroascorbic Acid," *Medical Science Research* 26.7 (1998): 461–63.

17. P. Arivazhagan et al., "Effect of DL-Alpha Lipoic Acid on Mitochondrial Enzymes in Aged Rats," *Chemico-Biological Interactions* 138.2 (2001): 189–98.

18. Ibid.

19. S. Jacob et al., "Oral Administration of Alpha Lipoic Acid Modulates Insulin Sensitivity in Patients with Type II Diabetes Mellitus: A Placebo-Controlled Pilot Trial," *Free Radicals in Biology and Medicine* 27.3–4 (1999): 309–14.

20. R. C. Eason et al., "Alpha Lipoic Acid Increases Glucose Uptake by Skeletal Muscles of Obese-Diabetic Ob/Ob Mice," *Diabetes, Obesity, and Metabolism* 4.1 (2002): 29–35.

21. J. L. Evans et al., "Pharmacokinetics, Tolerability, and Fructosamine-Lowering Effect of a Novel, Controlled-Release Formulation of Alpha Lipoic Acid," *Endocrine Practice* 8.1 (2002): 29–35.

22. D. Bonnefont-Rousselot, "Antioxidant and Anti-AGE Therapeutics: Evaluation and Perspectives," *Journal de la Société de Biologie* 195.4 (2001): 391–98.

23. Gideon Lim and K. Sushil Jain, "Lipoic Acid Decreases Lipid Peroxidation and Protein Glycosylation and Increases (NA+ + K+)- and CA++-ATPase Activities in High Glucose-Treated Human Erythrocytes," *Free Radical Biology and Medicine* 29.11 (2000): 1122–28.

24. S. Arslanian, "Type II Diabetes in Children: Clinical Aspects and Risk Factors," *Hormone Research* 57 Supplement 1 (2002): 19–28.

25. H. R. Mogul et al., "Syndrome W: A New Model of Hyperinsulinemia, Hypertension, and Midlife Weight Gain in Healthy Women with Normal Glucose Tolerance," *Heart Disease* 4.2: 78–85.

26. F. X. Pi-Sunyer, "The Medical Risks of Obesity," *Obesity Surgery*, 12 Supplement 1 (2002): 6S–11S.

27. M. J. Arkinstall et al., "Effect of Carbohydrate Ingestion on Metabolism During Running and Cycling," *Journal of Applied Physiology* 91.5 (2001): 2125–34.

28. S. M. Weltan et al., "Pre-Exercise Muscle Glycogen Content Affects Metabolism During Exercise Despite Maintenance of Hyperglycemia," *American Journal of Physiology* 274.1 Part 1 (1998): E83–E88.

29. S. K. Tsintzas and C. Williams, "Human Muscle Glycogen Metabolism During Exercise: Effect of Carbohydrate Supplementation," *Sports Medicine* (New Zealand) 25.1 (1998): 7–23.

30. M. J. Arkinstall et al., 2125–34.

31. M. Hargreaves, "Pre-Exercise Nutritional Strategies: Effects on Metabolism and Performance," *Canadian Journal of Applied Physiology* 26 Supplement (2001): S64–70.

32. D. C. Nieman, "Exercise Immunology: Nutritional Countermeasures," *Canadian Journal of Applied Physiology* 26 Supplement (2001): S45–55.

33. S. Claeyssens et al., "Effect of Enteral Glutamine on Leucine, Phenylalanine, and Glutamine Metabolism in Hypercortisolemic Subjects," *American Journal of Physiology: Endocrinology and Metabolism* 278.5 (2000): E817–24.

34. P. Keren et al., "Effect of Hyperglycemia and Hyperlipidemia on Atherosclerosis in LDL-Receptor-Deficient Mice: Establishment of a Combined Model and Association with Heat Shock Protein 65 Immunity," *Diabetes* 49.6 (2000): 1064–69.

35. P. C. Deedwania, "Mechanism of the Deadly Quartet," *Canadian Journal of Cardiology* 16E (2000): 17E–20E.

36. D. K. Levenhagen et al., "Post-Exercise Nutrient Intake Timing in Humans Is Critical to Recovery of Leg Glucose and Protein Homeostasis," *American Journal of Physiology: Endocrinology and Metabolism* 280.6 (2001): E982–93.

37. M. J. Gibala, "Nutritional Supplementation and Resistance Exercise: What Is the Evidence for Enhanced Skeletal Muscle Hypertrophy?" *Canadian Journal of Applied Physiology* 25.6 (2000): 524–35.

38. P. Schrauwen and M. Hesselink, "UCP2 and UCP3 in Muscle-Controlling Body Metabolism," *Journal of Experimental Biology* 205, Part 15 (2002): 2275–85.

39. P. Schrauwen et al., "Effect of Acute Exercise on Uncoupling Protein 3 Is a Fat Metabolism-Mediated Effect," *American Journal of Physiology: Endocrinology and Metabolism* 282.1 (2002): E11–7.

40. E. L. Greene et al., "Alpha Lipoic Acid Prevents the Development of Glucose-Induced Insulin Resistance in 3T3-L1 Adipocytes and Accelerates the Decline in Immunoreactive Insulin During Cell Incubation," *Metabolism: Clinical and Experimental* 50.9 (2001): 1063–69.

41. M. F. McCarty, "Complementary Measures for Promoting Insulin Sensitivity in Skeletal Muscle," *Medical Hypotheses* 51.6 (1998): 451–64.

42. D. Bursey and M. Freemark, "The Effects of Metformin on Body-Mass Index and Glucose Tolerance in Obese Adolescents with Fasting Hyperinsulinemia and a Family History of Type II Diabetes," *Pediatrics* 107.4 (2001): E55.

43. Todd J. Anderson et al., "Improved Endothelial Function with Metformin in Type II Diabetes Mellitus," *Journal of the American College of Cardiology* 37.5 (2001): 1344–50.

44. C. Saliou et al., "Antioxidants Modulate Acute Solar Ultraviolet Radiation-Induced NF-kappa-B Activation in a Keratinocyte Cell Line," *Free Radical Biology and Medicine* 26.1–2 (1999): 174–83.

45. T. K. Pandita et al., "Ataxia-Telangiectasia: Chronic Activation of Damage-Responsive Functions Is Reduced by Alpha Lipoic Acid," *Oncogene* 20.3 (2001): 289–294.

46. "Chernobyl Radiation Damage on Children Ameliorated with Alpha Lipoic Acid," *Likarska Sprava* 1 (2002): 24–26.

47. Jihun M. Lee, "A Possible Indirect Sympathomimetic Action of Metformin in the Arterial Vessel Wall of Spontaneously Hypertensive Rats," *Life Sciences* 69.9 (2001): 1085–92.

48. P. Kubes and D. M. McCafferty, "Nitric Oxide and Intestinal Inflammation," *American Journal of Medicine* 109.2 (2000): 150–58.

49. S. Cuzzocrea et al., "Peroxynitrite-Mediated DNA Strand Breakage Activates Poly (ADP-Ribose) Synthetase and Causes Cellular Energy Depletion in Carrageenan-Induced Pleurisy," *Immunology* 93.1 (1998): 96–101.

50. H. Nakagawa, et al., "Scavengers for Peroxynitrite: Inhibition of Tyrosine Nitration and Oxidation with Tryptamine Derivatives, Alpha Lipoic Acid, and Synthetic Compounds," *Chemical and Pharmaceutical Bulletin* (Tokyo) 48.2 (2000): 261–65.

51. "Effect of Melatonin on Cellular-Energy Depletion Mediated by Peroxynitrite and Poly (ADP-Ribose) Synthetase Activation in an Acute Model of Inflammation," *Journal of Pineal Research* 31.1 (2001): 76–84.

52. Ibid.

53. I. Ford et al., "The Effects of Treatment with Alpha Lipoic Acid or Evening Primrose Oil on Vascular Hemostatic and Lipid Risk Factors, Blood Flow, and Peripheral Nerve Conduction in the Streptozotocin-Diabetic Rat," *Metabolism: Clinical and Experimental* 50.8 (2001): 868–75.

54. James L. Groff and Sareen S. Gropper, *Advanced Nutrition and Human Metabolism*, 3rd ed. (Belmont, CA: West/Wadsworth, 2000) 91.

55. J. Miquel, "Can Antioxidant Diet Supplementation Protect Against Age-Related Mitochondrial Damage?" *Annals of the New York Academy of Sciences*, 959 (2002): 508–16.

56. P. Arivazhagan et al., "Effect of DL-Alpha Lipoic Acid on Mitochondrial Enzymes in Aged Rats," *Chemico-Biological Interactions* 138.2 (2001): 189–98.

Chapter 6: Revolutionary Scientific Developments

1. A. de Bruin, et al., "Involvement of Reactive Oxygen Species in TNF-Alpha-Mediated Activation of the Transcription Factor NF-kappa-B in Canine Dermal Fibroblasts," *Veterinary Immunology and Immunopathology* 71.2 (1999): 125–42.

2. B. S. Taylor et al., "Inhibition of Cytokine-Induced Nitric-Oxide-Synthase Expression by Gene Transfer of Adenoviral I-kappa-B Alpha," *Surgery* (Oxford) 126.2 (1999): 142–47.

3. F. Emmerich et al., "Overexpression of I-kappa-B Alpha Without Inhibition of NF-kappa-B Activity and Mutations in the I-kappa-B Alpha Gene in Reed-Sternberg Cells," *Blood* 94.9 (1999): 3129–34.

4. Ibid.

5. H. K. Wong et al., "Abnormal NF-kappa-B Activity in T Lymphocytes from Patients with Systemic Lupus Erythematosus Is Associated with Decreased P65-RelA Protein Expression," *Journal of Immunology* 163.3 (1999): 1682–89.

6. P. C. Cogswell et al., "Selective Activation of NF-kappa-B Subunits in Human Breast Cancer: Potential Roles for NF-kappa-B2/P52 and for BCL-3," *Oncogene* 19.9 (2000): 1123–31.

7. D. Javelaud et al., "Inhibition of Constitutive NF-kappa-B Activity Suppresses Tumorigenicity of Ewing Sarcoma EW7 Cells," *International Journal of Cancer* 98.2 (2002): 193–98.

8. P. L. Majano et al., "S-Adenosylmethionine Modulates Inducible Nitric-Oxide-Synthase Gene Expression in Rat Liver and Isolated Hepatocytes," *Journal of Hepatology* 35.6 (2001): 692–99.

9. W. Y. Almawi and O. K. Melemedjian, "Molecular Mechanisms of Glucocorticoid Anti-Proliferative Effects: Antagonism of Transcription-Factor Activity by Glucocorticoid Receptor," *Journal of Leukocyte Biology* 71.1 (2002): 9–15.

10. P. L. Majano et al.

11. B. S. Taylor, et al.

12. E. J. Dudek et al., "H_2O_2-Mediated Oxidative Stress Activates NF-kappa-B in Lens Epithelial Cells," *Free Radical Biology and Medicine* 31.5 (2001): 651–58.

13. L. Androne et al., "In Vivo Effect of Lipoic Acid on Lipid Peroxidation in Patients with Diabetic Neuropathy," *In Vivo* 14.2 (2000): 327–30.

14. S. Khanna et al., Alpha Lipoic Acid Supplementation: Tissue Glutathione Homeostasis at Rest and After Exercise," *Journal of Applied Physiology* 86.4 (1999): 1191–96.

15. Jadwiga Chroboczek et al., "Lipoic Acid–Derived Amphiphiles for Redox-Controlled DNA Delivery," *Chemistry and Biology* 7.10 (2000): 813–19.

16. T. M. Hagen et al., "(R) Alpha Lipoic Acid Reverses the Age-Associated Increase in Susceptibility of Hepatocytes to Tert-Butylhydroperoxide Both In Vitro and In Vivo," *Antioxidants and Redox Signaling* 2.3 (2000): 473–84.

17. S. E. Chaung et al., "Inhibition by Curcumin of Diethylnitrosamine-Induced Hepatic Hyperplasia, Inflammation, Cellular Gene Products, and Cell-Cycle-Related Proteins in Rats," *Food and Chemical Toxicology* 38.11 (2000): 991–95.

18. C. Jobin et al., "Curcumin Blocks Cytokine-Mediated NF-kappa-B Activation and Pro-Inflammatory Gene Expression by Inhibiting Inhibitory Factor I-kappa-B Kinase Activity," *Journal of Immunology* 163.6 (1999): 3474–83.

19. M. M. Chan et al., "In Vivo Inhibition of Nitric-Oxide-Synthase Gene Expression by Curcumin, a Cancer-Preventive Natural Product with Anti-Inflammatory Properties," *Biochemical Pharmacology* 55.12 (1998): 1955–62.

20. G. P. Lim et al., "The Curry Spice Curcumin Reduces Oxidative Damage and Amyloid Pathology in an Alzheimer Transgenic Mouse," *Journal of Neuroscience* 21.21 (2001): 8370–77.

21. M. G. Nair et al., "Cytotoxicity, Antioxidant, and Anti-Inflammatory Activities of Curcumins I–III from

Curcuma Longa," *Phytomedicine: International Journal of Phytotherapy and Phytopharmacology* 7.4 (2000): 303–308.

22. J. L. Arbiser et al., "Curcumin Is an In Vivo Inhibitor of Angiogenesis," *Molecular Medicine* 4.6 (1998): 376–83.

23. G. P. Lim et al.

24. A. Mazumder et al., "Curcumin Analogs with Altered Potencies Against HIV-1 Integrase as Probes for Biochemical Mechanisms of Drug Action," *Journal of Medicinal Chemistry* 40.19 (1997): 3057–63.

25. H. K. Wong et al.

26. H. Inano and M. Onoda, "Effect of Curcumin on the Production of Nitric Oxide by Cultured Rat Mammary Gland," *Nitric Oxide* 4.5 (2000): 505–515.

27. A. Mukhopadhyay et al., "Curcumin Down-Regulates Cell-Survival Mechanisms in Human Prostate Cancer Cell Lines," *Oncogene* 20.52 (2001): 7597–7609.

28. T. M. Hagen et al., "Feeding Acetyl-L-Carnitine and Lipoic Acid to Old Rats Significantly Improves Metabolic Function While Decreasing Oxidative Stress," *Proceedings of the National Academy of Sciences of the United States of America* 99.4 (2002): 1870–75.

29. P. J. Rani Arockia and C. Panneerselvam, "Carnitine as a Free Radical Scavenger in Aging," *Experimental Gerontology* 36.10 (2001): 1713–26

30. J. Liu et al., "Memory Loss in Old Rats Is Associated with Brain Mitochondrial Decay and RNA/DNA Oxidation: Partial Reversal by Feeding Acetyl-L-Carnitine and/or R-Alpha Lipoic Acid," *Proceedings of the National Academy of Sciences of the United States of America* 99.4 (2002): 2356–61.

31. B. Anuradha and P. Varalakshmi, "Protective Role of DL-Alpha Lipoic Acid Against Mercury-Induced Neural Lipid Peroxidation," *Pharmacological Research: The Official Journal of the Italian Pharmacological Society* 39.1 (1999): 67–80.

32. E. H. Sharman and S. C. Bondy, "Effects of Age and Dietary Antioxidants on Cerebral Electron Transport Chain Activity," *Neurobiology of Aging* 22.4 (2001): 629–34.

33. Y. Surh et al., "Molecular Mechanisms Underlying Chemo-Preventive Activities of Anti-Inflammatory Phytochemicals: Down-Regulation of COX2 and iNOS Through Suppression of NF-kappa-B Activation," *Mutation Research* 480–481.1–2: 243–68.

34. S. Rivest, "What Is the Cellular Source of Prostaglandins in the Brain in Response to Systemic Inflammation? Facts and Controversies," *Molecular Psychiatry* 4.6 (1999): 500–507.

35. Y. Surh et al.

36. A. Bierhaus et al., "Diabetes-Associated Sustained Activation of the Transcription Factor NF-kappa-B," *Diabetes* 50.12 (2001): 2792–2808.

37. D. Javelaud et al.

38. A. C. Chan et al., "Vitamin E Up-Regulates Arachidonic-Acid Release and Phospholipase A2 in Megakaryocytes," *Molecular and Cellular Biochemistry* 189.1-2 (1998):153–59.

39. K. R. Kim et al., "Effects of Vitamin E on Arachidonic-Acid Cascade in Platelets and Aorta of Acute Cadmium-Poisoned Rats," *Nutrition Research* 21.4 (2001): 657–66.

40. Phyllis A. Dennery et al., "Synergistic Inhibition of Cyclo-Oxygenase-2 Expression by Vitamin E and Aspirin," *Free Radical Biology and Medicine* 29.11 (2000): 1135–42.

41. N. Nand et al., "Lipid Peroxidation and Vitamin E in Ischemic Heart Disease," *Journal of the Association of Physicians of India* 45.11 (2001): 839–42.

42. Shiro Urano et al., "Aging and Oxidative Stress in Neuro-Degeneration," *BioFactors* 7.1–2 (1998): 103–112.

43. "Nutrition and Aging: Vitamin E Improves Microsomal Phospholipase A2 Activity and the Arachidonic-Acid Cascade in Kidney of Diabetic Rats," *Journal of Nutrition* 131.4 (2001): 1297–1301.

44. C. Y. Lee and J. M. Wan, "Immunoregulatory and Antioxidant Performance of Alpha Tocopherol and Selenium on Human Lymphocytes," *Biological Trace Element Research* 86.2 (2002): 123–36.

45. J. Lu et al., "The Metabolic Availability of Vitamin A Is Decreased at the Onset of Diabetes in Bio-Breeding Rats," *Journal of Nutrition* 130.8 (2000): 1958–62.

46. Y. Levy et al., "Dietary Supplementation of a Natural Isomer Mixture of Beta-Carotene Inhibits Oxidation Derived from Patients with Diabetes Mellitus," *Annals of Nutrition and Metabolism* 44.2 (2000): 54–60.

47. E. Bombardelli et al., "Botanical Derivatives for the Prostate," *Fitoterapia* (Milan) 71.1 (2000): S21–28.

48. W. B. Grant, "An Ecologic Study of Dietary Links to Prostate Cancer," *Alternative Medicine Review* 4.3 (1999): 162–69.

49. S. Agarwal and A. V. Rao, "Tomato Lycopene and Its Role in Human Health and Chronic Diseases," *Canadian Medical Association Journal* 163.6 (2000): 739–43.

50. S. M. Moeller et al., "The Potential Role of Dietary Xanthophylls in Cataract and Age-Related Macular Degeneration," *Journal of the American College of Nutrition* 19.5 (2001): 522S–52; and L. Crosbie et al., "Effects of Tomato Extract on Human Platelet Aggregation In Vitro," *Platelets* 12.4 (2001): 218–27.

51. Richard S. Bruno, "Lutein, Zeaxanthin, and Age-Related Macular Degeneration: Age-Related Macular Degeneration Is a Leading Cause of Blindness Among Individuals over the Age of 75," *Journal of Nutraceuticals, Functional and Medical Foods* 3.1 (2000): 79–86.

52. G. Dagnelie et al., "Lutein Improves Visual Function in Some Patients with Retinal Degeneration: A Pilot Study Via the Internet," *Optometry: Journal of the American Optometric Association* 71.3 (2000): 147–64.

53. Marie V. Krause and L. Kathleen Mahan, *Food, Nutrition, and Diet Therapy: A Textbook of Nutritional Care*, 7th ed. (Philadelphia: Saunders, 1984) 103.

54. Natacha S. Shaw et al., "Interphotoreceptor Retinoid-Binding Protein Contains Three Retinoid-Binding Sites," *Experimental Eye Research* 72.2 (2001): 183–90.

55. A. J. Fischer et al., "Localization of Retinoid-Binding Proteins, Retinoid Receptors, and Retinaldehyde Dehydrogenase in the Chick Eye," *Journal of Neurocytology* 28.7 (1999): 597–609.

56. N. M. Qtaishat et al., "Retinoid Kinetics in Eye Tissues of VPP Transgenic Mice and Their Normal Littermates," *Investigative Ophthalmology and Visual Science* 40.6: 1040.

57. T. Ogura et al., "Aldehyde Dehydrogenase 6, a Cytosolic Retinaldehyde Dehydrogenase Prominently Expressed in Sensory Neuroepithelia During Development," *Journal of Biological Chemistry* 275.52 (2000): 41210–18.

58. Robert S. Goodhart and Maurice E. Shils, eds., *Modern Nutrition in Health and Disease*, 5th ed. (Philadelphia: Lea and Febiger, 1973) 152.

59. Amy K. Harker-Murray, "Experimental Studies: The Role of Coenzyme Q10 in the Pathophysiology and Therapy of Experimental Congestive Heart Failure in the Dog," *Journal of Cardiac Failure* 6.3 (2000): 233–42.

60. D. Yu and Q Zhi, "Effects of Coenzyme Q10 on Myocardial Protection During Cardiac Valve Replacement and Scavenging Free-Radical Activity In Vitro," *Journal of Cardiovascular Surgery* 40.3 (1999): 355–61.

61. F. L. Rosenfeldt et al., "Coenzyme Q10 Improves the Tolerance of the Senescent Myocardium to Aerobic and Ischemic Stress: Studies in Rats and in Human Atrial Tissue," *BioFactors* 9.2-4 (1999): 291–99.

62. Ibid.

63. T. Ylikoski et al., "The Effect of Coenzyme Q10 on the Exercise Performance of Cross-Country Skiers," *Molecular Aspects of Medicine* 18.1 (1997): S283–90.

64. G. P. Littarru et al., "Coenzyme Q10 Blood Levels and Metabolic Demand," *International Journal of Tissue Reactions* 12.3 (1990): 145–48.

65. J. Karlson, "Heart and Skeletal Muscle Ubiquinone, or coQ10 as a Protective Agent Against Radical Formation in Man," *Advances in Myochemistry* (1987): 305–18.

66. Michael Colgan, *Optimum Sports Nutrition: Your Competitive Edge* (Ronkonkoma, NY: Advanced Research Press, 1993) 236.

67. Michael Colgan, "Antioxidants: The Real Story" (Unpublished Booklet, 1998) 13; and S. R. Thomas et al., "Dietary Co-Supplementation with Vitamin E and Coenzyme Q10 Inhibits Atherosclerosis in Apolipoprotein Egene Knockout Mice," *Arteriosclerosis, Thrombosis, and Vascular Biology* 21.4 (2001): 585–93.

68. Colgan, *Optimum Sports Nutrition*, 235.

69. O. T. Raitakari et al., "Coenzyme Q10 Improves LDL Resistance to Ex Vivo Oxidation But Does Not Enhance Endothelial Function in Hypercholesterolemic Young Adults," *Free Radical Biology and Medicine* 28.7 (2000): 1100–1105.

70. D. Mohr et al., "Dietary Supplementation with Coenzyme Q10 Results in Increased Levels of Ubiquinol-10 Within Circulating Lipoproteins and Increased Resistance of Human Low-Density Lipoprotein to the Initiation of Lipid Peroxidation," *Biochimica et Biophysica Acta* 1126.3 (1992): 247–54.

71. J. Bergemann et al., "Coenzyme Q10, a Cutaneous Antioxidant and Energizer," *BioFactors* 9.2–4 (1999): 371–78.

72. S. Echtay et al., "Coenzyme Q10 Is an Obligatory Co-Factor for Uncoupling Protein Function," *Nature* 408.6812 (2000): 609–12.

73. Ibid.

74. K. Sasaki et al., "Effects of Extract of Ginkgo Biloba Leaves and Its Constituents on Carcinogen-Metabolizing Enzyme Activities and Glutathione Levels in Mouse Liver," *Life Sciences* 70.14 (2002): 1657–67.

75. N. H. Al-Humadi et al., "Alteration of Intracellular Cysteine and Glutathione Levels in Alveolar Macrophages and Lymphocytes by Diesel-Exhaust Particle Exposure," *Environmental Health Perspectives* 110.4 (2002): 349–53.

76. Ibid.

77. E. Gitto et al., "Individual and Synergistic Antioxidative Actions of Melatonin: Studies with Vitamin E, Vitamin C, Glutathione, and Desferrioxamine (Desferoxamine) in Rat-Liver Homogenates," *Journal of Pharmacy and Pharmacology* 53.10 (2001): 1393–1401.

78. H. Shimpuku et al., "Effect of Vitamin E on the Degradation of Hydrogen Peroxide in Cultured Human Umbilical Vein Endothelial Cells," *Life Sciences* 68.3 (2000): 353–59.

79. P. Micke et al., "Effects of Long-Term Supplementation with Whey Proteins on Plasma Glutathione Levels of HIV-Infected Patients," *European Journal of Nutrition* 41.1 (2002): 12–8.

80. See Colgan, "Antioxidants: The Real Story."

81. G. Bounous and P. Gold, "The Biological Activity of Undenatured Dietary Whey Proteins: Role of Glutathione," *Clinical and Investigative Medicine* 14.4 (1991): 296–309.

82. Ibid.

83. C. K. Sen, "Cellular Thiols and Redox-Regulated Signal Transduction," *Current Topics in Cellular Regulation* 36 (2000): 1–30.

84. M. Sugimoto et al., "Effects of a New Anti-Rheumatic Drug KE-298 and Its Active Metabolite: -KE on Secretion of Thioredoxin and on the Level of Intracellular Glutathione in Human Monocytes and T Cells," *Molecular Immunology* 38.10 (2002): 793–99.

85. I. Manov et al., "Acetaminophen Hepatotoxicity and Mechanisms of Its Protection by N-Acetyl Cysteine: A Study of Hep3B Cells," *Experimental and Toxicological Pathology* 53.6 (2002): 489–500.

86. M. Sugimoto et al.

87. I. Manov et al.

88. L. E. Schmidt et al., "Acute Versus Chronic Alcohol Consumption in Acetaminophen-Induced Hepatotoxicity," *Hepatology* 35.4 (2002): 876–82.

89. S. Khanna et al.

90. K. Sasaki et al.

91. S. Ollagnier-de-Choudens and M. Fontecave, "The Lipoate Synthase from Escherichia Coli Is an Iron-Sulfur Protein," *FEBS Letters* 453.1–2 (1999): 25–28.

92. G. Le Flem et al., "Synthesis and Functional Properties of a Modified Human Insulin A-Chain: Implication in a 'Mini-Insulin' Structure Determination," *Bioorganic and Medicinal Chemistry* 10.7 (2002): 2111–17.

93. G. Bounous et al., "The Influence of Dietary Whey Protein on Tissue Glutathione and the Diseases of Aging," *Clinical and Investigative Medicine* 12.6 (1989): 343–49.

94. J. C. Anthony et al., "Leucine Supplementation Enhances Skeletal-Muscle Recovery in Rats Following Exercise," *Journal of Nutrition* 129.6 (1999): 1102–06.

95. J. S. Coombes and L. R. McNaughton, "Effects of Branched-Chain Amino Acid Supplementation on Serum Creatine Kinase and Lactate Dehydrogenase After Prolonged Exercise," *Journal of Sports Medicine and Physical Fitness* 40.3 (2000): 240–46.

96. C. Jodka et al., "Selective Amylin Inhibition of the Glucagon Response to Arginine Is Extrinsic to the Pancreas," *American Journal of Physiology: Endocrinology and Metabolism* 280.33 (2001): E443–49.

97. S. Nishida et al., "Long-Term Melatonin Administration Reduces Hyperinsulinemia and Improves the Altered Fatty-Acid Compositions in Type II Diabetic Rats Via the Restoration of Delta-5 Desaturase Activity," *Journal of Pineal Research* 32.1 (2002): 26–33.

98. O. J. Rimoldi et al., "Effects of Diabetes and Insulin on Hepatic Delta6 Desaturase Gene Expression," *Biochemical and Biophysical Research Communications* 283.2 (2001): 323–26.

99. H. Fujita et al., "Long-Term Ingestion of a Fermented Soybean-Derived Touchi Extract with Alpha-Glucosidase Inhibitory Activity Is Safe and Effective in Humans with Borderline and Mild Type II Diabetes," *Journal of Nutrition* 131.8 (2001): 2105–08.

100. J. Zhang and S. Kashket, "Inhibition of Salivary Amylase by Black and Green Teas and Their Effects on the Intraoral Hydrolysis of Starch," *Caries Research* 32.3 (1998): 233–38.

101. E. Z. Fisman et al., "Oral Anti-Diabetic Treatment in Patients with Coronary Disease: Time-Related Increased Mortality on Combined Glyburide/Metformin Therapy over a 7.7-Year Follow-Up," *Clinical Cardiology* 24.2 (2001): 151–58.

102. J. Olsson et al., "Increased Mortality in Type II Diabetic Patients Using Sulphonylurea and Metformin in Combination: A Population-Based Observational Study," *Diabetologia* 43.5 (2000): 558–60.

Chapter 7: Minerals: Stitches in the Biological Fabric

1. T. W. Kurtz and R. C. Morris, "Dietary Chloride as a Determinant of 'Sodium-Dependent' Hypertension," *Science* 222.4628 (1983): 1139–41.

2. F. C. Luft, et al., "Sodium Bicarbonate and Sodium Chloride: Effects on Blood Pressure and Electrolyte Homeostasis in Normal and Hypertensive Man," *Journal of Hypertension* 8.7 (1990): 663–70.

3. L. A. Martini et al., "High Sodium Chloride Intake Is Associated with Low Bone Density in Calcium Stone–Forming Patients," *Clinical Nephrology* 54.2 (2000): 85–93.

4. Z. Pan et al., "Effects of Oral Calcium Supplementation on Blood Pressure in Population," *Chinese Journal of Preventive Medicine* 34.2 (2000): 109–12.

5. Chun-Yah Yang, "Calcium and Magnesium in Drinking Water and Risk of Death from Cerebrovascular Disease," *Stroke* 29.2 (1998): 411–14.

6. Denise Pepin Marie-Pierre Sauvant, "Geographic Variation of the Mortality from Cardiovascular Disease and Drinking Water in a French Small Area (Puy de Dome)," *Environmental Research* 84.3 (1999): 219–27.

7. R. Masironi, "Geochemistry, Soils, and Cardiovascular Diseases," *Experientia* 43.1 (1987): 68–74.

8. M. Moser, "Current Recommendations for the Treatment of Hypertension: Are They Still Valid?" *Journal of Hypertension Supplement* 20.1 (2002): S3–10.

9. M. Raicu and S. Florea, "Deleterious Effects of Nifedipine on Smooth Muscle Cells Implies Alterations

of Intracellular Calcium Signaling," *Fundamental and Clinical Pharmacology* 15.6 (2001): 387–92.

10. L. Brambilla et al., "Potassium Depletion and Salt Sensitivity in Essential Hypertension," *Journal of Clinical Endocrinology and Metabolism* 86.6 (2001): 2857–62.

11. L. J. Beilin et al., "Lifestyle and Hypertension," *American Journal of Hypertension* 12.9, Part 1 (1999): 934–45.

12. A. Akbay et al., "Effect of Potassium Citrate Therapy on Stone Recurrence and Residual Fragments After Shockwave Lithotripsy in Lower Caliceal Calcium Oxalate Urolithiasis: A Randomized Controlled Trial," *Journal of Endourology* 16.3 (2002): 149–52.

13. D. E. Sellmeyer et al., "Potassium Citrate Prevents Increased Urine Calcium Excretion and Bone Resorption Induced by a High Sodium Chloride Diet," *Journal of Clinical Endocrinology and Metabolism* 87.5 (2002): 2008–12.

14. R. H. Dressendorfer et al., "Mineral Metabolism in Male Cyclists During High-Intensity Endurance Training," *International Journal of Sport Nutrition and Exercise Metabolism* 12.1 (2002): 63–72.

15. D. E. Sellmeyer et al.

16. T. D. Mickleborough et al., "Dietary Salt Alters Pulmonary Function During Exercise in Exercise-Induced Asthmatics," *Journal of Sports Science* 19.11 (2001): 865–73.

17. C. Hamelink et al., "Coincident Elevation of cAMP and Calcium Influx by PACAP-27 Synergistically Regulates Vasoactive Intestinal Polypeptide Gene Transcription Through a Novel PKA-Independent Signaling Pathway," *Journal of Neuroscience* 22.13 (2002): 5310–20.

18. H. Rhim et al., "Ginseng and Ginsenoside Rg3, a Newly Identified Active Ingredient of Ginseng, Modulate ca2+ Channel Currents in Rat Sensory Neurons," *European Journal of Pharmacology* 436.3 (2002): 151–58.

19. R. Liu et al., "Forskolin Upregulation of NOS I protein expression in Porcine Ciliary Processes: A New Aspect of Aqueous Humor Regulation," *Klinische Monatsblätter für Augenheilkunde* 219.4 (2002): 281–83.

20. W. C. van Staveren et al., "The Effects of Phosphodiesterase Inhibition on Cyclic GMP and Cyclic AMP Accumulation in the Hippocampus of the Rat," *Brain Research* 888.2 (2001): 275–86.

21. E. Bajna et al., "Dietary Calcium and Growth Modulation of Human Colon Cancer Cells: Role of the Extracellular Calcium-Sensing Receptor," *Cancer Detection and Prevention* 24.2 (2000): 127–36.

22. M. L. Powell et al., "The Role of Calcium in Health and Disease," *American Journal of Obstetrics and Gynecology* 181.6 (1999): 1560–69.

23. R. Rylander et al., "Moderate Alcohol Consumption and Urinary Excretion of Magnesium and Calcium," *Scandinavian Journal of Clinical Laboratory Investigation* 61.5 (2001): 401–05.

24. E. O. Ojuka et al., "Regulation of GLUT4 Biogenesis in Muscle: Evidence for Involvement of AMPK and ca(2+)," *American Journal of Physiology and Endocrinology Metabolism* 282.5 (2002): E1008–13.

25. R. P. Glahn et al., "Inhibition of Iron Uptake by Phytic Acid, Tannic Acid, and zncl2: Studies Using an In Vitro Digestion/Caco-2 Cell Model," *Journal of Agricultural and Food Chemistry* 50.2 (2002): 390–95.

26. Z. K. Roughead et al., "Initial Uptake and Absorption of Nonheme Iron and Absorption of Heme Iron

in Humans Are Unaffected by the Addition of Calcium as Cheese to a Meal with High Iron Bioavailability," *American Journal of Clinical Nutrition* 76.2 (2002): 419–25.

27. K. E. Scholz-Ahrens and J. Schrezenmeir, "Effects of Bioactive Substances in Milk on Mineral and Trace-Element Metabolism with Special Reference to Casein Phosphopeptides," *British Journal of Nutrition* 84, Supplement 1 (2000): S147–53.

28. F. Perez-Llamas et al., "Influence of Dietary Protein Type and Iron Source on the Absorption of Amino Acids and Minerals," *Journal of Physiology and Biochemistry* 57.4 (2001): 321–28.

29. M. Kamao et al., "Absorption of Calcium, Magnesium, Phosphorus, Iron, and Zinc in Growing Male Rats Fed Diets Containing Either Phytate-Free Soybean Protein or Soybean Protein Isolate or Casein," *Journal of Nutritional Science and Vitaminology* 46.1 (2000): 34–41.

30. D. J. Shaskey and G. A. Green, "Sports Haematology," *Sports Medicine* 29.1 (2000): 27–38.

31. H. C. Lukaski et al., "Interactions Among Dietary Fat, Mineral Status, and Performance of Endurance Athletes: A Case Study," *International Journal of Sport Nutrition and Exercise Metabolism* 11.2 (2002): 186–98.

32. J. Beard and B. Tobin, "Iron Status and Exercise," *American Journal of Clinical Nutrition* 72.2 Supplement (2000): 594S–97S.

33. D. J. Shaskey et al.

34. A. Paolicchi et al., "Gamma-Glutamyl Transpeptidase-Dependent Iron Reduction and LDL Oxidation: A Potential Mechanism in Atherosclerosis," *Journal of Investigative Medicine* 47.3 (1999): 151–60.

35. K. Chen et al., "Vitamin C Suppresses Oxidative Lipid Damage In Vivo, Even in the Presence of Iron Overload," *American Journal of Physiology: Endocrinology Metabolism* 279.6 (2000): E1406–12.

36. Anna Proteggente et al., "Iron Supplementation and Oxidative Damage to DNA in Healthy Individuals with High Plasma Ascorbate," *Biochemical and Biophysical Research Communications* 288.1 (2002): 245–51.

37. A. Rehman et al., "The Effects of Iron and Vitamin C Co-Supplementation on Oxidative Damage to DNA in Healthy Volunteers," *Biochemical and Biophysical Research Communications* 246.1 (1998): 293–98.

38. K. Summers, "Iron, Infection, and the Evolutionary Ecology of Heart Disease," *Medical Hypotheses* 56.5 (2001): 687–90.

39. C. Ratledge and L. G. Dover, "Iron Metabolism in Pathogenic Bacteria," *Annual Review of Microbiology* 54 (2000): 881–941.

40. S. A. Messina and R. Dawson, "Attenuation of Oxidative Damage to DNA by Taurine and Taurine Analogs," *Advances in Experimental Medicine and Biology* 483 (2000): 355–67.

41. M. A. Sochaski et al., "Lipid Peroxidation and Protein Modification in a Mouse Model of Chronic Iron Overload," *Metabolism* 51.5 (2002): 645–51.

42. P. P. Ward et al., "Lactoferrin and Host Defense," *Biochemistry and Cell Biology* 80.1 (2002): 95–102.

43. A. Marquet et al., "Biosynthesis of Biotin and Lipoic Acid," *Vitamins and Hormones* 61 (2001): 51–101.

44. Ananda S. Prasad, "Zinc in Human Health: An Update," *Journal of Trace Elements in Experimental Medicine* 11.2–3 (1998): 63–87.

45. A. Valencia-Sanchez et al., "Effectiveness of Calcium and Magnesium on Testicular Sulfatase Activity," *Archives of Andrology* 30.2 (1993): 129–36.

46. Ayhan O. Cavdar et al., "Blood Zinc (Plasma, Red Blood Cell Zinc) and Insulinike Growth Factor-1 in Children from an 'Impoverished' Area in Ankara," *Journal of Trace Elements in Experimental Medicine* 14.1 (2001): 31–34.

47. Ananda S. Prasad.

48. R. S. MacDonald, "The Role of Zinc in Growth and Cell Proliferation," *Journal of Nutrition* 130.5S Supplement (2000): 1500S–1508S.

49. J. Kumpulainen, "Selenium Status of Exclusively Breast-Fed Infants as Influenced by Maternal Organic or Inorganic Selenium Supplementation," *American Journal of Clinical Nutrition* 42.5 (1985): 829–35.

50. K. M. Brown and J. R. Arthur, "Selenium, Selenoproteins, and Human Health: A Review," *Public Health Nutrition* 4.2B (2001): 593–99.

51. Corinne H. Robinson, et al., *Normal and Therapeutic Nutrition*, 17th ed. (New York: Macmillan, 1986) 133.

52. S. Bolkent et al., "Protective Effects of DL-Alpha-Tocopherol Acetate and Sodium Selenate on the Liver of Rats Exposed to Gamma Radiation," *Biological Trace Element Research* 83.3 (2001: 263–73.

53. W. Li et al., "The Prevention of Primary Liver Cancer by Selenium in High-Risk Populations," *Chinese Journal of Preventive Medicine* 34.6 (2000): 336–38.

54. K. M. Brown and J. R. Arthur.

55. Marie V. Krause and L. Kathleen Mahan, *Food, Nutrition, and Diet Therapy*, 7th ed. (Philadelphia: Saunders, 1984) 177.

56. J. B. Vincent, "Elucidating a Biological Role for Chromium at a Molecular Level," *Accounts of Chemical Research* 33.7 (2000): 503–10.

57. R. A. Anderson, "Nutritional Factors Influencing the Glucose/Insulin System: Chromium," *Journal of the American College of Nutrition* 16.5 (1997): 404–10.

58. S. Davies et al., "Age-Related Decreases in Chromium Levels in 51,665 Hair, Sweat, and Serum Samples from 40,872 Patients: Implications for the Prevention of Cardiovascular Disease and Type II Diabetes Mellitus," *Metabolism* 46.5 (1997): 469–73.

59. S. M. Bahijiri et al., "The Effects of Inorganic Chromium and Brewer's Yeast Supplementation on Glucose Tolerance, Serum Lipids and Drug Dosage in Individuals with Type II Diabetes," *Saudi Medical Journal* 21.9 (2000): 831–37.

60. V. V. Snitynskyi, et al., "Biological Role of Chromium in Humans and Animals," *Ukrains'kyi biokhimichnyi zhurnal* 71.2 (1999): 5–9.

61. S. L. Volpe et al., "Effect of Chromium Supplementation and Exercise on Body Composition, Resting Metabolic Rate, and Selected Biochemical Parameters in Moderately Obese Women Following an Exercise Program," *Journal of the American College of Nutrition* 20.4 (2001): 293–306.

62. P. Amato et al., "Effects of Chromium Picolinate Supplementation on Insulin Sensitivity, Serum Lipids, and Body Composition in Healthy, Non-Obese, Older Men and Women," *Journals of Gerontology: Series A—Biological Sciences and Medical Sciences* 55.5 (2000): M260–63.

63. L. J. Farrell et al., "Effect of Resistance Training with or Without Chromium Picolinate Supplementation on Glucose Metabolism in Older Men and Women," *Metabolism* 48.5 (1999): 546–53.

64. J. B. Vincent, "The Biochemistry of Chromium," *Journal of Nutrition* 130.4 (2000): 715–18

65. W. Mertz, "Chromium in Human Nutrition: A Review," *Journal of Nutrition* 124.1 (1994): 117–19.

66. James L. Groff and Sareen Gropper, *Advanced Nutrition and Human Metabolism*, 3rd ed. (Belmont, CA: West/Wadsworth, 2000) 446–49.

67. W. Mertz, "Effects and Metabolism of Glucose Tolerance Factor," *Nutrition Reviews* (1975): 128–37.

68. J. B. Vincent, "Mechanisms of Chromium Action: Low-Molecular-Weight Chromium-Binding Substance," *Journal of the American College of Nutrition* 18.1 (1999): 6–12.

69. C. M. Davis and J. B. Vincent, "Chromium Oligopeptide Activates Insulin Receptor Tyrosine Kinase Activity," *Biochemistry* 36.15 (1997): 4382–85.

70. J. C. Molero et al., "Activation of MAP Kinase by Insulin and Vanadate in Adipocytes from Young and Old Rats," *Molecular and Cellular Endocrinology* 189.1–2 (2002): 77–84.

71. P. Arivazhagan et al., "Effect of DL-Alpha Lipoic Acid on Glutathione Metabolic Enzymes in Aged Rats," *Experimental Gerontology* 37.1 (2001): 81–87.

72. S. Khanna et al., "Alpha Lipoic Acid Supplementation: Tissue Glutathione Homeostasis at Rest and After Exercise," *Journal of Applied Physiology* 86.4 (1999): 1191–96.

73. B. Hultberg et al., "Lipoic Acid Increases Glutathione Production and Enhances the Effect of Mercury in Human Cell Lines," *Toxicology* 175.1-3 (2002): 103–10.

74. E. Senn et al., "Effects of Glutathione and of Cysteine on Intestinal Absorption of Selenium from Selenite," *Biological Trace Element Research* 33 (April-June 1992): 103–08.

75. L. J. Dahm and D. P. Jones, "Secretion of Cysteine and Glutathione from Mucosa to Lumen in Rat Small Intestine," *American Journal of Physiology* 267.2, Part 1 (1994): G292–300.

76. O. Benard and K. A. Balasubramanian, "Effect of Oxidant Exposure on Thiol Status in the Intestinal Mucosa," *Biochemical Pharmacology* 45.10 (1993): 2011–15.

77. S. M. Bahijiri, "Effect of Chromium Supplementation on Glucose Tolerance and Lipid Profile," *Saudi Medical Journal* 21.1 (2000): 45–50.

78. S. M. Bahijiri et al., "The Effects of Inorganic Chromium and Brewer's Yeast Supplementation," *Saudi Medical Journal* 21.9 (2000): 831–37.

79. M. Capellmann and H. M. Bolt, "Chromium (VI)–Reducing Capacity of Ascorbic Acid and of Human Plasma In Vitro," *Archives of Toxicology* 66.1 (1992): 45–50.

80. M. N. McLeod, "Chromium Potentiation of Antidepressant Pharmacotherapy for Dysthymic Disorder in Five Patients," *Journal of Clinical Psychiatry* 60.4 (1999): 237–40.

81. H. Nonaka et al., "Taurine Prevents the Decrease in Expression and Secretion of Extracellular Superoxide Dismutase Induced by Homocysteine: Amelioration of Homocysteine-Induced Endoplasmic Reticulum Stress by Taurine," *Circulation* 104.10 (2001): 1165–70.

82. X. Q. Liu and Y. H. Li, "Epidemiological and Nutritional Research on Prevention of Cardiovascular

Disease in China," *British Journal of Nutrition* 84, Supplement 2 (December 2000): S199–203.

83. J. Gustavsson et al., "Translocation of Insulin-Regulated Glucose Transporter Is Stimulated by Long-Chain 1,2-Diacylglycerol in Rat Adipocytes," *Experimental Cell Research* 221.2 (1995): 438–42.

84. S. Parcell, "Sulfur in Human Nutrition and Applications in Medicine," *Alternative Medicine Review* 7.1 (2002): 22–44.

85. R. Studer et al., "N-Acetyl Cysteine Down-Regulates Beta-Amyloid Precursor Protein Gene Transcription in Human Neuroblastoma Cells," *Biogerontology* 2.1 (2001): 55–60.

86. Ibid.

87. E. Barrager et al., "A Multicentered, Open-Label Trial on the Safety and Efficacy of Methylsulfonylmethane in the Treatment of Seasonal Allergic Rhinitis," *Journal of Alternative and Complementary Medicine* 8.2 (2002): 167–73.

88. M. S. Venikova et al., "Effect of Dimethylsulfoxide and Dimethylsulfone on a Destructive Process in the Joints of Mice with Spontaneous Arthritis," *Patologicheskaia Fiziologiia Eksperimentalnaia Terapiia* 2 (March-April 1991): 37–39.

89. S. J. Childs, "Dimethylsulfone (DMSO2) in the Treatment of Interstitial Cystitis," *Urologic Clinics of North America* 21.1 (1994): 85–88.

90. L. E. McGann and M. L. Walterson, "Cryoprotection by Dimethylsulfoxide and Dimethylsulfone," *Cryobiology* 24.1 (1987): 11–16

91. J. I. Morton and B. V. Siegel, "Effects of Oral Dimethylsulfoxide and Dimethylsulfone on Murine Autoimmune Lymphoproliferative Disease," *Proceedings of the Society for Experimental Biology and Medicine* 183.2 (1986): 227–30.

92. R. B. Jeppsen, "Toxicology and Safety of Ferrochel and Other Iron Amino-Acid Chelates," *Archivos Latinoamericanos Nutricion* 51.1, Supplement1 (2001): 26–34.

93. R. B. Jeppsen and J. F. Borzelleca, "Safety Evaluation of Ferrous Bisglycinate Chelate," *Food and Chemical Toxicology* 37.7 (1999): 723–31.

94. Oscar Pineda et al., "Effectiveness of Iron Amino-Acid Chelate on the Treatment of Iron Deficiency Anemia in Adolescents," *Journal of Applied Nutrition* 45.1–2 (1994).

95. Maggie Coplin et al., "Tolerability of Iron: A Comparison of Bisglycino Iron II and Ferrous Sulfate," *Clinical Therapeutics* 13.5 (1991).

96. E. J. Brink et al., "Interaction of Calcium and Phosphate Decreases Ileal Magnesium Solubility and Apparent Magnesium Absorption in Rats," *Journal of Nutrition* 122.3 (1992): 580–86.

97. T. Vaskonen et al., Diet Enrichment with Calcium and Magnesium Enhances the Cholesterol-Lowering Effect of Plant Sterols in Obese Zucker Rats," *Nutrition and Metabolism: Cardiovascular Disease* 11.3 (2001): 158–67.

98. Sally A. Schuette et al., "Bioavailability of Magnesium Diglycinate Versus Magnesium Oxide in Patients with Ileal Resection," *Journal of Parenteral and Enteral Nutrition* 18.5 (1994): 430–35.

99. M. Gawaz et al., "Platelet Function and Platelet-Leukocyte Adhesion in Symptomatic Coronary Heart Disease. Effects of Intravenous Magnesium," *Thrombosis Research* 83.5 (September 1996): 341–49.

100. L. S. Zijenah et al., "Platelet Adhesion to Collagen. Factors Affecting mg2(+)-Dependent and Bivalent-Cation-Independent Adhesion," *Biochemical Journal* 268.2 (1990): 481–86.

101. M. Gross, "Nutrition in Chronic Inflammatory Bowel Diseases: What Your Patient Tolerates Is Permitted," *mmw Fortschritte der Medizin* 144.3–4 (2002): 40–43.

Chapter 8: Minerals: Metabolic Miracles

1. S. Persson-Sjogren and G. Sjogren, "Effects of Dental Materials on Insulin Release from Isolated Islets of Langerhans," *Dental Materials* 18.1 (2002): 20–25.

2. A. Mohammad et al., "In Vivo Effects of Vanadium in Diabetic Rats Are Independent of Changes in pi-3 Kinase Activity in Skeletal Muscle," *Molecular and Cellular Biochemistry* 223.1–2 (2001): 103–08.

3. F. Chen et al., "Carcinogenic Metals and nf-kappa-b Activation," *Molecular and Cellular Biochemistry* 222.1–2 (2001): 159–71.

4. A. M. Evangelou, "Vanadium in Cancer Treatment," *Critical Reviews in Oncology/Hematology* 42.3 (2002): 249–65.

5. John H. McNeill et al., "Mechanisms of Vanadium Action: Insulin-Mimetic or Insulin-Enhancing Agent," published on the National Research Council Press Web site, September 14, 2000.

6. Allison B. Goldfine et al., "Metabolic Effects of Sodium Metavanadate in Humans with Insulin-Dependent and Non-Insulin-Dependent Diabetes Mellitus In Vivo and In Vitro Studies," *Journal of Clinical Endocrinology and Metabolism* 80: 3311–21.

7. Mayer Halberstam et al., "Oral Vanadyl Sulfate Improves Insulin Sensitivity in niddm but Not Obese Non-Diabetic Subjects," *Diabetes* 45 (May 1996): 659–66.

8. Neil Cohen et al., "Oral Vanadyl Sulfate Improves Peripheral Insulin Sensitivity in Patients with Non-Insulin-Dependent Diabetes Mellitus," *Journal of Clinical Investigation* 95 (June 1995): 2501–09.

9. Guenther Boden et al., "Effects of Vanadyl Sulfate on Carbohydrate and Lipid Metabolism in Patients with Non-Insulin-Dependent Diabetes Mellitus," *Metabolism* 45.9 (1996): 1130–35.

10. Allison Goldfine et al., "In Vivo and In Vitro Studies of Vanadate in Human and Rodent Diabetes Mellitus," *Molecular and Cellular Biochemistry* 153 (1995): 217–31.

11. J. Hajjar et al., "Effect of Vanadate on Amino-Acid Transport in the Rat Jejunum," *Proceedings of the Society for Experimental Biology and Medicine* 184 (1987): 403–09.

12. John H. McNeill et al.

13. Ibid.

14. Ibid.

15. Vlaire M. Steppan, "The Hormone Resistin Links Obesity to Diabetes," *Nature* 409.6818 (2001): 307–12.

16. Allison B. Goldfine et al., "Metabolic Effects of Sodium Metavanadate in Humans with Insulin-Dependent and Non-Insulin-Dependent Diabetes Mellitus In Vivo and In Vitro Studies," *Journal of Clinical Endocrinology and Metabolism* 80.11 (1995): 3311–20.

17. U. A. Shinde, "Effect of Chronic Treatment with Bis(Maltolato)Oxovanadium (IV) in Rat Model of Non-Insulin-Dependent Diabetes," *Indian Journal of Experimental Biology* 2001 39.9 (2001): 864–70.

Chapter 9: General Fat Facts

1. A. Drewnowski et al., "Taste Responses and Preferences for Sweet High-Fat Foods: Evidence for Opioid Involvement," *Physiology and Behavior* 51.2: 371–79.

2. M. E. Mercer and M. D. Holder, "Food Cravings, Endogenous Opioid Peptides, and Food Intake: A Review," *Appetite* 29.3 (1997): 325–52.

3. K. A. Gendall et al., "The Effects of Meal Composition on Subsequent Craving and Binge Eating," *Addictive Behaviors* 24.3 (1999): 305–15.

4. A. J. Hill et al., "Food Craving, Dietary Restraint, and Mood," *Appetite* 17.3 (1991): 187–97.

5. J. Harvey et al., "Effects on Food Cravings of a Very Low-Calorie Diet or a Balanced, Low-Calorie Diet," *Appetite* 21.2 (1993): 105–15.

6. L. Christensen and L. Pettijohn, "Mood and Carbohydrate Cravings," *Appetite* 3.2 (2001): 137–45.

7. J. J. Wurtman, "Carbohydrate Cravings: A Disorder of Food Intake and Mood," *Clinical Neuropharmacology* 11, Supplement 1 (1988): S139–45.

8. L. Christensen and S. Somers, "Comparison of Nutrient Intake Among Depressed and Nondepressed Individuals," *International Journal of Eating Disorders* 20.1 (1996): 105–09.

9. P. M. Kris-Etherton et al., "High-Monounsaturated Fatty-Acid Diets Lower Both Plasma Cholesterol and Triacylglycerol Concentrations," *American Journal of Clinical Nutrition* 70.6 (1999): 1009–15.

10. C. M. Williams, "Beneficial Nutritional Properties of Olive Oil: Implications for Postprandial Lipoproteins and Factor VII," *Nutrition and Metabolism: Cardiovascular Disease* 11.4, Supplement (2001): 51–56.

11. C. M. Kelly et al., "Dietary Monounsaturated Fatty Acids and Haemostasis," *Proceedings of the Nutrition Society* 60.2 (2001): 161–70.

12. F. F. Lauszus et al., "Effect of a High Monounsaturated Fatty-Acid Diet on Blood Pressure and Glucose Metabolism in Women with Gestational Diabetes Mellitus," *European Journal of Clinical Nutrition* 55.6 (2001): 436–43.

13. R. de la Puerta et al., "Protective Effects Upon Experimental Inflammation Models of a Polyphenol-Supplemented Virgin Olive Oil Diet," *Inflammation Research* 50.2 (2001): 102–06.

14. Ibid.

15. M. D. Herrera et al., "Effects of Dietary Oleic-Rich Oils (Virgin Olive and High-Oleic-Acid Sunflower) on Vascular Reactivity in Wistar-Kyoto and Spontaneously Hypertensive Rats," *British Journal of Nutrition* 86.3 (2001): 349–57.

16. F. Visiol and C. Galli, "Biological Properties of Olive Oil Phytochemicals," *Critical Reviews in Food Science and Nutrition* 42.3 (2002): 209–21.

17. M. Fito et al., "Postprandial and Short-Term Effects of Dietary Virgin Olive Oil on Oxidant/Antioxidant Status," *Lipids* 37.3 (2002): 245–51.

18. J. C. Lovejoy, "Dietary Fatty Acids and Insulin Resistance," *Current Atherosclerosis Reports* 1.3 (1999): 215–20.

19. R. N. Lemaitre et al., "Cell Membrane Trans Fatty Acids and the Risk of Primary Cardiac Arrest," *Circulation* 105.6 (2002): 697–701.

20. D. W. Lamson and S. M. Plaza, "Mitochondrial Factors in the Pathogenesis of Diabetes: A Hypothesis for Treatment," *Alternative Medicine Review* 7.2 (2002): 94–111.

21. J. B. Dictenberg et al., "Hyperlipidemic Effects of Trans Fatty Acids Are Accentuated by Dietary Cholesterol in Gerbils," *Journal of Nutritional Biochemistry* 6.7 (1995): 353–61.

22. A. Valenzuela and N. Morgado, "Trans Fatty Acid Isomers in Human Health and in the Food Industry," *Biological Research* 32.4 (1999): 273–87.

23. R. N. Lemaitre et al.

24. M. L. Slattery et al., "Trans Fatty Acids and Colon Cancer," *Nutrition and Cancer* 39.2 (2001): 170–75.

25. J. C. Lovejoy.

26. F. B. Hu et al., "Diet and Risk of Type II Diabetes: The Role of Types of Fat and Carbohydrate," *Diabetologia* 44.7 (2001): 805–17.

27. A. P. Simopoulos, "Is Insulin Resistance Influenced by Dietary Linoleic Acid and Trans Fatty Acids?" *Free Radical Biology and Medicine* 17.4 (1994): 367–72.

28. M. Taouis et al., "N-3 Polyunsaturated Fatty Acids Prevent the Defect of Insulin-Receptor Signaling in Muscle," *American Journal of Physiology: Endocrinology and Metabolism* 282.3 (2002): E664–71.

29. T. Shimura et al., "Docosahexaenoic Acid (DHA) Improved Glucose and Lipid Metabolism in KK-Ay Mice with Genetic Non-Insulin-Dependent Diabetes Mellitus (NIDDM)," *Biological and Pharmaceutical Bulletin* 20.5 (1997): 507–10.

30. Y. J. Huang et al., "Amelioration of Insulin Resistance and Hypertension in a Fructose-Fed Rat Model with Fish-Oil Supplementation," *Metabolism* 46.11 (1997): 1252–58.

31. D. R. Sullivan et al., "The Effects of Dietary N-3 Fatty Acid in Animal Models of Type I and Type II Diabetes," *Diabetes Research and Clinical Practice* 9.3 (1990): 225–30.

32. Shiro Urano et al., "Aging and Oxidative Stress in Neurodegeneration," *BioFactors* 7.1–2 (1998): 103–112.

33. P. Haban et al., "The Effect of N-3-Fatty-Acid Administration on Selected Indicators of Cardiovascular Disease Risk in Patients with Type II Diabetes Mellitus," *Bratislavske Lekarkse Listy* 99.1 (1998): 37–42.

34. M. Morishita et al., "The Dose-Related Hypoglycemic Effects of Insulin Emulsions Incorporating Highly Purified EPA and DHA," *International Journal of Pharmaceutics* 201.2 (2000): 175–85.

35. T. Raclot et al., "Site-Specific Regulation of Gene Expression by N-3 Polyunsaturated Fatty Acids in Rat White Adipose Tissues," *Journal of Lipid Research* 38.10 (1997): 1963–72.

36. R. W. Cook, "Incorporation, Metabolism, and Positional Distribution of Trans Unsaturated Fatty Acids in Developing and Mature Brain: Comparison of Elaidate and Oleate Administered Intracerebrally," *Biochimica et Biophysica Acta* 531.3 (1978): 245–56.

37. J. M. Bourre et al., "Peripheral Nerve Cells in Culture Rich in Schwann Cells Incorporate and Metabolize Trans Unsaturated Fatty Acid (Elaidic Acid) as Well as Physiological cis Isomer (Oleic Acid)," *Neuroscience Letters* 30.2 (1982): 173–78.

38. P. M. Kidd, "Multiple Sclerosis, an Autoimmune Inflammatory Disease: Prospects for Its Integrative Management," *Alternative Medicine Review* 6.6 (2001): 540–66.

39. I. Nordvik et al., "Effect of Dietary Advice and N-3 Supplementation in Newly Diagnosed MS Patients," *Acta Neurologica Scandinavica* 102.3 (2000): 143–49.

40. P. C. Calder, "N-3 Polyunsaturated Fatty Acids and Cytokine Production in Health and Disease," *Annals of Nutrition and Metabolism* 41.4 (1997): 203–34.

41. A. Kilkkinen et al., "Use of Oral Antimicrobials Decreases Serum Enterolactone Concentration," *American Journal of Epidemiology* 155.5 (2002): 472–77.

42. C. M. Bendel et al., "Cecal Colonization and Systemic Spread of Candida Albicans in Mice Treated with Antibiotics and Dexamethasone," *Pediatric Research* 51.3 (2002): 290–95.

43. Y. Takesue et al., "Changes in Intestinal Flora After Administration of Panipenem/Betamipron or Sulbactam/Cefoperazone for Treatment of Postoperative Infections in Gastrectomy Patients," *Journal of Infection and Chemotherapy* 5.1 (1999): 52–57.

44. A. Sullivan et al., "Effect of Antimicrobial Agents on the Ecological Balance of Human Microflora," *The Lancet: Infectious Diseases* 1.2 (2002): 101–14.

45. M. V. Valtonen et al., "Selection of Multi-Resistant Coliforms by Long-Term Treatment of Hypercholesterolaemia with Neomycin," *British Medical Journal* 1.6062 (1977): 683–84.

46. O. Feron et al., "Hypercholesterolemia Decreases Nitric-Oxide Production by Promoting the Interaction of Caveolin and Endothelial Nitric-Oxide Synthase," *Journal of Clinical Investigation* 103.6 (1999): 897–905.

47. P. Gorog and I. B. Kovacs, "Inhibition of Vascular Smooth Muscle Cell Migration by Intact Endothelium Is Nitric-Oxide-Mediated: Interference by Oxidized Low-Density Lipoproteins," *Journal of Vascular Research* 35.3 (1998): 165–69.

48. F. L. Crane, "Biochemical Functions of Coenzyme Q10," *Journal of the American College of Nutrition* 20.6 (2001): 591–98.

49. F. L. Rosenfeldt et al., "Coenzyme Q10 Protects the Aging Heart Against Stress: Studies in Rats, Human Tissues, and Patients," *Annals of the New York Academy of Sciences* 959 (April 2002): 355–59; discussion 463–65.

50. "Extra Coenzyme Q10 for Statin Users?" *TreatmentUpdate* 13.2 (2001): 4–7.

51. J. H. Cummings and G. T. Macfarlane, "Gastrointestinal Effects of Prebiotics," *British Journal of Nutrition* 87, Supplement 2: 145–51.

52. H. Haller et al., "The Role of Hyperglycemia and Hyperinsulinemia in the Pathogenesis of Diabetic Angiopathy," *Clinical Nephrology* 46.4 (1996): 246–55.

53. Marie V. Krause and L. Kathleen Mahan, *Food, Nutrition, and Diet Therapy*, 7th ed. (Philadelphia: Saunders, 1984) 566.

Chapter 10: Fats of Life

1. M. Hashimoto et al., "Docosahexaenoic Acid Provides Protection from Impairment of Learning Ability in Alzheimer's Disease Model Rats," *Journal of Neurochemistry* 81.5 (2002): 1084–91.

2. E. A. Mitchell et al., "Clinical Characteristics and Serum Essential Fatty-Acid Levels in Hyperactive Children," *Clinical Pediatrics* (Philadelphia) 26.8 (1987): 406–11.

3. J. R. Burgess et al., "Long-Chain Polyunsaturated Fatty Acids in Children with Attention-Deficit Hyperactivity Disorder," *American Journal of Clinical Nutrition* 71.1, Supplement (2000): 327S–30S.

4. M. T. Fillmore and C. R. Rush, "Impaired Inhibitory Control of Behavior in Chronic Cocaine Users," *Drug and Alcohol Dependence* 66.3 (2002): 265–73.

5. D. D. Martin et al., "The Fatty-Acid Composition of Human Gliomas Differs from That Found in Nonmalignant Brain Tissue," *Lipids* 31.12 (1996): 1283–88.

6. B. A. Stoll, "N-3 Fatty Acids and Lipid Peroxidation in Breast Cancer Inhibition," *British Journal of Nutrition* 87.3 (2002): 193–98.

7. J. L. Deferne and A. R. Leeds, "Resting Blood Pressure and Cardiovascular Reactivity to Mental Arithmetic in Mild Hypertensive Males Supplemented with Blackcurrant Seed Oil," *Journal of Human Hypertension* 10.8 (1996): 531–37.

8. J. M. Frenoux et al., "A Polyunsaturated Fatty-Acid Diet Lowers Blood Pressure and Improves Antioxidant Status in Spontaneously Hypertensive Rats," *Journal of Nutrition* 131.1 (2001): 39–45.

9. A. Colquhoun, "Gamma Linolenic Acid Alters the Composition of Mitochondrial Membrane Subfractions, Decreases Outer Mitochondrial Membrane Binding of Hexokinase, and Alters Carnitine Palmitoyltransferase I Properties in the Walker 256 Rat Tumor," *Biochimica et Biophysica Acta* 1583.1 (2002): 74–84.

10. U. N. Das, "Abrupt and Complete Occlusion of Tumor-Feeding Vessels by Gamma Linolenic Acid," *Nutrition* 18.7–8 (2002): 662–64.

11. J. A. Menendez et al., "Synergistic Interaction Between Vinorelbine and Gamma-Linolenic Acid in Breast Cancer Cells," *Breast Cancer Research and Treatment* 72.3 (2002): 203–19.

12. J. M. Parker-Barnes et al., "Identification and Characterization of an Enzyme Involved in the Elongation of N-6 and N-3 Polyunsaturated Fatty Acids," *Proceedings of the National Academy of Sciences of the United States of America* 97.15 (2000): 8284–89.

13. J. B. Barham et al., "Addition of Eicosapentaenoic Acid to Gamma-Linolenic-Acid-Supplemented Diets Prevents Serum Arachidonic-Acid Accumulation in Humans," *Journal of Nutrition* 130.8 (2000): 1925–31.

14. S. A. Metz, "Exogenous Arachidonic Acid Promotes Insulin Release from Intact or Permeabilized Rat Islets by Dual Mechanisms: Putative Activation of ca2+ Mobilization and Protein Kinase c," *Diabetes* 37.11 (1988): 1453–69.

15. E. Demcakova et al., "Delta-6 Desaturase Activity and Gene Expression, Tissue Fatty-Acid Profile, and Glucose Turnover Rate in Hereditary Hypertriglyceridemic Rats," *Endocrine Regulations* 35.4 (2001): 179–86.

16. B. Vessby, "Dietary Fat and Insulin Action in Humans," *British Journal of Nutrition* 83, Supplement 1 (2000): S91–96.

17. J. B. Barham et al.

18. K. P. Quoc and M. Pascaud, "Effects of Dietary Gamma Linolenic Acid on the Tissue Phospholipid Fatty-Acid Composition and the Synthesis of Eicosanoids in Rats," *Annals of Nutrition and Metabolism* 40.2 (1996): 99–108.

19. C. C. Miller and V. A. Ziboh, "Gamma-Linolenic-Acid-Enriched Diet Alters Cutaneous Eicosanoids," *Biochemical and Biophysical Research Communications* 154.3 (1988): 967–74.

20. D. F. Horrobin, "The Relationship Between Schizophrenia and Essential Fatty-Acid and Eicosanoid Metabolism," *Prostaglandins, Leukotrienes, and Essential Fatty Acids* 46.1 (1992): 71–77.

21. J. B. Barham et al.

22. S. Dalle et al., "Miniglucagon: A Local Regulator of Islet Physiology," *Annals of the New York Academy of Sciences* 865 (December 1998): 132–40.

23. C. L. Loizou et al., "The Effect of Insulin on Delta-5 Desaturation in HepG2 Human Hepatoma Cells and L6 Rat Muscle Myoblasts," *Prostaglandins, Leukotrienes, and Essential Fatty Acids* 61.2 (1999): 89–95.

24. B. Vessby.

25. L. C. Medeiros et al., "Insulin, But Not Estrogen, Correlated with Indexes of Desaturase Function in Obese Women," *Hormone and Metabolic Research* 27.5 (1995): 235–38.

26. T. Decsi et al., "Long-Chain Polyunsaturated Fatty Acids in Plasma Lipids of Obese Children," *Lipids* 31.3 (1996): 305–11.

27. S. el Boustani et al., "Direct In Vivo Characterization of Delta-5 Desaturase Activity in Humans by Deuterium Labeling: Effect of Insulin," *Metabolism* 38.4 (1989): 315–21.

28. D. Guigliano et al., "The Vascular Effects of L-Arginine in Humans: The Role of Endogenous Insulin," *Journal of Clinical Investigation* 99.3 (1997): 433–38.

29. P. Kubes et al., "Nitric Oxide and Intestinal Inflammation," *American Journal of Medicine* 109.2 (2000): 150–58.

30. O. Holian et al., "Inhibition of Gastric Cancer Cell Proliferation by Resveratrol: Role of Nitric Oxide," *American Journal of Physiology: Gastrointestinal and Liver Physiology* 282.5 (2002): G809–16.

31. K. Migita et al., "The Role of Peroxynitrite in Cyclo Oxygenase-2 Expression of Rheumatoid Synovium," *Clinical and Experimental Rheumatology* 20.1 (2002): 59–62.

32. Sergeeva Khramtsov, "Effect of Selenolipoic Acid on Peroxynitrite-Dependent Inactivation of NADPH-Cytochrome P450 Reductase," *Free Radical Research* 35.5 (2001): 491–97.

33. V. D. Belin et al., "Glucagon Decreases Cytokine Induction of Nitric-Oxide Synthase and Action on Insulin Secretion in RIN5F Cells and Rat and Human Islets of Langerhans," *Cytokine* 11.8 (1999): 585–92.

34. S. Nishida et al., "Long-Term Melatonin Administration Reduces Hyperinsulinemia and Improves the Altered Fatty-Acid Compositions in Type II Diabetic Rats Via the Restoration of Delta-5 Desaturase Activity," *Journal of Pineal Research* 32.1 (2002): 26–33.

35. Y. Yu et al., "Conjugated Linoleic Acid Decreases Production of Pro-Inflammatory Products in Macrophages: Evidence for a PPARgamma-Dependent Mechanism," *Biochimica et Biophysica Acta* 1581.3 (2002): 89–99.

36. J. B. Barham et al.

37. J. M. Parker-Barnes et al.

38. C. M. Nieuwenhuys et al., "Modulation of Rat-Platelet Activation by Vessel-Wall-Derived Prostaglandin and Platelet-Derived Thromboxane: Effects of Dietary Fish Oil on Thromboxane-Prostaglandin Balance," *Atherosclerosis* 154.2 (2001): 355–66.

39. C. Pirich et al., "Effects of Fish-Oil Supplementation on Platelet Survival and Ex Vivo Platelet Function in Hypercholesterolemic Patients," *Thrombosis Research* 96.3 (1999): 219–27.

40. E. Vericel et al., "The Influence of Low Intake of N-3 Fatty Acids on Platelets in Elderly People," *Atherosclerosis* 147.1 (1999): 187–92.

41. C. M. Fored et al., "Acetaminophen, Aspirin, and Chronic Renal Failure," *New England Journal of Medicine* 345.25 (2001): 1801–08.

42. P. Zhao and J. T. Slattery, "Effects of Ethanol Dose and Ethanol Withdrawal on Rat Liver Mitochondrial Glutathione: Implication of Potentiated Acetaminophen Toxicity in Alcoholics," *Drug Metabolism and Disposition* 30.12 (2002): 1413–17.

43. G. Wrathall et al., "Three Case Reports of the Use of Haemodiafiltration in the Treatment of Salicylate Overdose," *Human and Experimental Toxicology* 20.9 (2001): 491–95.

44. I. Manov et al., "Acetaminophen Hepatotoxicity and Mechanisms of Its Protection by N-Acetyl Cysteine: A Study of Hep3B Cells," *Experimental and Toxicologic Pathology* 53.6 (2002): 489–500.

45. S. D. Ray et al., "In Vivo Protection of DNA-Damage-Associated Apoptotic and Necrotic Cell Deaths During Acetaminophen-Induced Nephrotoxicity, Amiodarone-Induced Lung Toxicity and Doxorubicin-Induced Cardiotoxicity by a Novel IH636 Grapeseed Proanthocyanidin Extract," *Research Communications in Molecular Pathology and Pharmacology* 107.1–2 (2000): 137–66.

46. B. H. Lauterburg, "Analgesics and Glutathione," *American Journal of Therapeutics* 9.3 (2002): 225–33.

47. N. Vaisman and N. Arber, "The Role of Nutrition and Chemoprevention in Colorectal Cancer: from Observations to Expectations," *Best Practice and Research: Clinical Gastroenterology* 16.2 (2002): 201–17.

48. K. P. Wallace et al., "S-Adenosyl-L-Methionine (SAMe) for the Treatment of Acetaminophen Toxicity in a Dog," *Journal of the American Animal Hospital Association* 38.3 (2002): 246–54.

49. D. Bagchi et al., "Cellular Protection with Proanthocyanidins Derived from Grape Seeds," *Annals of the New York Academy of Sciences* 957 (May 2002): 260–70.

50. S. C. Lee et al., "Effects of Chinese Yam on Hepato-Nephrotoxicity of Acetaminophen in Rats," *Acta Pharmacologica Sinica* 23.6 (2002): 503–08.

51. S. Moalic et al., "A Plant Steroid, Diosgenin, Induces Apoptosis, Cell Cycle Arrest and COX Activity in Osteosarcoma Cell," *FEBS Letters* 506.3 (2001): 225–30.

Chapter 11: Clearing the Path

1. K. Migita et al., "The Role of Peroxynitrite in Cyclo-Oxygenase-2 Expression of Rheumatoid Synovium," *Clinical and Experimental Rheumatology* 20.1 (2002): 59–62.

2. M. D. Breyer et al., "Cyclo-Oxygenase-2 Selective Inhibitors and the Kidney," *Current Opinion in Critical Care* 7.6 (2001): 393–400.

3. J. Henao et al., "Celecoxib-Induced Acute Interstitial Nephritis," *American Journal of Kidney Diseases* 39.6 (2002): 1313–17.

4. K. E. Giercksky et al., "Selective Inhibitors of cox-2: Are They Safe for the Stomach?" *Scandinavian Journal of Gastroenterology* 35.11 (2000): 1121–24.

5. D. Baatar et al., "Selective Cyclo-Oxygenase-2 Blocker Delays Healing of Esophageal Ulcers in Rats and Inhibits Ulceration-Triggered C-Met/Hepatocyte Growth Factor Receptor Induction and Extracellular Signal-Regulated Kinase-2 Activation," *American Journal of Pathology* 160.3 (2002): 963–72.

6. O. M. Laudanno et al., "Celecoxib Vs. Indomethacin and Acute Gastric Lesions in Rats," *Medicina* (Buenos Aires) 60.2 (2000): 221–24.

7. O.M. Laudanno et al., "Gastrointestinal Damage Induced by Celecoxib and Rofecoxib in Rats," *Digestive Diseases and Sciences* 46.4 (2001): 779–84.

8. B. B. Fredholm and M. Hamberg, "Metabolism and Effect of Prostaglandin H2 in Adipose Tissue," *Prostaglandins* 11.3 (1976): 507–18.

9. B. Cannon et al., "Brown Adipose Tissue: More Than an Effector of Thermogenesis?" *Annals of the New York Academy of Sciences* 856 (September 1998): 171–87.

10. A. G. Dulloo et al., "Green Tea and Thermogenesis: Interactions Between Catechin-Polyphenols, Caffeine, and Sympathetic Activity," *International Journal of Obesity and Related Metabolic Disorders* 24.2 (2000): 252–58.

11. A. Astrup et al., "Pharmacology of Thermogenic Drugs," *American Journal of Clinical Nutrition* 55.1 Supplement (1992): 246S–48S.

12. A. G. Dulloo et al., "Peripheral Mechanisms of Thermogenesis Induced by Ephedrine 87.and Caffeine in Brown Adipose Tissue," *International Journal of Obesity* 15.5 (1991): 317–26.

13. R. Negrel, "Prostacyclin as a Critical Prostanoid in Adipogenesis," *Prostaglandins, Leukotrienes, and Essential Fatty Acids* 60.5–6 (1999): 383–86.

14. M. Monda et al., "NG Methyl-L-Arginine Increases the Hyperthermic Effects of Prostaglandin E1," *Journal of Physiology* (Paris) 90.2 (1996): 79–83.

15. P. Rohdewald, "A Review of the French Maritime Pine-Bark Extract (Pycnogenol), a Herbal Medication with a Diverse Clinical Pharmacology," *International Journal of Clinical Pharmacology and Therapeutics* 40.4 (2002): 158–68.

16. Lester Packer et al., "Enzyme Inhibition and Protein-Binding Action of the Procyanidin-Rich French Maritime Pine-Bark Extract, Pycnogenol: Effect on Xanthine Oxidase," *Journal of Agricultural and Food Chemistry* 48.11 (2000): 5630–39.

17. A. I. Schafer, "Effects of Nonsteroidal Anti-Inflammatory Therapy on Platelets," *American Journal of Medicine* 106.5B (1999): 25S–36S.

18. J. A. Mancini et al., "Nonsteroidal Anti-Inflammatory Drugs," *Molecular Pharmacology* 51.1 (1997): 52–60.

19. O. Boutaud et al., "Determinants of the Cellular Specificity of Acetaminophen as an Inhibitor of Prostaglandin H(2) Synthases," *Proceedings of the National Academy of Sciences of the United States of America* 99.10 (2002): 7130–35.

20. R. Amann and B. A. Peskar, "Anti-Inflammatory Effects of Aspirin and Sodium Salicylate," *European Journal of Pharmacology* 447.1 (2002): 1–9.

21. F. Giuliano et al., "Sodium Salicylate Inhibits Prostaglandin Formation Without Affecting the Induction of Cyclo Oxygenase-2 by Bacterial Lipopolysaccharide In Vivo," *Journal of Pharmacology and Experimental Therapeutics* 299.3 (2001): 894–900.

22. R. Amann and B. A. Peskar.

23. X. Shi et al., "Antioxidant Properties of Aspirin: Characterization of the Ability of Aspirin to Inhibit Silica-Induced Lipid Peroxidation, DNA damage, NF-kappa-B Activation, and TNF Alpha Production," *Molecular and Cellular Biochemistry* 199.1–2 (1999): 93–102.

24. J. Z. Haeggstrom and A. Wetterholm, "Enzymes and Receptors in the Leukotriene Cascade," *Cellular and Molecular Life Sciences* 59.5 (2002): 742–53.

25. M. Back, "Functional Characteristics of Cysteinyl-Leukotriene Receptor Subtypes," *Life Sciences* 71.6 (2002): 611–22.

26. R. M. McMillan, "Leukotrienes in Respiratory Disease," *Paediatric Respiratory Reviews* 2.3 (2001): 238–44.

27. M. Back, "Studies of Receptors and Modulatory Mechanisms in Functional Responses to Cysteinyl-Leukotrienes in Smooth Muscle," *Acta Physiologica Scandinavica: Supplementum* 648 (February 2002): 1–55.

28. L. Borish, "The Role of Leukotrienes in Upper and Lower Airway Inflammation and the Implications for Treatment," *Annals of Allergy, Asthma, and Immunology* 88.4, Supplement 1 (2002): 16–22.

29. H. Moini et al., "Enzyme Inhibition and Protein-Binding Action of the Procyanidin-Rich French Marine Pine-Bark Extract, Pycnogenol: Effect on Xanthine Oxidase," *Journal of Agricultural and Food Chemistry* 48.11 (2000): 5630–39.

30. T. Sun et al., "Study on Relationship Between Leukotrienes and Exercise-Induced Asthma," *Chinese Medical Journal* 82.1 (2002): 54–56.

31. K. W. Rundell and D. M. Jenkinson, "Exercise-Induced Bronchospasm in the Elite Athlete," *Sports Medicine* 32.9 (2002): 583–600.

32. T. D. Mickleborough et al., "Dietary Chloride as a Possible Determinant of the Severity of Exercise-Induced Asthma," *European Journal of Applied Physiology* 85.5 2001): 450–56.

33. G. A. MacGregor, "Salt: More Adverse Effects," *American Journal of Hypertension* 10.5, Part 2 (1997): 37S–41S.

Chapter 12: The Glycemic Factor

1. A. Katz and I. Raz, "Rapid Activation of Glycogen Synthase and Protein Phosphatase in Human Skeletal Muscle After Isometric Contraction Requires an Intact Circulation," *Pflugers Archive: European Journal of Physiology* 431.2 (1995): 259–65.

2. R. C. Hickner et al., "Muscle Glycogen Accumulation After Endurance Exercise in Trained and Untrained Individuals," *Journal of Applied Physiology* 83.3 (1997): 897–903.

3. F. Dela et al., "Insulin-Stimulated Muscle Glucose Clearance in Patients with NIDDM: Effects of One-Legged Physical Training," *Diabetes* 44.9 (1995): 1010–20.

4. R. Ilouz et al., "Inhibition of Glycogen Synthase Kinase-3Beta by Bivalent Zinc Ions: Insight into the Insulin-Mimetic Action of Zinc," *Biochemical and Biophysical Research Communications* 295.1 (2002): 102–06.

5. W. J. Ryves et al., "Glycogen Synthase Kinase-3 Inhibition by Lithium and Beryllium Suggests the Presence of Two Magnesium-Binding Sites," *Biochemical and Biophysical Research Communications* 290.3 (2002): 967–72.

6. K. Rooney et al., "Creatine Supplementation Alters Insulin Secretion and Glucose Homeostasis In Vivo," *Metabolism* 51.4 (2002): 518–22.

7. J. L. Ivy, "Dietary Strategies to Promote Glycogen Synthesis After Exercise," *Canadian Journal of Applied Physiology* 26 Supplement (2001): S236–45.

8. R. Maughan, "The Athlete's Diet: Nutritional Goals and Dietary Strategies," *Proceedings of the Nutrition Society* 61.1 (2002): 87–96.

9. A. Teuscher, "Carbohydrates and Dietary Fiber in the Diabetic Diet," *Schweizerische Medizinische Wochenschrift* 116.9 (1986): 282–87.

10. Chaturvedi A. Sreedevi, "Effect of Vegetable Fiber on Post-Prandial Glycemia," *Plant Foods for Human Nutrition* 44.1 (1993): 71–78.

11. D. J. Jenkins et al., "Starchy Foods and Fiber: Reduced Rate of Digestion and Improved Carbohydrate Metabolism," *Scandinavian Journal of Gastroenterology: Supplement* 129 (1987): 132–41.

12. J. Salmeron et al., "Dietary Fiber, Glycemic Load, and Risk of NIDDM in Men," *Diabetes Care* 20.4 (1997): 545–50.

13. U. Smith, "Carbohydrates, Fat, and Insulin Action," *American Journal of Clinical Nutrition* 59.3 Supplement (1994): 686S–89S.

14. T. M. Wolever et al., "The Glycemic Index: Methodology and Clinical Implications," *American Journal of Clinical Nutrition* 54.5 (1991): 846–54.

15. E. A. Richter et al., "Glucose, Exercise, and Insulin: Emerging Concepts," *Journal of Physiology* 535, Part 2 (2001): 313–22.

16. T. Kolter et al., "Contraction-Induced Translocation of the Glucose Transporter GLUT4 in Isolated Ventricular Cardiomyocytes," *Biochemical and Biophysical Research Communications* 189.2 (1992): 1207–14.

17. S. R. Wang et al., "The Effect of Sugar Cereal with and Without a Mixed Meal on Glycemic Response in Children with Diabetes," *Journal of Pediatric Gastroenterology and Nutrition* 13.2 (1991): 155–60.

18. M. C. Gulliford et al., "Differential Effect of Protein and Fat Ingestion on Blood-Glucose Responses to High- and Low-Glycemic-Index Carbohydrates in Noninsulin-Dependent Diabetic Subjects," *American Journal of Clinical Nutrition* 50.4 (1989): 773–77.

19. A. S. Rocca et al., "Monounsaturated Fatty-Acid Diets Improve Glycemic Tolerance Through Increased Secretion of Glucagon-Like Peptide-1," *Endocrinology* 142.3 (2001): 1148–55.

20. S. R. Wang et al.

21. M. Albert-Puleo, "Physiological Effects of Cabbage with Reference to Its Potential as a Dietary Cancer-Inhibitor and Its Use in Ancient Medicine," *Journal of Ethnopharmacology* 9.2–3 (1983): 261–72.

22. J. W. Fahey et al., "Sulforaphane Inhibits Extracellular, Intracellular, and Antibiotic-Resistant Strains of Helicobacter Pylori and Prevents Benzo[a]pyrene-Induced Stomach Tumors," *Proceedings of the National Academy of Sciences of the United States of America* 99.11 (2002): 7610–15.

23. R. P. Ferraris, "Dietary and Developmental Regulation of Intestinal Sugar Transport," *Biochemical Journal* 360, Part 2 (December 2001): 265–76.

24. B. A. Hirayama et al., "Common Mechanisms of Inhibition for the $Na+$/Glucose (hSGLT1) and $Na+$/cl-/GABA (hGAT1) Cotransporters," *British Journal of Pharmacology* 134.3 (2001): 484–95.

25. M. A. Ostos et al., "Fructose Intake Increases Hyperlipidemia and Modifies Apolipoprotein Expression in Apolipoprotein AI-CIII-AIV Transgenic Mice," *Journal of Nutrition* 132.5 (2002): 918–23.

26. J. Busserolles et al., "Rats Fed a High-Sucrose Diet Have Altered Heart Antioxidant Enzyme Activity and Gene Expression," *Life Sciences* 71.11 (2002): 1303–12.

27. J. Busserolles et al., "Short-Term Consumption of a High-Sucrose Diet Has a Pro-Oxidant Effect in Rats," *British Journal of Nutrition* 87.4 (2002): 337–42.

28. B. W. Wolf et al., "Glycemic and Insulinemic Responses of Nondiabetic Healthy Adult Subjects to an Experimental Acid-Induced Viscosity Complex Incorporated into a Glucose Beverage," *Nutrition* 18.7–8 (2002): 621–26.

29. T. Fushimi et al., "The Efficacy of Acetic Acid for Glycogen Repletion in Rat Skeletal Muscle After Exercise," *International Journal of Sports Medicine* 23.3 (2002): 218–22.

30. E. M. Ostman et al., "Barley Bread Containing Lactic Acid Improves Glucose Tolerance at a Subsequent Meal in Healthy Men and Women," *Journal of Nutrition* 132.6 (2002): 1173–75.

31. T. Fushimi et al.

32. D. Too et al., "Effect of a Precompetition Bodybuilding Diet and Training Regimen on Body Composition and Blood Chemistry," *Journal of Sports Medicine and Physical Fitness* 38.3 (1998): 245–52.

33. D. S. Kronfeld et al., "Dietary Protein Influences Acid-Base Responses to Repeated Sprints," *Equine Veterinary Journal Supplement* 30 (July 1999): 463–67.

34. N. G. de Santo et al., "Effect of an Acute Oral Protein Load on Renal Acidification in Healthy Humans and in Patients with Chronic Renal Failure," *Journal of the American Society of Nephrology* 8.5 (1997): 784–92.

35. L. A. Frassetto et al., "Estimation of Net Endogenous Noncarbonic Acid Production in Humans from Diet Potassium and Protein Contents," *American Journal of Clinical Nutrition* 68.3 (1998): 576–83.

36. D. Too et al.

37. I. Valencia, et al., "General Anesthesia and the Ketogenic Diet: Clinical Experience in Nine Patients," *Epilepsia* 43.5 (2002): 525–29.

38. T. Narita et al., "Determination of Optimal Protein Contents for a Protein-Restriction Diet in Type II Diabetic Patients with Microalbuminuria," *Tohoku Journal of Experimental Medicine* 193.1 (2001): 45–55.

39. L. A. Frassetto et al.

40. E. José-Cunilleras et al., "Glycemic Index of a Meal Fed Before Exercise Alters Substrate Use and Glucose Flux in Exercising Horses," *Journal of Applied Physiology* 92.1 (2002): 117–28.

41. A. G. Rassam et al., "The Mechanism of Glucose-Induced Catecholamine Stimulation," *Metabolism* 51.6 (2002): 761–64.

42. E. Bono-Gonzalez et al., "Glucose but Not Protein or Fat Load Amplifies the Cortisol Response to Psychosocial Stress," *Hormone Behavior* 41.3 (2002): 328–33.

43. M. A. Febbraio et al., "Pre-Exercise Carbohydrate Ingestion, Glucose Kinetics, and Muscle Glycogen Use: Effect of the Glycemic Index," *Journal of Applied Physiology* 89.5 (2000): 1845–51.

44. F. Pattou et al., "Enhancement of the Quality of Hepatic Graft by Restoration of Hepatic-Glycogen Reserves in the Donor," *La Presse medicale* 21.41 (1992): 2012–14.

45. A. M. Itinose et al., "N-Acetyl Cysteine Stimulates Hepatic-Glycogen Deposition in the Rat," Department of Clinical Sciences, University of Maringa, Brazil.

46. J. L. Sievenpiper et al., "Insulin Resistance: Concepts, Controversies, and the Role of Nutrition," *Canadian Journal of Dietetic Practice and Research* 63.1 (2002): 20–32.

47. A. Golay et al., "Progressive Defect of Insulin Action on Glycogen Synthase in Obesity and Diabetes," *Metabolism* 51.5 (2002): 549–53.

48. F. Dela et al., "Insulin-Stimulated Muscle Glucose Clearance in Patients with NIDDM: Effects of One-Legged Physical Training," *Diabetes* 44.9 (1995): 1010–20.

49. D. E. Jacks et al., "Effect of Exercise at Three Exercise Intensities on Salivary Cortisol," *Journal of Strength and Conditioning Research* 16.2 (2002): 286–89.

50. M. T. Lin, "The Effect of Glutamine-Supplemented Total Parenteral Nutrition on Nitrogen Economy Depends on Severity of Diseases in Surgical Patients," *Clinical Nutrition* 21.3 (2002): 213–18.

51. B. K. Pedersen et al., "Exercise and the Immune System: Influence of Nutrition and Aging," *Journal of Science and Medicine in Sport* 2.3 (1999): 234–52.

52. J. Neu et al., "Glutamine: Clinical Applications and Mechanisms of Action," *Current Opinion in Clinical Nutrition and Metabolic Care* 5.1 (2002): 69–75.

Chapter 13: Dieting Doesn't Work

1. Z. Fu et al., "Vitamin A Deficiency Reduces Insulinlike Growth Factor (IGF-1) Gene Expression and Increases IGF-1-Receptor and Insulin-Receptor Gene Expression in Tissue of Japanese Quail," *Journal of Nutrition* 131 (2001): 1189–94.

2. D. J. Shin and M. M. McGrane, "Vitamin A Regulates Genes Involved in Hepatic Gluconeogenesis in Mice," *Journal of Nutrition* 127 (1997): 1274–78.

3. C. Jousee et al., "Evidence for Multiple Signaling Pathways in the Regulation of Gene Expression by

Amino Acids in Human Cell Lines," *Journal of Nutrition* 130 (2000): 1555–60.

4. G. G. Meadows et al., "Specific Amino-Acid Deficiency Alters the Expression of Genes of Human Melanoma and Other Tumor Cell Lines," *Journal of Nutrition* 131 (2001): 3047–50.

5. N. Torres et al., "Histidine-Imbalanced Diets Stimulate Hepatic Histidase Gene Expression in Rats," *Journal of Nutrition* 129 (1999): 1979–83.

6. L. Rao et al., "Gene-Expression Profiling of Low Selenium Status in the Mouse Intestine: Transcriptional Activation of Genes Linked to DNA Damage, Cell Control, and Oxidative Stress," *Journal of Nutrition* 131 (2001): 3175–81.

7. H. Kudo et al., "Dietary Zinc Deficiency Decreases Glutathione S-Transferase Expression in the Rat Olfactory Epithelium," *Journal of Nutrition* 130 (2000): 38–44.

8. J. H. Choi and D. Kim, "Effects of Age and Dietary Restriction on Lifespan and Oxidative Stress of SAMP8 Mice with Learning and Memory Impairments," *Journal of Nutrition, Health, and Aging* 4.3 (2000): 182–86.

9. C. A. Jolly et al., "Life Span Is Prolonged in Food-Restricted Autoimmune-Prone (NZB x NZW)F(1) Mice Fed a Diet Enriched with (N-3) Fatty Acids," *Journal of Nutrition* 131.10 (2001): 2753–60.

10. D. P. Stanley and T. B. Kirkwood, "Calorie Restriction and Aging: A Life-History Analysis," *Evolution: International Journal of Organic Evolution* 54.3 (2000): 740–50.

11. J. H. Choi and D. Kim.

12. M. A. Lane et al., "Short-Term Calorie Restriction Improves Disease-Related Markers in Older Male Rhesus Monkeys (Macaca Mulatta)," *Mechanisms of Ageing and Development* 112.3 (2000): 185–96.

13. A. C. Gazdag et al., "Calorie Restriction Increases Insulin-Stimulated Glucose Transport in Skeletal Muscle from IRS-1 Knockout Mice," *Diabetes* 48.10 (1999): 1930–36.

14. J. L. Weed et al., "Activity Measures in Rhesus Monkeys on Long-Term Calorie Restriction," *Physiology and Behavior* 62.1 (1997): 97–103.

15. H. Y. Chung et al., "The Inflammation Hypothesis of Aging: Molecular Modulation by Calorie Restriction," *Annals of the New York Academy of Sciences* 928 (April 2001): 327–35.

16. C. A. Jolly et al.

17. M. Holecek, "Relation Between Glutamine, Branched-Chain Amino Acids, and Protein Metabolism," *Nutrition* 18.2 (2002): 130–33.

18. F. J. Andrews and R. D. Griffiths, "Glutamine: Essential for Immune Nutrition in the Critically Ill," *British Journal of Nutrition* 87, Supplement 1 (January 2002): S3–8.

19. E. Roth et al., "Regulative Potential of Glutamine: Relation to Glutathione Metabolism," *Nutrition* 18.3 (2002): 217–21.

20. O. Le Bacquer et al., "Effects of Glutamine Deprivation on Protein Synthesis in a Model of Human Enterocytes in Culture," *American Journal of Physiology: Gastrointestinal and Liver Physiology* 281.6 (2001): G1340–47.

21. A. B. Thomson et al., "Small Bowel Review: Diseases of the Small Intestine," *Digestive Diseases and Sciences* 46.12 (2001): 2555–66.

22. Y. Zhou et al., "Glutamine-Dipeptide-Enriched Enteral Nutrition Improving Gut Permeability in Severe Burns, *Chinese Medical Journal* 79.11 (1999): 825–27.

23. P. E. Wischmeyer et al., "Glutamine Reduces Cytokine Release, Organ Damage, and Mortality in a Rat Model of Endotoxemia," *Shock* 16.5 (2001): 398–402.

24. Y. Hu et al., "The Colonic Response to Genotoxic Carcinogens in the Rat: Regulation by Dietary Fiber," *Carcinogenesis* 23.7 (2002): 1131–37.

25. R. K. Leu et al., "Effects of Resistant Starch and Nonstarch Polysaccharides on Colonic Luminalenvironment and Genotoxin-Induced Apoptosis in the Rat," *Carcinogenesis* 23.5 (2002): 713–19.

26. A. L. Sesink et al., "Red Meat and Colon Cancer: Dietary Haem, but Not Fat, Has Cytotoxic and Hyperproliferative Effects on Rat Colonic Epithelium," *Carcinogenesis* 21.10 (2000): 1909–15.

27. V. G. Rios, article in *Revista Neurologia* 33.10 (2001): 909–15.

28. D. J. Bihari, "Metabolic Acidosis," *British Journal of Hospital Medicine* 35.2 (1986): 89–90, 92, 94–95.

29. A. S. al-Mudallal et al., "Diet-Induced Ketosis Does Not Cause Cerebral Acidosis," *Epilepsia* 37.3 (1996): 258–61.

30. L. L. Thiol et al., Ketone Bodies Do Not Directly Alter Excitatory or Inhibitory Hippocampal Synaptic Transmission," *Neurology* 54.2 (2000): 325–31.

31. E. C. Wirrell et al., "Is a Fast Necessary When Initiating the Ketogenic Diet?" *Journal of Child Neurology* 17.3 (2002): 179–82.

32. M. Nakazawa et al., "Effects of Ketogenic Diet on Electroconvulsive Threshold and Brain Contents of Adenosine Nucleotides," *Brain Development* 5.4 (1983): 375–80.

33. J. C. McGrogan et al., "The Implementation and Maintenance of the Ketogenic Diet in Children," *Journal of Neuroscience Nursing* 31.5 (1999): 294–302.

34. D. R. Nordli, Jr., et al., "Experience with the Ketogenic Diet in Infants," *Pediatrics* 108.1 (2001): 129–33.

35. S. Yehuda et al., "Essential Fatty-Acid Preparation (SR-3) Raises the Seizure Threshold in Rats," *European Journal of Pharmacology* 254.1–2 (1994): 193–98.

36. S. Schlanger et al., "Diet Enriched with Omega-3 Fatty Acids Alleviates Convulsion Symptoms in Epilepsy Patients," *Epilepsia* 43.1 (2002): 103–04.

37. I. Lauritzen et al., "Polyunsaturated Fatty Acids Are Potent Neuroprotectors," *EMBO Journal* 19.8 (2000): 1784–93.

38. R. A. Voskuyl et al., "Anticonvulsant Effect of Polyunsaturated Fatty Acids in Rats, Using the Cortical Stimulation Model," *European Journal of Pharmacology* 341.2–3 (1998): 145–52.

39. J. D. McGarry and D. W. Foster, "Hormonal Control of Ketogenesis. Biochemical Considerations," *Archives of Internal Medicine* 137.4 (1977): 495–501.

40. C. A. Horswill, "Weight Loss and Weight Cycling in Amateur Wrestlers: Implications for Performance and Resting Metabolic Rate," *International Journal of Sport Nutrition* 3.3 (1993): 245–60.

41. K. D. Tipton, "Muscle Protein Metabolism in the Elderly: Influence of Exercise and Nutrition," *Canadian Journal of Applied Physiology* 26.6 (2001): 588–606.

42. I. G. Fatouros et al., "The Effects of Strength Training, Cardiovascular Training, and Their Combination on Flexibility of Inactive Older Adults," *International Journal of Sports Medicine* 23.2 (2002): 112–19.

43. P. Schrauwen et al., "Effect of Acute Exercise on Uncoupling Protein 3 Is a Fat Metabolism-Mediated Effect," *American Journal of Physiology: Endocrinology and Metabolism* 282.1 (2002): E11–17.

44. B. Cannon et al., "Brown Adipose Tissue. More Than an Effector of Thermogenesis?" *Annals of the New York Academy of Sciences* 856 (September 1998): 171–87.

Chapter 14: State of Mind Matters

1. C. A. Gitto et al., "The Patient with Alzheimer's Disease," *Quintessence International* 32.3 (2001): 221–31.

2. Y. Lecrubier, "The Burden of Depression and Anxiety in General Medicine," *Journal of Clinical Psychiatry* 62, Supplement 8 (2001): 4–9; discussion 10–11.

3. M. C. Bralet et al., "Cause of Mortality in Schizophrenic Patients: Prospective Study of Years of a Cohort of 150 Chronic Schizophrenic Patients," *L'Encephale* 26.6 (2000): 32–41.

4. L. M. Furlanetto et al., "Association Between Depressive Symptoms and Mortality in Medical Inpatients," *Psychosomatics* 41.5 (2000): 426–32.

5. L. E. Hollister, "Electrocardiographic Screening in Psychiatric Patients," *Journal of Clinical Psychiatry* 56.1 (1995): 26–29.

6. S. P. Roose, "Depression, Anxiety, and the Cardiovascular System: The Psychiatrist's Perspective," *Journal of Clinical Psychiatry* 62, Supplement 8 (2001): 19–22; discussion 23.

7. C. R. Sharpe et al., "The Effects of Tricyclic Antidepressants on Breast-Cancer Risk," *British Journal of Cancer* 86.1 (2002): 92–97.

8. S. O. Dalton et al., "Antidepressant Medications and Risk for Cancer," *Epidemiology* 11.2 (2000): 171–76.

9. M. Cotterchio et al., "Antidepressant Medication Use and Breast-Cancer Risk," *American Journal of Epidemiology* 151.10 (2000): 951–57.

Chapter 15: Applying Ageless Performance

1. D. E. Jacks et al., "Effect of Exercise at Three Exercise Intensities on Salivary Cortisol," *Journal of Strength and Conditioning Research* 16.2 (2002): 286–89.

2. D. J. Jenkins et al., "Effects of High- and Low-Isoflavone Soy Foods on Blood Lipids, Oxidized LDL, Homocysteine, and Blood Pressure in Hyperlipidemic Men and Women," *American Journal of Clinical Nutrition* 76.2 (2002): 365–72.

3. T. A. Sanders et al., "Moderate Intakes of Intact Soy Protein Rich in Isoflavones Compared with Ethanol-Extracted Soy Protein Increase HDL but Do Not Influence Transforming Growth Factor Beta(1) Concentrations and Hemostatic Risk Factors for Coronary Heart Disease in Healthy Subjects," *American Journal of Clinical Nutrition* 76.2 (2002): 373–77.

4. S. Tonstad et al., "A Comparison of the Effects of Two Doses of Soy Protein or Casein on Serum Lipids,

Serum Lipoproteins, and Plasma Total Homocysteine in Hypercholesterolemic Subjects," *American Journal of Clinical Nutrition* 76.1 (2002): 78–84.

5. P. Chowdhury and M. Soulsby, "Lipid Peroxidation in Rat Brain Is Increased by Simulated Weightlessness and Decreased by a Soy-Protein Diet," *Annals of Clinical and Laboratory Science* 32.2 (2002): 188–92.

6. C. Nagata et al., "Hot Flushes and Other Menopausal Symptoms in Relation to Soy-Product Intake in Japanese Women," *Climacteric* 2.1 (1999): 6–12.

7. R. Mackey and J. Eden, "Phytoestrogens and the Menopause," *Climacteric* 1.4 (1998): 302–08.

8. S. Dudasova and E. Grancicova, "Influence of Casein and Soy Flour Proteins on Amino-Acid Content in the Liver of Experimental Animals," *Physiological Research* 41.6 (1992): 411–16.

9. J. D. Radcliffe and D. M. Czajka-Narins, "Use of Arginine to Reduce the Severity of Retinoid-Induced Hypertriglyceridemia," *Nutrition and Cancer* 36.2 (2000): 200–06.

10. D. K. Levenhagen et al., "Post-Exercise Protein Intake Enhances Whole-Body and Leg Protein Accretion in Humans," *Medicine and Science in Sports and Exercise* 34.5 (2002): 828–37.

11. K. S. Nair et al., "Failure of Carbohydrate to Spare Leucine Oxidation in Obese Subjects," *International Journal of Obesity* 11.5 (1987): 537–44.

12. M. U. Yang et al., "Metabolic Effects of Substituting Carbohydrate for Protein in a Low-Calorie Diet: A Prolonged Study in Obese Patients," *International Journal of Obesity* 5.3 (1981): 231–36.

13. Y. Segev et al., "Involvement of the Skeletal GH-IGF System in an Experimental Model of Diabetes-Induced Growth Retardation," *Acta Diabetologica* 39.2 (2002): 61–67.

14. K. Ramstad and J. H. Loge, "Melatonin Treatment of Sleep Disorders in Disabled Children," *Tidsskrift for den Norske Laegeforening* 122.10 (2002): 1009–11.

15. E. Gitto et al., "Individual and Synergistic Antioxidative Actions of Melatonin: Studies with Vitamin E, Vitamin C, Glutathione, and Desferrioxamine (Desferoxamine) in Rat-Liver Homogenates," *Journal of Pharmacy and Pharmacology* 53.10 (2001): 1393–401.

16. S. Nishida et al., "Long-Term Melatonin Administration Reduces Hyperinsulinemia and Improves the Altered Fatty-Acid Compositions in Type II Diabetic Rats Via the Restoration of Delta-5 Desaturase Activity," *Journal of Pineal Research* 32.1 (2002): 26–33.

17. G. Saab et al., "Changes in Human Muscle Transverse Relaxation Following Short-Term Creatine Supplementation," *Experimental Physiology* 87.3 (2002): 383–89.

18. M. J. Gibala, "Nutritional Supplementation and Resistance Exercise: What Is the Evidence for Enhanced Skeletal Muscle Hypertrophy?" *Canadian Journal of Applied Physiology* 25.6 (2000): 524–35.

19. G. Parise et al., "Effects of Acute Creatine Monohydrate Supplementation on Leucine Kinetics and Mixed-Muscle Protein Synthesis," *Journal of Applied Physiology* 91.3 (2001): 1041–47.

20. A. J. Carter et al., "Preincubation with Creatine Enhances Levels of Creatine Phosphate and Prevents Anoxic Damage in Rat Hippocampal Slices," *Journal of Neurochemistry* 64.6 (1995): 2691–99.

21. C. P. Bolotte, "Creatine Supplementation in Athletes: Benefits and Potential Risks," *Journal of the Louisiana State Medical Society* 150.7 (1998): 325–27.

22. J. R. Poortmans and M. Francaux, "Long-Term Oral Creatine Supplementation Does Not Impair Renal Function in Healthy Athletes," *Medicine and Science in Sports and Exercise* 31.8 (1999): 1108–10.

23. J. M. Lawler et al., "Direct Antioxidant Properties of Creatine," *Biochemical and Biophysical Research Communications* 290.1 (2002): 47–52.

24. L. Gianotti et al., "Arginine Counteracts the Inhibitory Effect of Recombinant Human Insulinlike Growth Factor I on the Somatotroph Responsiveness to Growth-Hormone-Releasing Hormone in Humans," *Journal of Clinical Endocrinology and Metabolism* 85.10 (2000): 3604–08.

25. T. C. Welbourne, "Increased Plasma Bicarbonate and Growth Hormone After an Oral Glutamine Load," *American Journal of Clinical Nutrition* 61.5 (1995): 1058–61.

26. T. R. Ziegler et al., "Safety and Metabolic Effects of L-Glutamine Administration in Humans," *JPEN: Journal of Parenteral and Enteral Nutrition* 14.4 Supplement (1990): 137S–146S.

27. P. Furst, "New Developments in Glutamine Delivery," *Journal of Nutrition* 131.9 Supplement (2001): 2562S–68S.

28. C. Moinard et al., "Involvement of Glutamine, Arginine, and Polyamines in the Action of Ornithine Alpha-Ketoglutarate on Macrophage Functions in Stressed Rats," *Journal of Leukocyte Biology* 67.6 (2000): 834–40.

29. M. D. Vukovich and G. D. Dreifort, "Effect of Beta-Hydroxy-Beta-Methylbutyrate on the Onset of Blood-Lactate Accumulation and v(o)(2) Peak in Endurance-Trained Cyclists," *Journal of Strength and Conditioning Research* 15.4 (2001): 491–97.

30. A. E. Knitter et al., "Effects of Beta-Hydroxy-Beta-Methylbutyrate on Muscle Damage After a Prolonged Run," *Journal of Applied Physiology* 89.4 (2000): 1340–44.

31. W. Pliml et al., "Effects of Therapeutic Ribose Levels on Human Lymphocyte Proliferation In Vitro," *Clinical Investigations* 71.10 (1993): 770–73.

32. P. E. May et al., "Reversal of Cancer-Related Wasting Using Oral Supplementation with a Combination of Beta-Hydroxy-Beta-Methylbutyrate, Arginine, and Glutamine," *American Journal of Surgery* 183.4 (2002): 471–79.

33. R. H. Clark et al., "Nutritional Treatment for Acquired Immunodeficiency Virus–Associated Wasting Using Beta-Hydroxy-Beta-Methylbutyrate, Glutamine, and Arginine: A Randomized, Double-Blind, Placebo-Controlled Study," *JPEN: Journal of Parenteral and Enteral Nutrition* 24.3 (2000): 133–39.

34. Y. C. Kao et al., "Molecular Basis of the Inhibition of Human Aromatase (Estrogen Synthetase) by Flavone and Isoflavone Phytoestrogens: A Site-Directed Mutagenesis Study," *Environmental Health Perspectives* 106.2 (1998): 85–92.

35. M. I. Kosovskii et al., "The Effect of Nerobol and Ecdysterone on Insulin-Dependent Processes Linked Normally and in Insulin Resistance," *Problemy Endokrinologii* 35.5 (1989): 77–81.

36. A. M. Fulghesu et al., "N-Acetyl Cysteine Treatment Improves Insulin Sensitivity in Women with Polycystic Ovary Syndrome," *Fertility and Sterility* 77.6 (2002): 1128–35.

37. Robert S. Goodhart and Maurice E. Shils, eds., *Modern Nutrition in Health and Disease*, 5th ed. (Philadelphia: Lea and Febiger, 1973) 83.

38. G. Sarwar et al., "Influence of Feeding Alkaline/Heat Processed Proteins on Growth and Protein and Mineral Status of Rats," *Advances in Experimental Medicine and Biology* 459 (1999): 161–77.

39. I. E. Liener, "Implications of Anti-Nutritional Components in Soybean Foods," *Critical Reviews in Food Science and Nutrition* 34.1 (1994): 31–67.

40. G. Sarwar, "Amino-Acid Ratings of Different Forms of Infant Formulas Based on Varying Degrees of Processing," *Advances in Experimental Medicine and Biology* 289 (1991): 389–402.

41. Goodhart and Shils, 92.

42. J. Mauron, "Influence of Processing on Protein Quality," *Journal of Nutritional Science and Vitaminology* (Tokyo) 36, Supplement 1 (1990): S57–69.

43. H. Jing and D. D. Kitts, "Chemical and Biochemical Properties of Casein-Sugar Maillard Reaction Products," *Food and Chemistry Toxicology* 40.7 (2002): 1007–15.

44. J. J. Boza et al., "Effect of Glutamine Supplementation of the Diet on Tissue Protein Synthesis Rate of Glucocorticoid-Treated Rats," *Nutrition* 17.1 (2001): 35–40.

45. A. M. Davison et al., "Water-Supply Aluminium Concentration, Dialysis Dementia, and Effect of Reverse-Osmosis Water Treatment," *The Lancet* 2.8302 (1982): 785–87.

46. G. Pickering, "Hydration and Exercise in the Elderly," *Revue de la Société Française de Médecine du Sport* 13.1 (1998): 5–9.

47. P. Mita et al., "Epidemiology of Male Infertility," *Archivio Italiano di Urologia, Andrologia* 70.2 (1998): 85–91.

48. B. Adelusi et al., "Correlation of Smoking and Coffee-Drinking with Sperm Progressive Motility in Infertile Males," *African Journal of Medicine and Medical Science* 27.1–2 (1998): 47–50.

49. R. L. Ferrini et al., "Caffeine Intake and Endogenous Sex Steroid Levels in Post-Menopausal Women: The Rancho Bernardo Study," *American Journal of Epidemiology* 144.7 (1996): 642–44.

50. W. R. Lovallo et al., "Stress-Like Adrenocorticotropin Responses to Caffeine in Young Healthy Men," *Pharmacology, Biochemistry, and Behavior* 55.3 (1996): 365–69.

51. T. E. Graham, "Caffeine, Coffee, and Ephedrine: Impact on Exercise Performance and Metabolism," *Canadian Journal of Applied Physiology* 26 Supplement (2001): S103–19.

52. B. Mackness et al., "Low Paraoxonase Activity in Type II Diabetes Mellitus Complicated by Retinopathy," *Clinical Science* (London) 98.3 (2000): 355–63.

53. K. S. Sidhu and M. B. Collisi, "A Case of an Accidental Exposure to a Veterinary Insecticide Product Formulation," *Veterinary and Human Toxicology* 31.1 (1989): 63–64.

54. T. R. Sobha and O. Prakash, "Glycosuria in Organophosphate and Carbamate Poisoning," *Journal of the Association of Physicians of India* 48.12 (2000): 1197–99.

55. M. Guven et al., "Endocrine Changes in Patients with Acute Organophosphate Poisoning," *Human and Experimental Toxicology* 18.10 (1999): 598–601.

56. M. Nag and N. Nandi, "Effect of Three Organophosphates on Respiration in Rat Brain and Liver Tissue," *Bioscience Reports* 11.1 (1991): 7–10.

57. D. E. Ray and P. G. Richards, "The Potential for Toxic Effects of Chronic, Low-Dose Exposure to Organophosphates," *Toxicology Letters* 120.1–3 (2001): 343–51.

58. L. J. Fourtes et al., "Cholinesterase-Inhibiting Insecticide Toxicity," *American Family Physician* 47.7 (1993): 1613–20.

59. F. E. Samson et al., "Soman-Induced Changes in Brain Regional Glucose Use," *Fundamental and Applied Toxicology* 4.2, Part 2 (1984): S173–83.

60. A. Trotter et al., "Growth of the Uterus and Mammary Glands and Vaginal Cytologic Features in Extremely Premature Infants with Postnatal Replacement of Estradiol and Progesterone," *American Journal of Obstetrics and Gynecology* 186.2 (2002): 184–88.

61. C. J. Henry and B. Emery, "Effect of Spiced Food on Metabolic Rate," *Human Nutrition: Clinical Nutrition* 40.2 (1986): 165–68.

62. D. Laurent et al., "Effects of Caffeine on Muscle Glycogen Utilization and the Neuroendocrine Axis During Exercise," *Journal of Clinical Endocrinology and Metabolism* 85.6 (2000): 2170–75.

63. S. Ryu et al., "Caffeine as a Lipolytic Food Component Increases Endurance Performance in Rats and Athletes," *Journal of Nutritional Science and Vitaminology* (Tokyo) 47.2 (2001): 139–46.

64. B. G. Pollock et al., "Inhibition of Caffeine Metabolism by Estrogen-Replacement Therapy in Post-Menopausal Women," *Journal of Clinical Pharmacology* 39.9 (1999): 936–40.

65. D. C. May et al., "Effects of Cimetidine on Caffeine Disposition in Smokers and Nonsmokers," *Clinical Pharmacology and Therapeutics* 31.5 (1982): 656–61.

66. C. Hartisch et al., "Dual Inhibitory Activities of Tannins from HamamelisVirginiana and Related Polyphenols on 5-Lipoxygenase and Lyso-PAF: Acetyl-COA Acetyltransferase," *Planta Medica* 63.2 (1997): 106–10.

67. A. M. Fine, "Oligomeric Proanthocyanidin Complexes: History, Structure, and Phytopharmaceutical Applications," *Alternative Medicine Review* 5.2 (2000): 144–51.

68. E. M. van Hoeyveld et al., "Allergenic and Antigenic Activity of Peptide Fragments in a Whey Hydrolysate Formula," *Clinical and Experimental Allergy* 28.9 (1998): 1131–37.

69. S. Halken et al., "Comparison of a Partially Hydrolyzed Infant Formula with Two Extensively Hydrolyzed Formulas for Allergy Prevention: A Prospective, Randomized Study," *Pediatric Allergy and Immunology* 11.3 (2000): 149–61.

70. S. Makinen-Kiljunen and R. Sorva, "Bovine Beta-Lactoglobulin Levels in Hydrolyzed Protein Formulas for Infant-Feeding," *Clinical and Experimental Allergy* 23.4 (1993): 287–91.

71. T. S. Popova et al., "Role of Glutamine in Enteral Nutrition in Intestinal Insufficiency," *Voprosy Pitaniia* 69.5 (2000): 51–55.

72. J. Neu et al., "Glutamine: Clinical Applications and Mechanisms of Action," *Current Opinion in Clinical Nutrition and Metabolic Care* 5.1 (2002): 69–75.

73. J. Carrier et al., "Effect of Oral Iron Supplementation on Oxidative Stress and Colonic Inflammation in Rats with Induced Colitis," *Alimentary Pharmacology and Therapeutics* 15.12 (2002): 1989–99.

Chapter 16: Condition-Specific Therapies

1. T. Stein et al., "Energy Metabolism Pathways in Rat Muscle Under Conditions of Simulated Microgravity," *Journal of Nutritional Biochemistry* 13.8 (2002): 471.

2. Y. S. Cha et al., "Effects of Carnitine-Coingested Caffeine on Carnitine Metabolism and Endurance Capacity in Athletes," *Journal of Nutritional Science and Vitaminology* (Tokyo) 47.6 (2001): 378–84.

3. F. Brouns and G. J. van der Vusse, "Utilization of Lipids During Exercise in Human Subjects: Metabolic and Dietary Constraints," *British Journal of Nutrition* 79.2 (1998): 117–28.

4. D. Branca et al., "Carnitine Effect on Heart Steatosis Induced in Rats by Rapeseed Oil," *International Journal for Vitamin and Nutritional Research* 47.2 (1977): 162–66.

5. F. Maccari et al., "The Effect of Exogenous L-Carnitine on Biochemical Parameters in Serum and in Heart of the Hyperlipidaemic Rat," *Basic Research in Cardiology* 82, Supplement 1 (1987): 75–81.

6. R. N. Iyer et al., "L-Carnitine Moderately Improves the Exercise Tolerance in Chronic Stable Angina," *Journal of the Association of Physicians of India* 48.11 (2000): 1050–52.

7. C. Stefanutti et al., "Effect of L-Carnitine on Plasma Lipoprotein Fatty Acids Pattern in Patients with Primary Hyperlipoproteinemia," *Clinica Terapeutica* 149.2 (1998): 115–19.

8. E. S. Stroes et al., "Folic Acid Reverts Dysfunction of Endothelial Nitric-Oxide Synthase," *Circulation Research* 86.11 (2000): 1129–34.

9. W. C. Ko et al., "Mechanisms of Relaxant Action of 3-o-Methylquercetin in Isolated Guinea Pig Trachea," *Planta Medica* 68.1 (2002): 30–35.

10. Y. C. Wang et al., "Effects of Neutrophils on Histamine Release from Mast Cells," *Zhongguo Yao Li Xue Bao* 11.3 (1990): 285–88.

11. P. Affinito et al., "Post-Menopausal Osteoporosis: Therapeutic Approaches," *Minerva Ginecologica* 49.3 (1997): 109–20.

12. K. Katase et al., "Effects of Ipriflavone on Bone Loss Following a Bilateral Ovariectomy and Menopause: A Randomized Placebo-Controlled Study," *Calcified Tissue International* 69.2 (2001): 73–77.

13. H. Ohta et al., "Effects of One-Year Ipriflavone Treatment on Lumbar Bone Mineral Density and Bone Metabolic Markers in Post-Menopausal Women with Low Bone Mass," *Hormone Research* 51.4 (1999): 178–83.

14. F. Dalais et al., "Effects of Dietary Phytoestrogens in Post-Menopausal Women," *Climacteric* 1.2 (1998): 124–29.

15. P. B. Clifton-Bligh et al., "The Effect of Isoflavones Extracted from Red Clover (Rimostil) on Lipid and Bone Metabolism," *Menopause* 8.4 (2001): 259–65.

16. S. Genedani et al., "Influence of SAMe on the Modifications of Brain Polyamine Levels in an Animal Model of Depression," *Neuroreport* 12.18 (2001): 3939–42.

17. A. di Rocco et al., "S-Adenosyl-Methionine Improves Depression in Patients with Parkinson's Disease in an Open-Label Clinical Trial," *Movement Disorders* 15.6 (2000): 1225–29.

18. B. D. Sloley et al., "Identification of Kaempferol as a Monoamine-Oxidase Inhibitor and Potential Neuroprotectant in Extracts of Ginkgo Biloba Leaves," *Journal of Pharmacy and Pharmacology* 52.4 (2000): 451–59.

19. M. Rosler et al., "Free Radicals in Alzheimer's Dementia: Currently Available Therapeutic Strategies," *Journal of Neural Transmission: Supplementum* 54 (1998): 211–19.

20. Y. Lecrubier et al., "Efficacy of St. John's Wort Extract ws 5570 in Major Depression: A Double-Blind, Placebo-Controlled Trial," *American Journal of Psychiatry* 159.8 (2002): 1361–66.

21. S. Ando et al., "Enhancement of Learning Capacity and Cholinergic Synaptic Function by Carnitine in Aging Rats," *Journal of Neuroscience Research* 66.2 (2001): 266–71.

22. J. Liu et al., "Delaying Brain Mitochondrial Decay and Aging with Mitochondrial Antioxidants and Metabolites," *Annals of the New York Academy of Sciences* 959 (April 2002): 133–66.

23. C. Dabrosin et al., "Flaxseed Inhibits Metastasis and Decreases Extracellular Vascular Endothelial Growth Factor in Human Breast Cancer Xenografts," *Cancer Letters* 185.1 (2002): 31–37.

24. D. D. Kitts et al., "Antioxidant Activity of the Flaxseed Lignan Secoisolariciresinol Diglycoside and Its Mammalian Lignan Metabolites Enterodiol and Enterolactone," *Molecular and Cellular Biochemistry* 202.1–2 (1999): 91–100.

25. C. Gonzalez et al., "Effect of Treatment with Different Doses of 17-Beta-Estradiol on Insulin-Receptor Substrate-1," *Journal of the Pancreas* 2.4 (2001): 140–49.

26. W. Li and J. F. Fitzloff, "Simultaneous Determination of Terpene Lactones and Flavonoid Aglycones in Ginkgo Biloba by High-Performance Liquid Chromatography with Evaporative Light-Scattering Detection," *Journal of Pharmaceutical and Biomedical Analysis* 30.1 (2002): 67–75.

27. L. Selloum et al., "Effects of Flavonols on the Generation of Superoxide Anion Radicals by Xanthine Oxidase and Stimulated Neutrophils," *Archives of Biochemistry and Biophysics* 395.1 (2001): 49–56.

28. L. A. Kozhemiakin et al., "Xanthine-Oxidase Activity in Mononuclear Cells of Human Blood," *Biulleten' Eksperimental'noi Biologii i Meditsiny* 113.2 (1992): 138–39.

29. P. I. Hsu et al., "Risk Factors for Ulcer Development in Patients with Non-Ulcer Dyspepsia: A Prospective Two-Year Follow-Up Study of 209 Patients," *Gut* 51.1 (2002): 15–20.

30. N. D. Yeomans, "Management of Peptic Ulcer Disease Not Related to Helicobacter," *Journal of Gastroenterology and Hepatology* 17.4 (2002): 488–94.

31. J. W. Fahey et al., "Sulforaphane Inhibits Extracellular, Intracellular, and Antibiotic-Resistant Strains of Helicobacter Pylori and Prevents Benzo[a]pyrene-Induced Stomach Tumors," *Proceedings of the National Academy of Sciences of the United States of America* 99.11 (2002): 7610–15.

32. T. Fukai et al., "Anti–Helicobacter Pylori Flavonoids from Licorice Extract," *Life Sciences* 71.12 (2002): 1449–63.

33. Ibid.

34. R. C. Schiavi et al., "Diabetes Mellitus and Male Sexual Function: A Controlled Study," *Diabetologia* 36.8 (1993): 745–51.

35. M. S. Choo et al., "Functional Evaluation of Tadenan on Micturition and Experimental Prostate Growth Induced with Exogenous Dihydrotestosterone," *Urology* 55.2 (2000): 292–98.

36. W. H. Goldman et al., "Saw-Palmetto-Berry Extract Inhibits Cell Growth and Cox2-Expression in Prostatic Cancer Cells," *Cell Biology International* 25.11 (2001): 1117–24.

37. K. Gauthaman et al., "Aphrodisiac Properties of Tribulus Terrestris Extract (Protodioscin) in Normal and Castrated Rats," *Life Sciences* 71.12 (2002): 1385–96.

38. A. Adimoelja, "Phytochemicals and the Breakthrough of Traditional Herbs in the Management of Sexual Dysfunctions," *International Journal of Andrology* 23, Supplement 2 (2000): 82–84.

39. J. C. Chen et al., "Effects of Ginsenoside Rb2 and RC on Inferior Human Sperm Motility In Vitro," *American Journal of Chinese Medicine* 29.1 (2001): 155–60.

40. L. L. Murphy and T. J. Lee, "Ginseng, Sex Behavior, and Nitric Oxide," *Annals of the New York Academy of Sciences* 962 (May 2002): 372–77.

41. S. Randolph, "When Candida Turns Deadly," *RN* 2002 65.3: 41–44; quiz 45.

42. J. D. Sobel, "Treatment of Vaginal Candida Infections," *Expert Opinion on Pharmacotherapy* 3.8 (2002): 1059–65.

43. L. Hovi et al., "Invasive Fungal Infections in Pediatric Bone-Marrow-Transplant Recipients: Single Center Experience of 10 Years," *Bone Marrow Transplant* 26.9 (2000): 999–1004.

44. M. de Micheli et al., "A Common Drug-Responsive Element Mediates the Upregulation of the Candida Albicans ABC Transporters CDR1 and CDR2, Two Genes Involved in Anti-Fungal Drug Resistance," *Molecular Microbiology* 43.5 (2002): 1197–214.

45. Y. C. Kao et al., "Molecular Basis of the Inhibition of Human Aromatase (Estrogen Synthetase) by Flavone and Isoflavone Phytoestrogens: A Site-Directed Mutagenesis Study," *Environmental Health Perspectives* 106.2 (1998): 85–92.

46. D. R. Campbell and M. S. Kurzer, "Flavonoid Inhibition of Aromatase Enzyme Activity in Human Preadipocytes," *Journal of Steroid Biochemistry and Molecular Biology* 46.3 (1993): 381–88.

47. Y. C. Kao et al.

48. B. M. Collins et al., "The Estrogenic and Anti-Estrogenic Activities of Phytochemicals with the Human Estrogen Receptor Expressed in Yeast," *Steroids* 62.4 (1997): 365–72.

49. T. A. Roy et al., "Interrelationships of Serum-Testosterone and Free-Testosterone Index with FFM and Strength in Aging Men," *American Journal of Physiology: Endocrinology and Metabolism* 283.2 (2002): E284–94.

50. C. Schulman and B. Lunenfeld, "The Ageing Male," *World Journal of Urology* 20.1 (2002): 4–10.

51. S. J. Winters et al., "Testosterone, Sex-Hormone-Binding Globulin, and Body Composition in Young Adult African American and Caucasian Men," *Metabolism* 50.10 (2001): 1242–47.

52. K. Satoh et al., "Inhibition of Aromatase Activity by Green-Tea-Extract Catechins and Their Endocrinological Effects of Oral Administration in Rats," *Food and Chemistry Toxicology* 40.7 (2002): 925–33.

53. T. Kalme et al., "Estradiol Increases the Production of Sex-Hormone-Binding Globulin but Not Insulinlike-Growth-Factor-Binding Protein-1 in Cultured Human Hepatoma Cells," *Fertility and Sterility* 72.2 (1999): 325–29.

54. K. Yaffe et al., "Sex Hormones and Cognitive Function in Older Men," *Journal of the American Geriatric Society* 50.4 (2002): 707–12.

55. V. Flynn and W. J. Hellstrom, "Androgen Deficiency in the Aging Male: Pathophysiology, Diagnosis, and Treatment Alternatives," *Current Urology Reports* 2.6 (2001): 473–79.

56. G. A. Brown et al., "Effects of Androstenedione-Herbal Supplementation on Serum Sex Hormone Concentrations in 30- to 59-Year-Old Men," *International Journal for Vitamin and Nutrition Research* 71.5 (2001): 293–301.

57. L. Dehennin et al., "Human Nutritional Supplements in the Horse—Dehydroepiandrosterone Versus Androstenedione: Comparative Effects on the Androgen Profile and Consequences for Doping Analysis," *Journal of Analytical Toxicology* 25.8 (2001): 685–90.

58. J. D. Veldhuis et al., "Muting of Androgen Negative Feedback Unveils Impoverished Gonadotropin-Releasing Hormone/Luteinizing Hormone Secretory Reactivity in Healthy Older Men," *Journal of Clinical Endocrinology and Metabolism* 86.2 (2001): 529–35.

59. M. Numazawa et al., "Aromatization of 16Alpha-Hydroxyandrostenedione by Human Placental Microsomes: Effect of Pre-Incubation with Suicide Substrates of Androstenedione Aromatization," *Journal of Steroid Biochemistry and Molecular Biology* 81.2 (2002): 165–72.

60. G. A. Brown et al., "Endocrine and Lipid Responses to Chronic Androstenediol-Herbal Supplementation in 30- to 58-Year-Old Men," *Journal of the American College of Nutrition* 20.5 (2001): 520–28.

61. P. G. Adaikan et al., "Proerectile Pharmacological Effects of Tribulus Terrestris Extract on the Rabbit Corpus Cavernosum," *Annals of the Academy of Medicine* (Singapore) 29.1 (2000): 22–26.

62. B. Allolio and W. Arlt, "DHEA Treatment: Myth or Reality?" *Trends in Endocrinology and Metabolism* 13.7 (2002): 288.

63. M. Vallee et al., "Role of Pregnenolone, Dehydroepiandrosterone, and Their Sulfate Esters on Learning and Memory in Cognitive Aging," *Brain Research: Brain Research Reviews* 37.1-3 (2001): 301–12.

64. F. Labrie et al., "DHEA and Its Transformation into Androgens and Estrogens in Peripheral Target Tissues: Intracrinology," *Frontiers in Neuroendocrinology* 22.3 (2001): 185–212.

65. Ibid.

66. Ibid.

67. F. Labrie et al., "Intracrinology and the Skin," *Hormone Research* 54.5-6 (2000): 218–29.

68. T. Nagai et al., "Neuroactive Steroid and Stress Response," *Nihon Shinkei Seishin Yakurigaku Zasshi* 21.5 (2001): 157–62.

69. M. F. Ribeiro and L. M. Garcia-Segura, "Dehydroepiandrosterone Regulates Insulinlike-Growth-Factor-1 System in Adult Rat Hypothalamus," *Endocrine* 17.2 (2002): 129–34.

INDEX

336, 337, 436, 462
thiamine (B$_1$), 76, 77, 83–91, 124, 459, *487*
thromboxane, 7, 25, 66, 151, 158, *159*, 160,
184, 256, 257, 261, 270, 271, 281, *284*, 285,
288, 289, 291, 431
thyroxine, 7 25, 164, 256
tobacco, 239, 341, 464
trans fat, 233–45, 330, 425
Tribulus terrestris, 60, 392, 393, 451, 465–67,
471–76
tumor necrosis factor (TNF), 25, 155, 223
turmeric, *178*, 437

ulcer, 218, 283, 306, 464, 465
uncoupling protein (UCP3), 137, 138, *286*, 336
uric acid, 287, 463, 464

vegetarian, 187, 188, 423
visualization, 62, 68, 348, 350, 351, 356–60,
363, 446, 457, 464
vitamin, 2, 4, 45–48, 56, 64, 65, 75, 77, 83–85,
87, 89, 90, 92, 118–120, 135, 139, *178*, 180,
183, 187, 193, 200, 202, 203, 217, 228, 244,
257, 272, 277–79, 299, 305–07, 322, 331, 334,
364, 365, 367, 370, 372, 384, *388–90*, 407,
422, *427*, *428*, *437*, *438*, 449, 456, 459–61,
486, *487*
A, 108, 163–65, 323, *389*, *428*, *438*,
457, *487*
Bs, 83, 85, 88, 89, 91, 92, 202, 203,
334, 384, 394, 397, *487*
C, 4, 47, 48, 50, 77, 83, 85, 92, 108, 109,
110, 111–14, 116–21, 123, 126, 162,
168, 187–89, 199, 201, 357, *388*, *389*,
391, 397, *427–30*, 432, *437–38*, 445,
457, *486–87*
D, 35, 165, 456, *486–87*
E, 20, 50, 85, 92, 101, 108, 109, *110*,
126, 160–64, 166, 168, 192, 193, 199,
242, 249, *250*, 254, 271, 279, *389*,
391, *427–28*, *430*, *438*, 457, *486–87*

water, importance of, 222–23, 326, 331, 334,
371, 377, *388–90*, 395, 396, 401, 411, 426,
427–30, 464, 483, *485*, *492*
weight management, 21, 40, 44, 58, 70, 128,
129, 132, 137, 185, 229, 257, 286, 296, 309,

323–25, 330, 333, 335, 363, 402, 405, 415
Weil, Dr. Andrew, 135
Western Gym, 64
wheat germ oil, 162
whey, 68, 138, 168, 170, 189, 198, 199, 215,
278, 311, 312, 316, 320, 328, 367, 378–81,
384, 387, *388–90*, 391, 393, 394, 411–14, 416,
418, 422, 423, *427–30*, 431, 438, 442, 443,
445, *485*, *489*
Whitaker, Dr. Julian, 220
white willow bark, 463
wild-yam extract, 273
World Health Organization (WHO), 112, 118

xanthine oxidase, 287, 463

yohimbe, 467
yo-yo dieting, 329–30